E. Gramer · F. Grehn (Eds.)

Pathogenesis and Risk Factors of Glaucoma

Springer

Berlin
Heidelberg
New York
Barcelona
Hong Kong
London
Milan
Paris
Singapore
Tokyo

E. Gramer · F. Grehn (Eds.)

Pathogenesis and Risk Factors of Glaucoma

With 93 Figures, some in Color, and 50 Tables

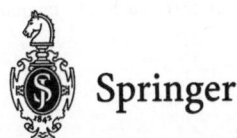

Springer

Professor Dr. med. Dr. jur. Eugen Gramer
Professor Dr. med. Dr. hc. Franz Grehn

Bayerische Julius-Maximilians-Universität Würzburg
Augenklinik im Kopfklinikum
Josef-Schneider-Straße 11
97080 Würzburg, Germany

Library of Congress Cataloging-in-Publication Data
Pathogenesis and risk factors of glaucoma / ed.: E. Gramer ; F. Grehn. – Berlin ;
Heidelberg ; New York ; Barcelona ; Hong Kong ; London ; Milan ; Paris ;
Singapore ; Tokyo : Springer 1999
ISBN-13: 978-3-642-64302-6   e-ISBN-13: 978-3-642-60203-0
DOI: 10.1007/978-3-642-60203-0

Production: PRO EDIT GmbH, 69126 Heidelberg, Germany
Cover design: design & production, 69121 Heidelberg, Germany
Typesetting: Mitterweger Werksatz, 68723 Plankstadt, Germany
SPIN: 10725717   24/3135-5 4 3 2 1 0 – Printed on acid-free paper

Preface

The pathogenesis and risk factors of glaucoma were the subject of a closed international Glaucoma Symposium of the University Eye Hospital, Wuerzburg, held in the castle of Friedrichsruhe in Friedrichsruhe, Germany, from 3–5 September, 1998.

This volume contains 25 contributions presented at the symposium by well-known glaucoma experts from different countries. New insights into the pathomechanisms of glaucomas, glaucoma detection and causal treatment of risk factors were discussed. At this symposium and the social events there was a lively exchange of scientific knowledge between participants who came from many different countries, all with a common interest in glaucoma. We would like to thank all speakers for making the long journeys to Germany and for their contributions which serve to update the present state of knowledge and provide the basis for further glaucoma research.

This book ties together current topics such as compliance with medical therapy, wound healing, genetic risk factors, gene therapy, optic nerve damage in relation to visual field loss, disc hemorrhages, intraocular pressure, low blood pressure, retinal ischemia, and treatment of causal factors of glaucoma. The reader thus is given to participate and profit from the new information on many aspects of glaucoma.

We thank CHIBRET Pharmazeutische GmbH, Haar, Germany, and especially Harald Schwarz for their help in organizing this meeting and for their financial support of the symposium, the social program and the publication of the proceedings.

Wuerzburg, July 1999   Eugen Gramer · Franz Grehn

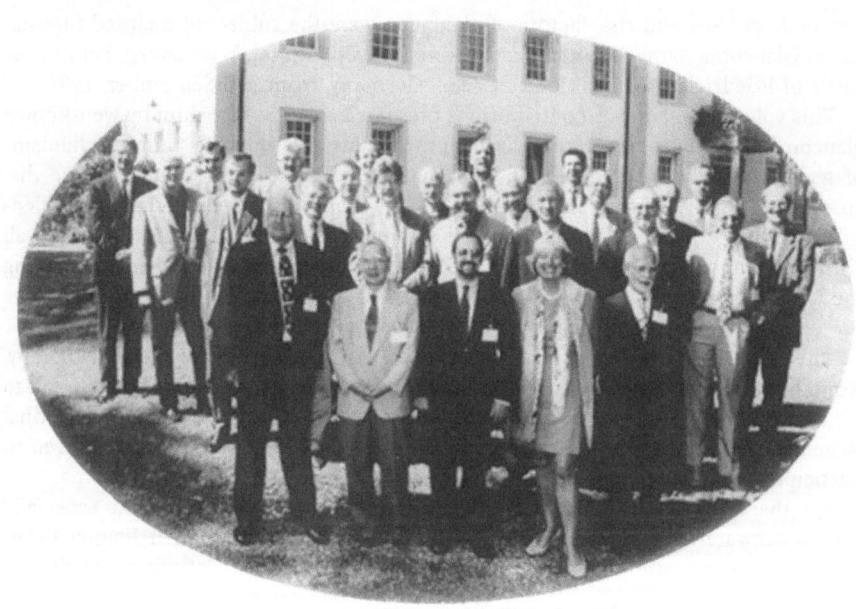

Participants of the closed international glaucoma symposium
"Pathogenesis and Risk Factors of Glaucoma",
3–5 September 1998 in Friedrichsruhe/Germany

Contents

List of Contributors

Bartz-Schmidt, K. U., Dr. Priv.-Doz.
  Universitäts-Augenklinik, Joseph-Stelzmann-Straße 9, 50931 Köln, Germany
Bechetoille, A., Prof.
  Director, Service d'Ophthalmologie, Centre Hospitalier Universitaire, D'Angers 4,
  rue Larrey, 49033 Angers Cedex 01, France
Becker, C. M., Prof. Dr.
  Institut für Biochemie, Lehrstuhl I der Universität Erlangen, Fahrstraße 17,
  91054 Erlangen, Germany
Bodis-Wollner, I., M.D., D.Sc.
  Professor of Neurology and Ophthalmology
  State University of New York, Department of Neurology, 450 Clarkson Avenue,
  Box 213, Brooklyn, NY 11203, USA
Brandt, C. R., Ph.D.
  University of Wisconsin-Madison, Department of Ophthalmology and Visual
  Sciences and Medical Microbiology and Immunology, Clinical Science Center,
  600 Highland Ave F4/336, Madison, WI 53792–3220, USA
Bresson-Dumont, H., M.D.
  Service d'Ophthalmologie, Centre Hospitalier Universitaire, D'Angers 4,
  rue Larrey, 49033 Angers Cedex 01, France
Dawson, A.
  University of Southern California, School of Medicine,
  Department of Ophthalmology, Doheny Eye Institute, 1450 San Pablo Street,
  Los Angeles, CA 90033, USA
Donnelly, S.
  University of Southern California, School of Medicine,
  Department of Ophthalmology, Doheny Eye Institute, 1450 San Pablo Street,
  Los Angeles, CA 90033, USA
Fauss, D. J.
  University of California, Department of Ophthalmology, 10 Kirkham St,
  Box 0130, Room K 301, San Francisco, CA 941143, USA
Gabelt, B. T., M.S.
  University of Wisconsin-Madison, Department of Ophthalmology
  and Visual Sciences, Clinical Science Center, 600 Highland Ave F4/336,
  Madison, WI 53792–3220, USA

Garchon, H.-J., M.D. Ph.D.
  Hôpital Necker, Department of Human Genetics, 161, rue de Sèvres,
  75743 Paris Cedex 15, France
Geiger, B., M.D.
  Department of Molecular Cell Biology, Weizmann Institute of Science,
  Rehovot, Israel 76100
Gloor, B., Prof. Dr.
  Direktor der Universitäts-Augenklinik, Universitätsspital, Frauenklinikstraße 24,
  8091 Zürich, Switzerland
Goldberg, I., M.D., M.B., B.S. (Syd), FRACO, FRACS
  Director, Glaucoma Service, Department of Ophthalmology, Prince of Wales
  Hospital and University of New South Wales, 187 Macquarie Street, Sydney,
  NSW 2000 Australia
Gomes, M., M.D.
  Wills Eye Hospital, 900 Walnut Street, Philadelphia, PA 19107, USA
Gramer, E., Prof. Dr. Dr.
  Universitäts-Augenklinik, Josef-Schneider-Straße 11, 97080 Würzburg, Germany
Gramer, G.
  An den Mühltannen 16, 97080 Würzburg, Germany
Grehn, F., Prof. Dr. Dr. h.c.
  Direktor der Universitäts-Augenklinik, Josef-Schneider-Straße 11,
  97080 Würzburg, Germany
Heimann, K., Prof. Dr.
  Universitäts-Augenklinik, Joseph-Stelzmann-Straße 9, 50931 Köln, Germany
Hetherington, J., M.D., FACS
  Professor of Ophthalmology, University of California Medical, Center K-301,
  University of California, Box 0352, San Francisco, CA 94143, USA
Hitchings, R., M.D.
  Professor of Ophthalmology, Director of Research, Moorfields Eye Hospital,
  City Road, London EC1V2PD, UK
Hwang, S.
  Wills Eye Hospital, 900 Walnut Street, Philadelphia, PA 19107, USA
Ishida, K., M.D.
  Gifu University, School of Medicine, 40 Tsukasa-Machi, Gifu 500, Japan
Kaufmann, P.L., M.D.
  Professor of Ophthalmology, University of Wisconsin-Madison,
  Department of Ophthalmology and Visual Sciences, Clinical Science Center,
  600 Highland Ave F4/336, Madison, WI 53792–3220, USA
Kitazawa, Y., M.D., Ph.D.
  Professor of Ophthalmology and Chairman, Gifu University, School of Medicine,
  40 Tsukasa-Machi, Gifu 500, Japan
Krieglstein, G. K., Prof. Dr.
  Direktor der Unversitäts-Augenklinik, Joseph-Stelzmann-Straße 9, 50931 Köln,
  Germany
Küchle, M., Prof. Dr.
  Universitäts-Augenklinik Erlangen, Schwabachanlage 6, 91054 Erlangen, Germany

Labree, L.
University of Southern California, School of Medicine,
Department of Ophthalmology, Doheny Eye Institute, 1450 San Pablo Street,
Los Angeles, CA 90033, USA

Liu, X., M.D.
University of Wisconsin-Madison, Department of Ophthalmology and Visual
Sciences, Clinical Science Center, 600 Highland Ave F4/336, Madison,
WI 53792–3220, USA

Lütjen-Drecoll, E., Prof. Dr.
Vorstand des Anatomischen Instituts, Lehrstuhl II der Universität Erlangen,
Universitätsstraße 19, 91054 Erlangen, Germany

Mills, R. P., M.D.
Professor of Ophthalmology and Chairman, University of Washington
School of Medicine, Mailstop RJ-10, Box 356485, Seattle, WA 98195–6485, USA

Minckler, D. S., M.D.
Professor of Ophthalmology and Director Glaucoma Service, University of
Southern California, School of Medicine, Department of Ophthalmology,
Doheny Eye Institute, 1450 San Pablo Street, Los Angeles, CA 90033, USA

Nass, J. U.
Institut für Klinische Physiologie, Universitäts-Klinikum Benjamin Franklin,
Freie Universität Berlin, Hindenburgdamm 30, 12200 Berlin, Germany

Naumann, G. O. H., Prof. Dr.
Direktor der Universitäts-Augenklinik Erlangen, Schwabachanlage 6,
91054 Erlangen, Germany

Nixon, S.
University of Southern California, School of Medicine,
Department of Ophthalmology, Doheny Eye Institute, 1450 San Pablo Street,
Los Angeles, CA 90033, USA

Peterson, J. A., B.S.
University of Wisconsin-Madison, Department of Ophthalmology
and Visual Sciences, Clinical Science Center, 600 Highland Ave F4/336,
Madison, W1 53792–3220, USA

Pfeiffer, N., Prof. Dr.
Direktor der Universitäts-Augenklinik, Langenbeckstraße 1, 55131 Mainz,
Germany

Picht, G., Dr.
Universitäts-Augenklinik, Josef-Schneider-Straße 11, 97080 Würzburg, Germany

Polansky, J. R., M.D.
University of California, Department of Ophthalmology, 10 Kirkham St,
Box 0130, Room K 301, San Francisco, CA 94143, USA

Psichias, A., Dr.
Unviersitäts-Augenklinik, Joseph-Stelzmann-Straße 9, 50931 Köln, Germany

Schlötzer-Schrehardt, U., Dr. Priv.-Doz.
Universitäts-Augenklinik Erlangen, Schwabachanlage 6, 91054 Erlangen, Germany

Spaeth, G. L., M.D.
Professor of Ophthalmology, Director Glaucoma Service, Wills Eye Hospital,
900 Walnut Street, Philadelphia, PA 19107, USA

Stumpff, F., Dr.
  Institut für Klinische Physiologie, Universitäts-Klinikum Benjamin Franklin,
  Freie Universität Berlin, Hindenburgdamm 30, 12200 Berlin, Germany
Thieme, H., Dr.
  Institut für Klinische Physiologie, Universitäts-Klinikum Benjamin Franklin,
  Freie Universität Berlin, Hindenburgdamm 30, 12200 Berlin, Germany
Thumann, G., Dr.
  Universitäts-Augenklinik, Joseph-Stelzmann-Straße 9, 50931 Köln, Germany
Thygesen, J., M.D.
  Professor of Ophthalmology, Department of Ophthalmology 2061, Copenhagen,
  University Hospital, Rigshospitalet, Blegdamsvej 9, 2100 Copenhagen, Denmark
Tian, B., M.D.
  University of Wisconsin-Madison, Department of Ophthalmology
  and Visual Sciences, Clinical Science Center, 600 Highland Ave, F4/336,
  Madison, WI 53792-3220, USA
Traverso, C.E., Prof., M.D.
  Department of Ophthalmology, Universita di Genova, San Martino Pad 9,
  16132 Genova, Italy
Varma, R., M.D.
  University of Southern California, School of Medicine,
  Department of Ophthalmology, Doheny Eye Institute, 1450 San Pablo Street,
  Los Angeles, CA 90033, USA
Welge Lüssen, U., Dr.
  Anatomisches Institut, Lehrstuhl II der Universität Erlangen,
  Universitätsstraße 19, 91054 Erlangen, Germany
Wiederholt, M., Prof. Dr.
  Direktor des Instituts für Klinische Physiologie,
  Institut für Klinische Physiologie, Universitäts-Klinikum Benjamin Franklin,
  Freie Universität Berlin, Hindenburgdamm 30, 12200 Berlin, Germany
Yamamoto , T., M.D.
  Gifu University, School of Medicine, 40 Tsukasa-Machi, Gifu 500, Japan
Zeyen, T., M.D. Ph.D.
  Director Glaucoma Service, Middelheim Hospital, Lindendreef 1,
  2020 Antwerp, Belgium
Zimmerman, C. C., M.D.
  University of California, Department of Ophthalmology, 10 Kirkham St,
  Box 0130, Room K 301, San Francisco, CA 941143, USA

Ophthalmology's Contributions to Clinical Research and Glaucoma – Study Designs Utilized in Journal Publications During the Last Decade

D. Minckler, R. Varma, A. Dawson, S. Nixon, S. Donnelly, and L. Labree

Introduction

This study was undertaken to ascertain what trends, if any, may be occurring in the utilization of various study designs during the last 10 years of clinical vision research manuscripts published in Ophthalmology. Besides providing a baseline for future analyses, this process provided an excellent opportunity to test the application of a new study design scheme developed for the journal (Table 1).

Ophthalmology first began requiring an abstract after transitioning from the Transactions of the American Academy of Ophthalmology and Otolaryngology to a peer-reviewed journal in 1978. A four-part structured abstract (purpose, methods, results and conclusions) was required after January 1992 [1]. Transition to a seven-part structured abstract, including additional sections on study design, participants/controls, and main outcome measures, was begun in late 1995 (Fig. 1). The new requirements were based on recent recommendations of the Journal of the American Medical Association (JAMA) and the expectation that an expanded abstract format would substantially improve readers' ability to rapidly assess the nature and quality of the study being described [2]. The new requirements for identifying the study design in abstracts, using standard terms or phrases, resulted initally in remarkably varied responses from authors and led to the conclusion that an acceptable study design terminology should be developed for use in the journal's abstracts.

Over the last 2 years, a Study Design Interest Group[1], including members of the Editorial Board, developed a study design scheme (Table 1) and related glossary. The scheme allows the majority of papers received to be categorized as to study design with a reasonable degree of accuracy. When manuscripts include mixed types of studies, more than one category may apply. In any case, the scheme includes the categories of interventional or observational case series and experimental (investigational)

---

[1] Chairman: Don Minckler Editorial Board Writing Committee Members: Douglas R. Anderson, Roy W. Beck, Robert C. Drews, Yoshiaki Kitazawa, Richard Alan Lewis, Maureen G. Maguire, Joel S. Mindel, David C. Musch, Joan O'Brien, Denis M. O'Day, William H. Spencer, Richard A. Stone, Alan Sugar, Rohit Varma.
Editorial Board Reviewers: George B. Bartley, Mark S. Blumenkranz, James D. Brandt, Susan Day, Robert Folberg, William R. Freeman, Peter Hamilton, Glenn J. Jaffe, Robert E. Kalina, Ronald Klein, Roger F. Steinert, Andrea C. Tongue, Thomas A. Weingeist.
Outside Reviewers: Daniel Albert, Stanley Azen, Kay Dickersin, Curtis Meinert, Paul Lichter, Paul Mitchell, Harry Quigley, Alfredo Sadun, Alfred Sommer, Bradley Staatsman, Richard Wormald, Bernard Schwartz, Janet Sunness, Susan Vitale.

Table 1. Ophthalmology JOURNAL STUDY DESIGN SCHEME. Editorial board study design interest group: [Appendix to instructions for authors] Ophthalmology 1990, 106:185–206. # 1–11 Correspond to available worksheets

I. Clinical interventional studies (clinical trials):
  A. Comparative trials:
    1. Randomized controlled trial (#1)
    2. Non-randomized comparative trial (#2)[a]
  B. Non-comparative case series (#3)
  C. Interventional case report (#4)
II. Observational studies:
  A. Case-control study (#5)[b]
  B. Cross-sectional study (#6)[c]
  C. Cohort study (#7)[d]
  D. Case series (#8)
  E. Observational case report (#9)
III. Other study types:
  A. Systematic review and meta-analyses (#10)
  B. Experimental (investigation) study (#11)
  C. Review[e]
  D. Historical manuscript[e]

[a] May include: 1. prospective study with concurrent control group; 2. prospective study with non-concurrent control group; 3. retrospective study with concurrent control group; 4. retrospective study with non-concurrent control group.
[b] An observational (non-interventional, usually retrospective) study that begins by identifying individuals with a disease (cases) for comparison to individuals without a disease (controls). The research typically proceeds from effect to cause.
[c] An observational study that identifies individuals with and without the condition being studied in a defined population at the same point in time (synonymous with prevalence study); may or may not be population-based.
[d] An observational study that begins by identifying individuals with (study group) and without (control group) a factor being investigated. Study and control groups may be concurrent or non-concurrent; almost always *prospective* and longitudinal with regard to data collection; may or may not be population-based.
[e] Worksheets not necessary.

Ophthalmology's Required Structured Abstract Sections: [see Instructions for Authors, July 1998 issue or www.eyenet.org/ophthalmology for additional explanation, definitions] (maximum 350 words total)

Objective/Purpose: (States the goals or reasons for performing the study)
Design: (Designates the type of study using a few words or a phrase, such as randomized controlled trial, non-randomized comparative trial, etc. [see Study Design Scheme] and modifiers such as prospective, rerospective, multi-center etc. as appropriate)
Participants/Controls: (Indicates the numbers of participants or eyes and control subjects)
Intervention/Methods/Testing: (Describes the principal surgical or non-surgical treatments, tests or procedures utilized during the study)
Main Outcome Measures: (Indicates the primary and/or secondary outcome measurements assessed during the study, such as visual acuity, intraocular pressure, infection rate, using single words or phrases)
Results: (Summarizes the data accumulated during the study)
Conclusions: (States and interprets the most important conclusions derived from the study data)

Fig. 1. Ophthalmology's structured abstract

studies, classification flexible enough to include most manuscripts not otherwise easily labeled as to study design. As a measure of reproducibility of the scheme, repeat categorizations of the same issue's papers at different times by the Editor have resulted in an essentially identical classification.

As part of this inter-related effort the Study Design Group has also generated study design worksheets (Table 1), modeled after the Consolidated Standards of Reporting Trials (CONSORT) agreement [3], corresponding to all major types of studies published by the journal. These worksheets are intended as guidelines for authors to use during the preparation of manuscripts for submission and may eventually be required, as is the CONSORT agreement for randomized controlled trials. Completed worksheets received with manuscripts by the editorial office will be sent to reviewers to aid in the peer review process.

Methods

Five hundred forty one papers, representing 21.3 % of the total of 2541 published from January through June for the years 1987, 1990, 1994, and 1998, were reviewed and categorized using the newly developed study design scheme. Every manuscript was assigned one code indicating the study type, and a second code indicating the number of subjects studied, and whether it had been retrospective or prospective. Retrospective is defined for this purpose as indicating the data were collected after all measurements or events (i.e., chart review). Prospective is defined as indicating that data were collected going forward in time before all measurements or events according to a pre-defined protocol (i.e., randomized controlled trial). Study size and whether the sequence of data collection had been retrospective or prospective were indicated by one of six categories: retrospective small ($n \leq 10$), medium ($n \leq 30$), or large ($n > 30$), and prospective small ($n \leq 10$), medium ($n \leq 30$), and large ($n > 30$). In addition to coding all manuscripts for study design type, size and sequence of data collection, the number of authors for each was tabulated and a mean number of listed authors for each 6-month period calculated. Glaucoma papers published in the same four intervals ($n = 62$) were tabulated separately for study design type.

Electronically stored data in the Editorial Office database were analyzed to determine the geographic origin of all accessioned and published papers for each year between 1987 and 1998.

Data were analyzed statistically (Table 2) and graphically (Figs. 1–5) to evaluate trends in various study design categories.

Results

Case reports (observational and interventional combined) showed a downward trend from 13.4 % in 1987 and 13.5 % in 1990 to 7.5 % and 5.1 % in 1994 and 1998, respectively (Table 2) (Fig. 2). Combined non-comparative interventional case series and observational case series remained relatively level at 56.3 %, 52.1 %, and 46.2 %, respectively (Fig. 3). Combined randomized controlled clinical trials and non-randomized comparative trials increased over each interval from 7.5 % in 1987 to

Table 2. Study types in published manuscripts

Study type	1987	1990	1994	1998	Annualized change	R^2	P
Case reports (observational and interventional)	13.4%	13.5%	7.5%	5.1%	-0.85±0.18	0.91	0.04
Case series (non-comparative interventional and observational)	56.3%	52.1%	57.1%	46.2%	-0.69±0.55	0.43	0.34
Randomized controlled trials	2.5%	0	6.1%	7%	0.55±0.28	0.66	0.19
Non-randomize comparative trials	5%	10.9%	7.5%	8.9%	0.20±0.34	0.14	0.62
Randomized controlled clinical trials and non-randomized comparative trials	7.5%	10.9%	13.6%	15.9%	0.75±0.08	0.98	0.01
Case control, cross-sectional and cohort studies	3.3%	10.1%	14.9%	20.8%	1.54±0.14	0.98	0.008
Retrospective studies							
All	44.2%	51.2%	74.7%	57.3%	1.64±1.54	0.36	0.40
Small ($n \leq 10$)	14.2%	24.4%	21%	18%	0.16±0.63	0.03	0.83
Medium ($10 < n \leq 30$)	11.7%	12.6%	34%	17.4%	1.01±1.35	0.22	0.53
Large ($n > 30$)	18.3%	14.2%	19.7%	21.9%	0.47±0.34	0.48	0.30
Prospective studies							
All	20.8%	33.6%	8.1%	32.2%	0.21±1.75	0.01	0.91
Small ($n \leq 10$)	2.5%	6.7%	3.4%	2.6%	-0.11±0.28	0.07	0.74
Medium ($10 < n \leq 30$)	5.8%	12.6%	0.7%	6.4%	0.47±0.34	0.09	0.70
Large ($n > 30$)	12.5%	14.3%	4%	23.2%	0.62±1.08	0.14	0.62
Human tissue/autopsy	22.2%	16.8%	11.6%	4.5%	-1.57±0.07	0.996	0.002
Experimental studies	11.8%	11.8%	4%	7%	-0.60±0.38	0.56	0.23
Comparative studies	8.3%	16.8%	22.4%	22.8%	1.29±0.40	0.84	0.08
Non-comparative studies	79.9%	71.6%	73.6%	70.2%	-.69±0.41	0.59	0.23

R^2 correlation coefficient; P value for linear regression.

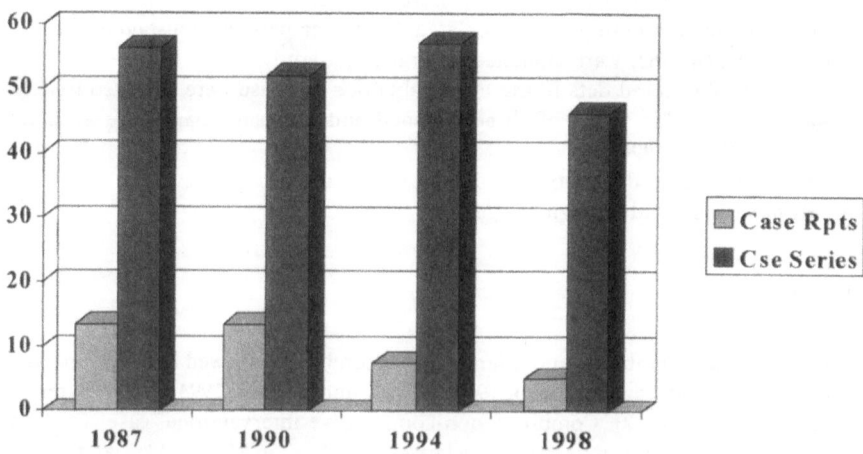

Fig. 2. Published observational and interventional cas reports and case series (% of total). *Ophthalmology*; Jan–June 1987, 1990, 1994, 1998

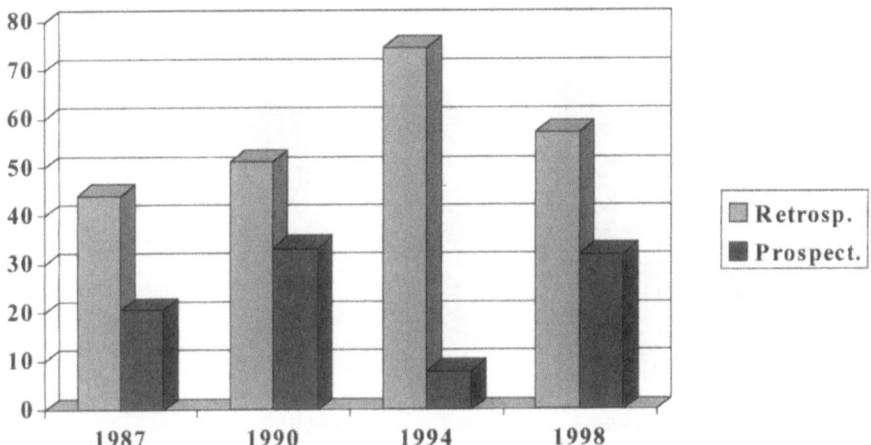

Fig. 3. Percentages of comparative and non-comparative case series. *Ophthalmology,* Jan–June 1987, 1990, 1994, 1998

10.9 %, 13.6 %, and 15.9 %, respectively (Table 2). Combined case-control, cross-sectional, and cohort studies increased from 3.3 % to 10.1 %, 14.9 %, and 20.8 %, respectively (Table 2).

Large ($n > 30$) retrospective studies (data collected after all measurements, interventions or events) remained stable at 18.3 %, 14.2 %, 19.7 %, and 21.9 %. Large ($n > 30$) prospective studies (data collected before and after measurements, interventions, or events according to a pre-planned protocol) varied between 12.5 % in 1987 to 14.3 %, 4.0 %, and 23.2 %, respectively, across the intervals (Fig. 4).

Study designs utilized in glaucoma topics generally paralleled those across all tropics (Fig. 5). Trends in the geographic origins of accessioned and published papers

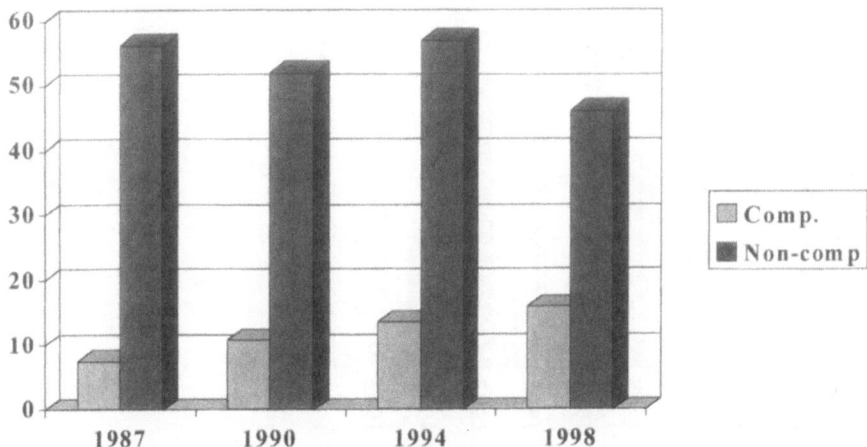

Fig. 4. All retrospective and prospective studies. *Ophthalmology;* Jan–June 1987, 1990, 1994, 1998

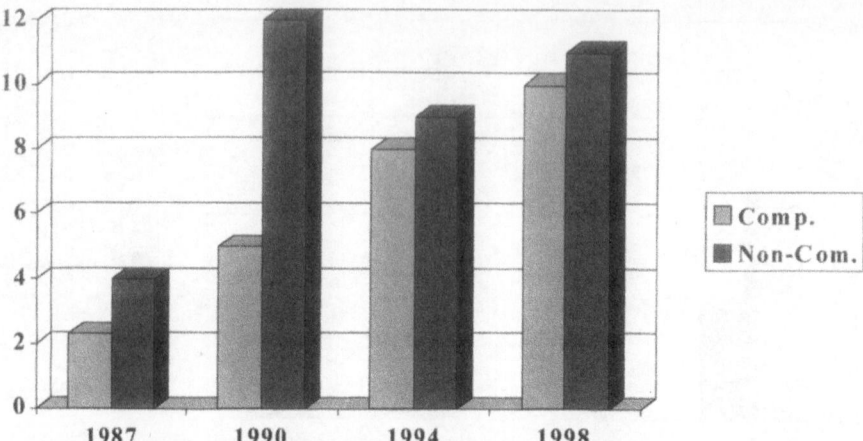

Fig. 5. Study design in published glaucoma papers: all comparative (RCT, NRCT, Exp.) vs non-comparative series. *Ophthalmology*; Jan–June 1987, 1990, 1994, 1998

indicate increasing submissions by non-North American authors (Fig. 6). Human tissue and autopsy-based papers are in decline (Fig. 7). The number of authors listed per paper shows an upward trend (Fig. 8).

Discussion

These data, from a sample representing 21.3 % of the total papers published during the years 1987/1998, provide us with clear trends in the use of various study designs, as defined for this one clinical vision journal (Figs. 2–5). Non-comparative studies,

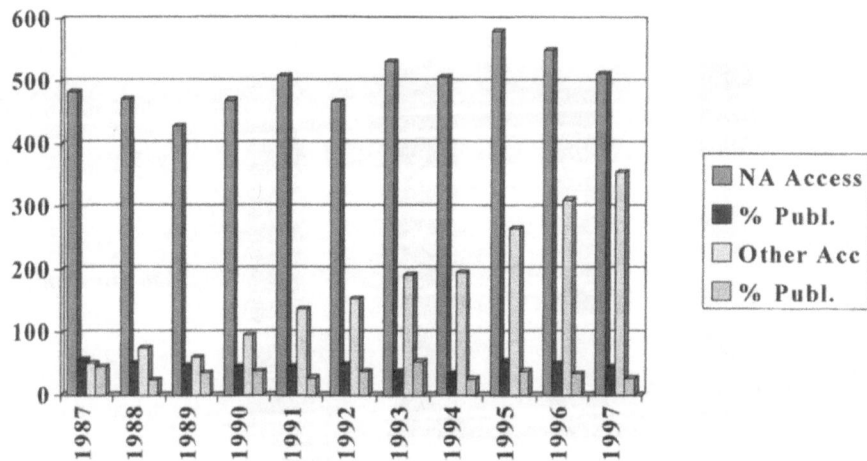

Fig. 6. *Ophthalmology*; 1987–1997: number of North American vs other accessions and percentages of each published

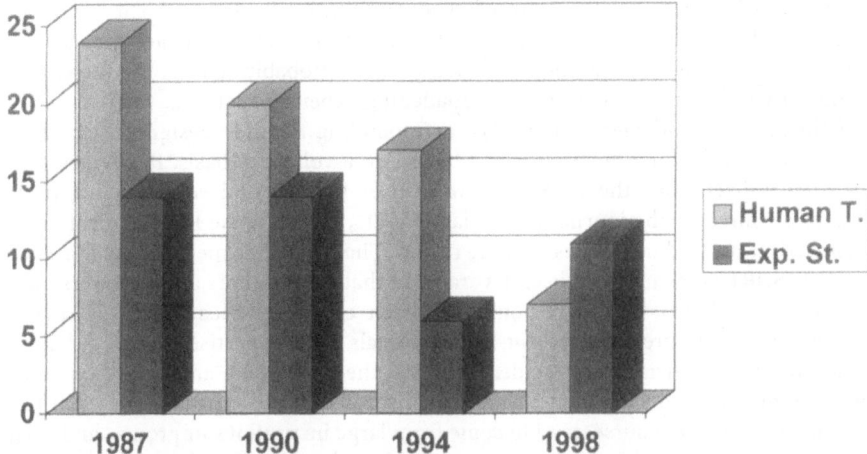

Fig. 7. Human tissue/autopsy studies and experimental studies. *Ophthalmology*; Jan–June 1987, 1990, 1994, 1998

including case reports and non-comparative case series, are declining, while comparative studies that include controls are increasing. Future studies, using these data as a baseline, should enable ascertainment of whether or not the trends toward increasingly sophisticated study designs are continuing. Glaucoma, as a specific sub-topic, has enjoyed the same general trend (Fig. 5) of increasingly rigorous study design types over the same period.

The growth in accessioned manuscripts originating from non-North American sites (Fig. 6) indicates that Ophthalmology is increasingly international in its appeal to authors, consistent with similar trends in membership for the American Academy of Ophthalmology. The relative stability in the percentages of accepted papers from

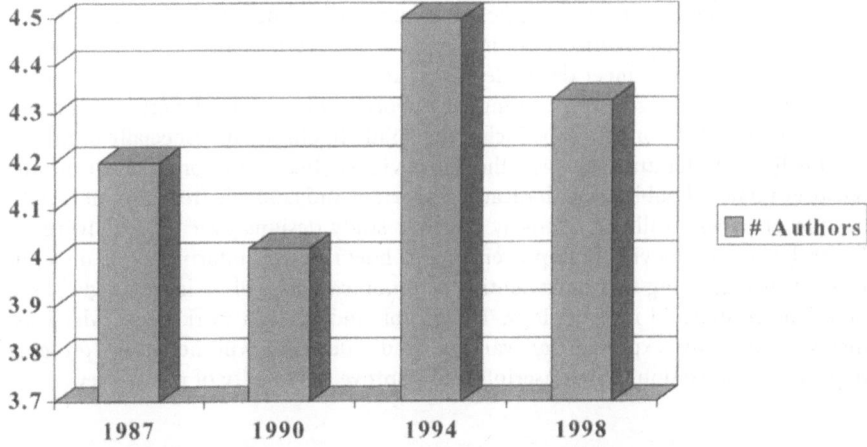

Fig. 8. Number of listed authors. *Ophthalmology*; Jan–June 1987, 1990, 1994, 1998

outside North America, in the face of exponential growth in non-North American accessions, hopefully indicates fairness and lack of geographic bias in acceptance. The trend toward increasing numbers of listed authors probably reflects the increasing complexity of clinical studies and the broadening expertise required.

Utilization of worksheets (Table 1), corresponding to study designs in Ophthalmology's study design scheme, has just begun on a voluntary basis. It is hoped that these worksheets, like the CONSORT worksheet for randomized controlled trials (RCTs), required by the journal for the last 2 years, will facilitate the organization of manuscripts and aid the process of peer review. The journal's experience to data with the CONSORT agreement has been favorable in that both authors and reviewers have found it useful. This initial response has been especially encouraging as review requests for RCTs are usually sent to individuals with expertise in study design, including biostatisticians and epidemiologists, the least likely among reviewers to need a reminder as to what issues should be discussed in this type of manuscript [4]. RCT manuscripts, of course, tend to come from large institutions or groups, and such studies have usually been organized, conducted, and analyzed with input by experts in clinical research and study design, rendering completion of the worksheet a relatively simple task.

The study design scheme and related worksheets are intended to aid authors in the organization of manuscripts and reviewers in their evaluation of the scientific validity of the research described. The scheme is intended to apply only to the study types received by the journal, and its hierarchical organization is not meant as a rating of the scientific importance of various study types. The scheme, by its organization, however, does emphasize the importance of controls, by definition a necessary aspect of randomized controlled trials, comparative trials, case-control studies, and cohort studies.

It is expected that author-reviewer feedback will result in continual evolution of the worksheets and their application [5,6]. Only time and comparisons of large numbers of published papers before and after institution of this process will demonstrate whether or not the utilization of study design worksheets has positively affected the overall quality of published papers. At the very least, the worksheets will expose authors and reviewers to a scientifically rigorous methodology for organizing and evaluating manuscripts, incorporating current expert opinion as to what items should be included to meet desirable standards for various study designs. It seems likely that case series, still constituting the majority of published papers in most peer reviewed clinical vision journals, including Ophthalmology, will especially profit.

This limited literature review, although obviously biased by confinement to only one peer reviewed publication, indicated important and laudable trends towards publication of papers utilizing relatively rigorous study designs over the last 10 years. Regardless of the inevitable improvements in how research information is disseminated, it is reassuring that our scientific communications will be increasingly based on scientifically valid methodology. The use of study design worksheets, which list inclusion ususally expected for various study designs, will hopefully promote improved organization of manuscripts and improve the quality of peer review.

References

1. Lichter PR (1991) Structured abstracts now required for all submission to the journal [Editorial]. Ophthalmology 98:1611–1612
2. Haynes RB, Mulrow CD, Huth EJ, et al. (1990) More informative abstracts revisited. Ann Intern Med 113:69–76
3. Begg C, Cho M, Eastwood S, et al. (1996) Improving the quality of reporting of randomized controlled trials: the CONSORT statement. JAMA 276:637–639
4. Meinert CL (1996) Clinical trials: the gold standard for evaluation of therapy [Editorial]. Ophthalmology 1996; 103:869–870
5. Meinert CL (1998) Beyond CONSORT: need for improved reporting standards for clinical trials [Editorial]. JAMA 279:1487–1489
6. Moher D (1989) CONSORT: an evolving tool to help improve the quality of reports of randomized controlled trials. [Editorial]. JAMA 279:1489–1491.

CHAPTER 2

Glaucoma – The Metamorphosis of the Content of a Term During the Course of Time

B. P. Gloor

Introduction

For almost 300 years the term glaucoma meant elevated intraocular pressure. Detection of elevated pressure was essential for the diagnosis, but this was not always the case. Because the meaning of this word has been questioned over the last years, it seemed worthwhile to examine the metamorphosis of the content of this term over time. At the beginning of written tradition "glaucoma" described the green color of the pupil; "glaucoma" was the name of a color. Later, for many centuries, glaucoma simply became a describing an undefined blinding disease. With the beginning of the seventeenth century, until 1855, the word glaucoma encompassed one causative agent of damage of ocular tissues, and this agent was intraocular pressure. When the ophthalmoscope became avaiblabe, it became evident, that damage to the optic nerve head and field loss were the other two markers of the disease, tied together as cause and effect. With another 100 years of growing knowledge of intraocular fluid exchange, histopathology, findings of slit lamp biomicroscopy and gonioscopy it became apparent, that there exists not one glaucoma, but many different glaucomas. Glaucoma thus became a generic name. For a considerable part of these glaucomas, increased outflow resistance is responsible for elevated pressure and damage to the optic disc. This is also the case in a large part of the primary open-angle glaucoma. Some turmoil arose when glaucomatous optic neuropathy was found in eyes with normal pressure. From this time on the term glaucoma became somewhat vague. Glaucoma became defined as the result of a synergism of many risk factors leading to optic neuropathy. The concept "Glaucoma is optic neuropathy" followed. But only if the disc and optic neuropathy become the defining markers of glaucoma, does the etiology of glaucoma appear to be so multifactorial. The disadvantage, or maybe the advantage, of the term glaucoma is that it names neither an organ, nor a tissue, nor a fluid, nor a virus, nor a metabolic defect, nor a single gene. The term glaucoma remains a vessel which can be filled or emptied arbitrarily, but the term should not be filled with so many diseases that it becomes meaningless. It could again become the term for a single damaging force or provocative agent, and that is pressure, which has to be present, if the other markers, such as field loss and optic neuropathy, can also be found or can be expected. Hoskins and Kass in Becker and Shaffers textbook state (1989): "... glaucoma will be defined as a disturbance of the structure or functional integrity of the eye that can be arrested or diminished by adequate lowering of intraocular pressure." Even when Anderson [2] had to summarize the recent (1997) symposium in Basel on „Nitric oxide and Endothelin in the Pathogenesis of Glaucoma" he named intraocular

Table 1. Glaucoma – The Metamorphosis of the Content of a term during the course of time

- Color / aspect of the pupil
- Pressure
- Pressure, cupping, field loss (1855)
- The glaucomas
  - Secondary glaucomas
  - Primary glaucoma(s) →
  - Pupillary block / angle closure
  - POAG →
    - Elevated pressure
- Glaucoma is increased resistance of outflow
  - Normal pressure (NPG)
- Glaucoma is a basket full of risk factors leading to optic neuropathy
- Glaucoma is optic Neuropathy
- Glaucoma is a vascular disease
- Glaucoma is a disease determined by specific genes (1955)
- PRESSURE AGAIN – the essential mediator of damage

For eye diseases, in which pressure is not involved, the name glaucoma should be dropped.

pressure the culprit: "We probably all accept, almost as a definition of the disease, that in glaucoma an introcular pressure (IOP) higher that an eye can tolerate results in the type of optice nerve damage and visual dysfunction that we recognize as characteristic of glaucoma." It is somehow a paradox, that in not established glaucoma, this is ocular hypertension – the term pressure is predominant! Diseases which need a therapy other than one that lowers pressure have to be sorted out, even of there is always a relation between perfusion pressure and intraocular pressure. Recognizing optic neuropathy should not obscure the view on the anterior segment of the eye. Table 1 summarizes the metamorphosis of the content of the term glaucoma.

To emphasize the topic, two quite different definitions or clues for the diagnosis of glaucoma are quoted: In the *Swiss Textbook of Ophthalmology,* Goldmann [27] made the following statement in 1954: "Under the term glaucoma (green cataract) diseases are summarized, which are the consequence of rise of intraocular pressure and of which the essential is this rise of intraocular pressure". Some 41 years later, Hirvelä, Tuulonen and Laatikainen [35] wrote "The diagnosis of glaucoma was based upon the presene of glaucomatous optic nerve head damage observed in photographs or on ophthalmoscopy regardless of the IOP level". These two different views make clear that a term like glaucoma can change its content even in a short period of time. But the back and forth between these two poles is even much older! It started as soon the ophthalmoscope revolutioned ophthalmology. The middle of ninetecuth century, when the ophthalmoscope was presented by Helmholtz in 1850 [60] and 1851 [33], was, in fact, the start of the modern age of ophthalmology. But what did the word glaucoma mean in earlier times?

At the time of Hippocrates [50,51], there was no clear differentiation between cataract and glaucoma. Both terms, cataract (hypokyma; υποκυμα, or suffusio) and glaucoma (γλαυκωμα), were used to name blinding diseases. With time cataract was more often used for curable, and glaucoma for uncurable eye diseases. Already in antiquity glaukos (γλαυκοσ) described the color of the pupil as shimmering, sea-colored, green. And for a long time, the aspect of the pupil remained the distinctive mark to classify eye diseases (Table 2).

Table 2. Differentiation of eye diseases by the color of the pupil

STAR, COLOR, ASPECT OF THE PUPIL

Star: to stare	staraplint	staerblind
• schwarzer Star	Black star	Black pupil with amaurosis
• weisser Star	White star	Leukoma
• grauer Star	Grey star	Cataract
• grüner Star	Green star	Glaucoma

The German word *star* has the same root as the English "to stare". It comes from the old high German "staraplint", the Anglo-Saxon "staerblind", the Middle Netherlands "staerblind". "Starren", in german, stands for a lifeless look. "Black star" means black pupil and stands for amaurosis, "white star" for leukoma, "grey star" for cataract and "green star" for glaucoma [51].

Slowly, but not unanimously, from the seventeenth century on, the term glaucoma became reserved for a disease characterized by elevated pressure, measured by fingers. Table 3 lists the most important names [34, 51, 16]; but in many textbooks of the eighteenth century glaucoma was still not clearly differentiated from cararact, e.g., O'Holloran 1750 [53]. In the middle of the eighteenth century cataract became definitely situated in the lens and established as a disease of the lens by Brisseau and Maître-Jan [51]. Glaucoma was thought to be a disease of the vitreous, e.g., as described by Rowley (1790)[56].

A statement made by Bowman 1862 may highlight this period: "As a practitionar, having to releave disease, I call all undue tension of the eye glaucomatous tension" [13].

Table 3. Glaucoma characterized by elevated pressure. (From [34]

1622	Richard Banister [34]
1705	Brisseau and Maître-Jan localize "cataract in the lens," glaucoma in the vitreous. Pressure (Druck, Tensio = spannung, tension) differentiates Glaucoma ("false cataract", Saint-Yves) from cataract [34]
1726	Woolhouse [34]
1745	Platner (eye hard by pressure with finger) [34]
1813	Beer (classical description of acute Glaucoma) [34]
1821	Desmarres [34]
1823	Guthrie [34]
1830	Mackenzie [50]
1855	v. Graefe [28–30]
1862	Bowman (grades pressure measured by finger) [11]
1862	Donders
1884	Arlt [3]
1890	Knies [40]
1893	Schweigger [63]
1894	Fick, Zurich [22]
1898	Vossius [76]
1903	Fuchs [22]
1915	Axenfeld [4]
....	
....	
1950	Goldmann [27]
1969	Duke-Elder [17, 18]
1989	Hoskins and Kass in Becker-Shaffers textbook [37]
1998	Anderson [2]

Already v. Graefe (1858) considered the definition of glaucoma by the characteristic optic neuropathy; but finally he rejected this definition. He wrote, "To define the glaucomatous disease I consider definition by the disease of the optic nerve as insufficient ... Similar changes can be found in other diseases (amaurosis with excavation of the disc"[29,30]. Thus:

(1) The disease of the optic nerve is only a symptom but does not merit the term glaucoma by itself. (2) The excavation of the optic nerve is not present in early stages of glaucoma, but develops over time. If we would base the diagnosis on glaucomatous excavation of the optic nerve, we forego treating the disease at a time when treatment is most effective. (3) The complex of pressure symptoms alone defines the term glaucoma as analyzed in a previous paper.

The diseases v. Graefe was dealing with mainly were what is currently defined as angle-closure glaucomas with pupillary block. Patients with primary open-angle glaucoma (POAG) as now defined, probably very seldom went to the ophthalmologist before end-stage disease was reached. Iridectomy was a true beaktrough; v. Graefe accomplished it without having understood the pathomechanism of acute angle-closure glaucoma! *Not seldom, wrong imaginations may lead to a surgical procedure that works.* But v. Graefes observation, that secondary glaucomas with iris bombé can be cured by the procedure called transfixio, paved the way. Although, at least for a while he missed the special nature of POAG: "Some colleagues maintain that in cases which are without manifest inflammatory signs, iridectomy is unsuccessful"[30]. Nevertheless he mentions "simple chronic excavation." The pathogenesis of acute and subacute glaucoma remained an enigma for v. Graefe and his contemporaries: "Arthritic", hypersecretion, inflammation, congestion (of the ciliary processes), angioneurosis, closure of the vortex veins, malresorption, "Lymphstauung", stress, etc. were acused of being the cause. Donders probably recognized POAG and spoke of "simple secretory neurosis"[36].

After v. Graefe, another 100 years were necessary to sort out of the mist of a presumed entity the many different diseases we still subsume under the term glaucoma. But progress was already made in 1855, when glaucoma consisted not only of increased pressure, but also of field loss and cupping of the disc.

These three signs of the disease are considered as essential features and called for instruments to measure them and to comprehend the etiology. Theories lead to the invention of tools and instruments. The instruments may prove or disprove the theories, may restrict or enlarge the content of a term and can change the understanding of a disease. Instruments can also narrow the view and hide the details. Instruments may become very misleading, if the scope and the exactitude of measurement are outside the critical range. This was the case e.g. with Donders' tonometer [16]. After the invention of the ophthalmoscope, the next steps were the development of instruments to measure field loss and pressure. Histopathology, slit-lamp biomicroscopy, gonioscopy, electron microscopy, angiography, and new imaging techniques with laser light, instruments to measure color, blood flow, pulse frequency and amplitude, etc., followed. The story of the development of these instruments and the progress made in anatomy, histology, physiology, pathophysiology, biochemistry, molecular biology and the genetics of the eye is also the story of what we presume is glaucoma.

Field Loss

It look a long time to specify and quantify field loss. Arcuate defects were described by Landsberg in 1869 [23] and recognized as nerve fibre bundle defects by Bjerrum in 1890 [23]. It was Bjerrum who established the **specific pattern** of field loss in glaucoma. His pupil, Rönne, added important details in 1909 [23]. Good quantification became possible only after Goldmann introduced his perimeter, in 1945 [25]. Harms and Aulhorn [23] added static perimetry, and another step forward was made with computerization. This was done by two groups of researchers, one in Bern, with Frankhauser, Spahr and Bebie, and the other in Sweden, with Krakau and Heijl, starting around 1972–1977 [23].

What Added Perimetry to our Understanding and Definition of Glaucoma

Perimetry measures what is essential for the patient! Perimetry shows the specific pattern and time course of the disease process in the ganglion cells of the retina. Perimetry led to a staging of field loss. What is the result of the fine-tuning by computerized perimetry? At least it showed the limits of perimetry: (1) Fluctuations of sensitivity are limiting factors for follow-up. (2) Even with computerized perimetry, we catch not the beginning but the beginning of the end of the disease.

Pressure and Tonometry

During the time v. Graefe and Donders, the instruments available suggested that normal pressure in the eye is 40 mm Hg. Donders instrument measured from 40 to 200 mm Hg [16]. This has to be considered when somebody claims that low-pressure glaucoma was already recognized in those days. Improvement came with the introduction of tonometry by aplanation. Weber (1867), Maklakoff (1885), and Fick (1888) were the pioneers [16]. Fick considered 29 mm Hg as normal, POAG as having 24–34 mm Hg, and absolute glaucoma as having 50–60 mm Hg [21]. The instruments were not very reliable and did not find their way into daily practice, except in eastern Europe. It is remarkable that an instrument theoretically loaded with many drawbacks became the first tool to deliver quite consistent knowledge of intraocular pressure. A reliable indentation-tonometer was introduced by Schioetz in 1905. This kind of tonometer dominated the scence for more than half a century. Only after he despaired "messing around" to improve this type of instrument, did Goldmann again grasp the idea of measuring intraocular pressure by aplanation and presented, in 1954, a useful aplanation tonometer [26].

What Added Exact Tonometry to the View in Glaucoma?

Distribution curves of intraocular pressure in large populations was established. These allow, or at least suggest, separation between low, normal and high pressure, and demonstrate that there is something like normal pressure glaucoma, or at least an optic neuropathy resembling glaucomatous optic neuropathy without elevated intraocular pressure. Therefore, tonometry is an example of how instruments and exact measurement can change the view of diseases. Furthermore, exact tonometry became, and is still, a cornerstone of adjusting pressure-lowering therapy. The term "target pressure" reflects the contemporary thinking that every single glaucoma patient has his or her own tolerable pressure or – overstated – own glaucoma.

Etiology of Pressure Rise

Pressure rise became slowly understood after it was recognized that there is production and outflow of aqueous (Lymphcirculation [61]) and that outflow may be blocked. Essential contributions came from Leber, who worked on fluid exchange in the eye from 1873 until 1900. He and his pupil Deutschmann [14] recognized that aqueous is formed by the ciliary processes, passes Fontana's space (the trabecular meshwork) and leaves the eye through Schlemm's canal [47–49]. This was still challenged, until World War I, e.g., by Hamburger [32]. Even in 1945, Duke-Elder still discussed the iris and/or ciliary body as sources of the aqueous [17]. In the years 1918, 1921 and 1923, Seidel delivered definite proof that aqueous is formed by the ciliary body [64–66]. At the same time as Leber looked at production of aqueous. Weber (1877) recognized, in pathology specimens, blockage of the outflow pathways [77]. He thought that congestion of the ciliary body was responsible for pressing the iris forward toward the cornea. J.P. Smith (1888), when he described the narrowing of the anterior chamber, still thought that a congestion of the ciliary body triggered acute glaucoma [45]. In 1897 Czermak [13] already understood angle-closure glaucoma, almost in the same way as Curran [12], in Kansas City, and Seidel in Heidelberg. In 1920 [45] both recognized the pupillary block – angle closure mechanism. At this time, tools became available to understand several forms of pressure rise by clinical observation: slit-lamp biomicroscopy and gonioscopy.

Slit Lamp Biomicroscopy and Gonioscopy

Slit-lamp biomicroscopy was invented by Gullstrand in 1911 [31], but it was Vogt who recognized the impact of this instrument. He collected almost all possible findings in the anterior segment of the eye into a textbook and atlas which remains unsurpassed and still up to date [73–75]; but he did not recognized what did not grow in his own garden [52]. After he he had several disputes with Koeppe, another expert in slit-lamp biomicroscopy, he wrote in a footnote (!) to the introduction of this work: "Several years ago Koeppe developed instruments to bring parts of the fundus of the eye (disc and macula) in the reach of slit lamp examination. This method is not taken into account, because it is without practical relevance. This is also the reason not to consider microscopy of the chamber angle and ultramicroscopy"[73]. It may be comforting that giants also can suffer from scotomas.

Increasing knowledge on outflow pathways stimulated invention of optical instruments to view the chamber angle. Trantas, in 1907 [67] (and again in 1935 [68]), Salzmann in 1914 and 1915 [58, 59], Koeppe, in 1919 and 1920 [42–44] and Troncoso, in 1925 [70], led the fundaments of gonisoscopy. But it took almost 20 years until the method of Koeppe found its way into clinical practice – not in Europe but in the US – when Barkan in 1936 [5–7], combined the Koeppelens with a binocular microscope hanging on a tripod. With Barkan, the distintion between pupillary block-angle-closure glaucoma and POAG became established [8,9], but gonloscopy found its way into daily practice only after Goldmann presented his goniolens at the 15th International Congress of Ophthalmology in Cairo in 1937 [24]. He introduced his one-mirror contact lens to combine goniscopy with slit-lamp biomicroscopy. Classification of the width of the chamber angle followed (see [71]). Barkan found the advantages of his method of gonioscopy in the visibility of large areas of the chamber angle. The undisputed advantage of Goldmanns method is that the optical slit is available to evaluate the structures in and around the chamber angle.

What Did Slit Lamp Biomicroscopy and Gonioscopy Add to the View on Glaucoma?

From now on slit-lamp biomicroscopy and gonioscopy allowed an appearingly clear cut separation of the glaucomas into two groups: **The first one can be defined by visible changes in the outflow pathways responsible for elevated pressure leading to optic neuropathy, field loss and other changes in the tissues of the eye.** This group contains pupillary block-angle-closure glaucoma, congenital glaucoma, developmental glaucomas, pseudoexfoliation glaucoma, pigmentary glaucoma, neovascularisation glaucoma, and most of the other secondary glaucomas. In this group there is little doubt that the cause of the rise of intraocular pressure is the key feature of the disease. **The second group is what sails under the flag of POAG.** In this group, containing about 90 % of all glaucoma patients, instruments for precise measurement of intraocular pressure made it possible to sort out low tension glaucoma (LTG) or normal pressure glaucoma (NPG). This also let us recognize that there may be etiologies other than elevated pressure of optic atrophies with cupping. At least in name, low pressure glaucoma pressure still ekes out its existence. For some time, the proportion of LTGs was overestimated as being one third to a half of all POAGs. Newer population studies show that, if ocular hypertensives are included, $5/6$ of them have pressure above 22 mm Hg, and $1/6$ have pressures below 22 mm Hg; a quarter of the established POAG patients have elevated pressure [19,39]. To what extent this proportion becames smaller if pressure is measured in the supine position in the morning before the patient gets up – and for this the doctor also has to leave his or her bed earlier than most ophthalmologists do – is not essential for the present discussion. However, patients with elevated pressure and usually classified as having POAG also form a heterogenous group. For example when we were looking at a sample of 100 patients in whom glaucoma or ocular hypertension developed before the age of 40, 77 % of 200 eyes showed developmental changes in the chamber angle [41]. The fact, that in

POAG no convincingly explaining pathology could be found in the outflow pathways and that pressure elevation is not always present in eyes harboring optic nerve heads with glaucomatous-like excavation led van Buskirck and Cioffi [72] to look for an other identification or definition of glaucoma: "Screening patients by measuring intraocular pressure will identify only about half of the patients with glaucoma. However, the one clinical finding of all patients with glaucoma is the characteristic optic neuropathy." Obviously it was a small step to transform this definition into the single criterion for diagnosis, by Hirvelä, Tuulonen and Laatikainen, who wrote in 1995, as mentioned above: "The diagnosis of glaucoma was based upon the presence of glaucomatous optic nerve head damage observed in photographs or by ophthalmoscopy regardless of the IOP level" [35]. By the time it became fashionable to diagnose glaucoma by the aspect of the optic nerve head, the statement **"glaucoma is optic neuropathy"** again won great acceptance. This statement is at least incomplete or unprecise and has drawbacks. A term or the name of a disease usually comprises a definition of this disease, separates the disease from other diseases and/or names the etiology or main agent leading to the disease, or names the common features of a group of diseases. The statement **"glaucoma is optic neuropathy"** brings no separation from other diseases of the optic nerve. If it is the only criterion for diagnosis, many ongoing glaucomas will be missed e.g., developmental glaucomas, because it is a definition or diagnosis or description of a feature near or at the endpoint and not at the beginning of the disease. In my opinion, this is some sort of capitulation. Also, many pseudoglaucomas will be declared as glaucoma [69]. And one important point: The same morphology is not identical with the same pathogenesis. Nonetheless, this definition stimulated the development of new tools to examine and measure changes in the optic nerve head. This was pioneered by Elschnig (1907) [19]. Photogrammetry was introduced by Holm and Krakau in 1970 [36], Saheb, Drance and Nelson in 1972 [57], and Portney in 1973 [54]. Photometry, planimetry, stereoplanimetry are connected with the names of Read and Spaeth [55], Schwartz [62], Airaksinen, Jonas, Dannheim, and many others; stereochronoscopy by Goldmann and Lothmar; flicker comparison by Bengtson and Krakau in 1977; photometry by Robert in 1982; laser ophthalmoscopy by Zinser, Weinreb, Klingbeil, Zeimer, Michelson. Follow-up documentation of the optic nerve head, at least by fundus photographs, stereoplanimetry and/or topographical mapping with laser ophthalmoscopes became standard in many glaucoma centers.

What Did Revival of the Concept "Glaucoma Is Optic Neuropathy" Add to the View of Glaucoma?

At least it forced a new look at what is going on at the optic nerve head. The search for correlation between field loss and cupping showed no strong association [15, 55] and change of cupping became an important parameter for follow-up. It diluted, somehow, what should be understood under the term glaucoma. To some extent it narrowed the view of glaucoma to what is going on at the optic nerve head, to the other extent it enlarged the content of the term glaucoma and also stimulated ideas, concepts and theories about possible factors leading to, or saving from, damage of the optic nerve – which all still have to be substantiated!

The (presumend) existence of LTG suggested defining (elevated) intraocular pressure as only one risk factor among other risk factors and not as the causative agent, and the step was small to define glaucoma as a vascular and circulatory disease. Much research has focused on ocular blood flow. Measurement of pulsatile ocular blood flow is the newest trend [46]. For this the most exciting new instrument is the SMART-LENS, a multifunctional ophthalmodynamic tonometer built into a contact lens which allows measurement of intraocular pressure, pulse amplitude and simultaneous observation of the eye. It is an invention of Robert and Kanngiesser [20]. Because perfusion pressure always has to overcome intraocular pressure, vascular components are always involved, but the question is: If vascular disease is the main cause of optic neuropathy, is this still glaucoma or is it really helpful to call this glaucoma?

Focusing on the optic nerve head and on ocular blood flow let us almost forget intraocular fluid exchange and outflow pathways, but the pendulum has swung back: research on what is going on in the anterior segment of the eye is again taking place. Molecular biology and molecular genetics bring a new aspect into efforts to understand and define glaucoma. Different glaucomas could be diseases caused by defects of specific genes. To correlate genotypes and phenotypes is the task for the coming years.

Why is Glaucoma Such a Vague Affair?

One reason is that although one speaks about glaucoma, only POAG – still a very large basket – is meant. Confusion arised regarding POAG after it became obvious that the diagnosis could not be made by just looking for a single facet of the disease, especially not only by measuring intraocular pressure. This is like "throwing out the baby with the bath water." We have to differentiate between screening, making the diagnosis, and tyring to find a definition.

In screening for glaucoma, we cannot rely on one single indicator or parameter. For every single marker or parameter there is a huge overlap between normal and diseased. This applies for pressure, cup, nerve fibre loss, field and all the different functions of the visual system.

In the diagnosis of glaucoma, intraocular pressure, disc, nerve fibre layer, field, chamber angle and the whole anterior segment have to be considered. As in many other diseases, in many cases of POAG the diagnosis is a matter of follow-up and time.

Conclusion

The question is: would it not be wise to drop the term glaucoma for diseases in which pressure is not the dominant, but only a marginal, risk factor, even if there is always a relation between perfusion pressure and intraocular pressure? Aging of the optic nerve head only is not a disease! Age-related apoptosis is also not a disease! So called arteriosclerotic glaucoma is most of the time not a glaucoma. When it comes to health economics our task will be to sort out all optic neuropathies which do not respond to pressure-lowering therapy. This is an enormous enterprise. If one adheres to the sentence: "Glaucoma is optic neuropathy" at least some qualifications are necessary: "Glaucoma begins as a disease of the anterior segment with increased outflow resistance leading to increased intraocular pressure or a pressure too high for the eye of a single individuum, and which damages the optic nerve".

References

1. Albert DM, Edwards DD ed (1996) The History of Ophthalmology. Blackwell Science, Cambridge Mass. p. 211–212
2. Anderson DR (1998) How should glaucoma patients be handled. In: Haefliger IO, Flammer J (ed) Nitric oxide and endothelin in the pathogenesis of glaucoma. Lippincott-Raven, Philadelphia, New York, pp. 242–253
3. Arlt F (1884) Zur Lehre vom Glaucom. Wilhelm Braumüller, Wien
4. Axenfeld Th (1915) Lehrbuch der Augenheilkunde, 4. Aufl. G. Fischer, Jena
5. Barkan O (1936) The function and structure of the angle of the anterior chamber and Schlemms canal. Arch Opthal 15:101–110
6. Barkan O (1936) On the genesis of glaucoma. Am J Ophthalmol 19:209–215
7. Barkan O (1936) A new operation for chronic glaucoma. Am J Ophthalmol 19:951–966
8. Barkan O (1938) Glaucoma: classification, causes and surgical control. Am J Ophthalmol 21:1099–1117
9. Barkan O (1954) Pupillary block and the narrow angle mechanisms. Am J Ophthalmol 37:332–349
10. Bonomi L, G Marchini, M Marraffa et al (1998) Prevalence of glaucoma and intraocular pressure. Distribution in a defined population. The Egna-Neumarkt Study. Ophthalmology 105:209–215
11. Bowman W (1862) On glaucomatous affections and their treatment by Iridectomy. Br Med J 377–382. In: The collected papers of Sir W. Bowman. J. Burdon-Sanderson, J.W. Huke (eds) Vol. II Harrison, London 1892. Printed by The Classics of Ophthalmology, Gryphon Editions, Birmingham Alabama, 1984
12. Curran EJ (1920) A new operation for glaucoma involving a new principle in the etiology and treatment of chronic primary glaucoma. Arch Ophthalmol 49:131–155
13. Czermak W (1897) Einiges zur Lehre von der Entstehung und zum Verlaufe des prodomalen und akuten Glaukomanfalles. Prager Med Wochenschrif 22:15–17
14. Deutschmann R (1880) Über die Quellen des Humors aqueus. v. Graefes Arch F Ophth XXVI 3:117–133
15. Dimitrakos SA, Fey U, Gloor B, Jäggi P (1985) Correlation or non-correlation between glaucomatous field loss as determined by automated perimetry and changes in the surface of the optic disc. In: Greve EL, Leydhecker W, Raitta C (eds) Second European Glaucoma Symposium, Helsinki, DW Junk, Dordrecht pp. 23–33
16. Draeger J (1966) Tonometry – physical fundamentals, development of methods and clinical application. S. Karger, Basel, New York
17. Duke-Elder WSt (1945) Textbook of ophthalmology, vol. III. Henry Kimpton, London pp. 3355–3368
18. Duke-Elder WSt (1996) Glaucoma and hypotony. In: System of ophthalmology, vol. XI, ff Henry Kimpton, London chapter VI p 379
19. Elschnig A (1907) Über physiologische, atrophische und glaukomatöse Exkavation. Ber Ophthalmol Ges Heidelberg 34:2–7
20. Entenman B, Robert YCA, Pirani P, Kanngiesser H, Dekker PW (1997) Contact lens tonometry – application in humans. Invest Ophthalmol Vis Sci 38: 2447–2451
21. Fick AE (1894) Lehrbuch der Augenheilkunde, Leipzig
22. Fuchs E (1903) Lehrbuch der Augenheilkunde, 9. Aufl. Leipzig, Wien
23. Gloor B, Stürmer J (1993) Entwicklung der Perimetrie. In: Gloor B (ed) Perimetrie 2. Aufl., Bücherei des Augenarztes Band 110 F. Enke, Stuttgart, pp. 1–7
24. Goldmann H (1938) Zur Technik der Spaltlampenmikroskopie. Ophthalmologica 96:90–97
25. Goldmann H (1945) Grundlagen exakter Perimetrie. Ophthalmologica 109:57–70
26. Goldmann H (1955) Un nouveau tonomètre a l'applanation. Bull Mém Soc Franç Ophtal 67:474–477
27. Goldmann H (1954) Das Glaukom. In: Amsler M, Brückner A, Franceschetti A, Goldmann H, Streiff EB: Lehrbuch der Augenheilkunde, 2. Aufl. S. Karger, Basel p 398
28. Graefe A (1857) Über die Iridektomie bei Glaukom und über den glaukomatösen Prozess. Arch Ophthalm 3, 2., Abt. aus Sattler, Hrsg., Albrecht von Graefe's grundlegende Arbeiten über den

Heilwert der Iridektomie beim Glaukom, Amr. Barth, Leipzig 1911, Nachdruck Zentralantiquariat Leipzig 1968, 8–37

29. v. Graefe A (1858) Weitere klinische Bemerkungen über Glaukom, glaukomatöse Krankheiten und über die Heilwirkung der Iridektomie. Arch Ophthalm 4, 2. Abt. p 1, aus Sattler, Hrsg., Albrecht von Graefe's grundlegende Arbeiten über den Heilwert der Iridektomie beim Glaukom, Amr. Barth, Leipzig 1911, Nachdruck Zentralantiquariat Leipzig 1968, 38–63

30. v. Graefe A (1862) Über die Resultate der Iridektomie und über einige Formen von konsektutivem und kompliziertem Glaukom. Arch Ophthalm 8, 2, Abt. p 1862, aus Sattler, hersg. Albrecht von Graefe's grundlegende Arbeiten über die Heilwerte der Iridektomie beim Glaukom, Amr. Barth, Leipzig 1911, Nachdruck Zentralantiquariat Leipzig 1968, 64–77

31. Gullstrand A (1911) Demonstration der Nernstspaltlampe. Verslg ophthalm. Ges. Heidelberg 374

32. Hamburger C (1914) Beiträge zur Ernährung des Auges. Leipzig

33. Helmholtz H (1851) Beschreibung eines Augenspiegels zur Untersuchung der Netzhaut im lebenden Auge. Berlin

34. Hirschberg J (1918) Geschichte der Augenheilkunde Bd I–X; Bd VII Allgemeines Inhalts- und -Verzeichnis p. 171

35. Hirvelä A, Tuulonen A, Laatikainen L (1995) Intraocular pressure prevalence in glaucoma in elderly people in Finland. Int. Ophthalmol 18:299–307

36. Holm O, Krakau CET (1970) A photographic method for measuring volume of papillary excavations. Ann Ophthalmol 1:327–332

37. Hoskins HD, Kass MA (1989) Becker-Shaffers Diagnosis and Therapy of the Glaucomas, 6th edition, Mosby, St. Louis

38. Jaeger E (1855/56) Beiträge zur Pathologie des Auges (Fol 56 S, Wien, KK Hof- und Stattsdruckerei)

39. Klein BEK, Klein R, Sponsel WE et al. (1992) Prevalence of glaucoma. The Beaver Dam Eye Study. Ophthalmology 99:1499–1504

40. Knies M (1890) Grundriss der Augenheilkunde. 2. Aufl. JF Bergmann, Wiesbaden

41. Kniestedt Chr, Kammann MT, Stürmer J, Gloor B (1998) Dysgenetic changes in the chamber angle in patients with glaucoma or in glaucoma suspects developed under the age of 40. XXVIIIth International Congress of Ophthalmology, Amsterdam, Book of Abstracts 135

42. Koeppe L (1919) Die Theorie und Anwendung der Stereomikroskopie des lebenden menschlichen Kammerwinkels im fokalen Licht des Gullstrandschen Nernstspaltlampe. Münch Med Wschr 66 708–709

43. Koeppe L (1919) Die Mikroskopie des lebenden Kammerwinkels im fokalen Licht der Gullstrandschen Nernstspaltlampe. v. Graefe's Arch Ophthal 101:48–66

44. Koeppe L (1920) Das stereomikroskopische Bild des lebenden Kammerwinkels an der Nernstspaltlampe beim Glaukom. Klin Mbl Augenheilk 65:389

45. Kronfeld PC (1996) Glaucoma. In: Albert DM, Edwards Dd (ed) The history of ophthalmology. Blackwell Science, Cambridge MA, pp 211–212

46. Langham ME, Farrell RA, O'Brien V et al (1989) Blood flow in the human eye. Acta Ophthalmol (Suppl) 191:9–13

47. Leber Th (1894) Der gegenwärtige Stand unserer Kenntnis vom Flüssigkeitswechsel des Auges. Ergebn Anatomie u. Entwicklungsgeschichte. Hrsg. V. Merkel u. Bonnet, VII, p 143–196

48. Leber Th (1895) Über den Flüssigkeitswechsel in der vorderen Kammer. Arch. F. Augenheilkunde. XXXI. S. 309. Ber. 24. Vers. D. ophthalm. Gesellsch. Heidelberg S. 83

49. Leber Th, Bentzen, ChrG (1895) Der Circulus venosus Schlemmii steht nicht in offener Verbindung mit der vorderen Augenkammer. Arch f Ophthalm. XLI 1, S. 235

50. Mackenzie W (1835) A practical treatise on the diseases of the eye. London, Longman, Reese, Orme, Brown and Green, p 822 ff

51. Münchow W (1984) Geschichte der Augenheilkunde, Separatdruck aus „Der Augenarzt" Band 9, 2. Aufl. F. Enke Stuttgart

52. Niederer H-M (1989): Alfred Vogt (1879–1943) – Seine Zürcher Jahre 1923–1943. Zürcher Medizingeschichtliche Abhandlungen, Nr. 207, hrsg. HM Koelbing et al. Juris Druck + Verlag, Zürich

53. O'Hollroan S (1750) A new treatise on the glaucoma or cataract, Powell, Dublin

54. Portney GL (1974) Photogrammetric categorial analysis of the optic nerve head. Trans AM Acad Oph Otol 78:275–289

55. Read RM, Spaeth GL (1874) The practical clinical appraisal of the optic disc in glaucoma: The natural history of cup progression and some specific disc-field correlation. Trans Am Acas Ophthalmol Otolaryngol 78:255–274

56. Rowley W (1790) A treatise on one hundred and eighteen principal diseases of the eyes and eyelids. Wingrave, London

57. Saheb NE, Drance SM, Nelson A: The use of photogrammetry in evaluating the cup of the optic nervehead for study in chronic simple glaucoma. Can J Ophthalmol 7:466–471

58. Salzmann M (1914) Die Ophthalmoskopie der Kammerbucht I. Z. Augenheilk. 31:1–19.
59. Salzmann M (1915) Die Ophthalmoskopie der Kammerbucht II. Z. Augenheilk. 34:26–69
60. Schett A (1996) The Ophthalmascope – Der Augenspiegel, JP Wayenborgh, Oostende Belgium, p 20
61. Schoute GJ, Koster-Gzn W (1901): Lymphcirkulation und Glaukom (Die Physiologie und Pathologie des Flüssigkeitswechsels im Auge) Bericht über die Jahre 1895–1900 in Th. Axenfeld et al. Ergebnisse der Allgemeinen Pathologie und Pathologischen Anatomie des Auges, Hrsg O Lubarsch, Ostertag, JF Bergmann, Wiesbaden
62. Schwartz B (1973) Cupping and pallor of the optic disc. Arch Ophthalmol 89:272–277
63. Schweigger C (1893) Handbuch der Augenheilkunde, 6. Aufl. A. Hirschwald, Berlin
64. Seidel E (1918) Experimentelle Untersuchungen über die Quelle und den Verlauf der intraokularen Saftströmung. v. Graefes Arch. Ophthal, 95:1–72
65. Seidel E (1921) Weitere experimentelle Untersuchungen über die Quelle und den Verlauf der intraokularen Saftströmung: IX. Mitteilung über den Abfluß des Kammerwassers aus der vorderen Augenkammer. v. Graefes Arch. Ophthal, 104:357–402
66. Seidel E (1923) Weitere experimentelle Untersuchungen über die Quelle und den Verlauf der intraokularen Saftströmung: XX. Mitteilung: Die Messung des Blutdrucks in dem episkleralen Venengeflecht, den vorderen Ciliar- und den Wirbekvenen normaler Augen (Messungen am Tier- und Menschenauge). v. Graefes Arch. Ophthal 112:252–259
67. Trantas A (1907) Ophthalmoscopie de la region ciliaire et retrociliaire. Arch ophthal (franç) 27:581–606
68. Trantas A (1935) Alterations gonioscopiques dans différentes affections oculaires. Bull soc Héllénique d'Opht 1:3
69. Trobe JD, Glaser JS, Janet C, Cassady MS (1980) Optic Atrophy – Differential Diagnosis by Fundus Observation Alone. Arch Ophthalmol 98:1040–1050
70. Troncoso MU (1925) Gonioscopy and clinical application. A gonoscopical study of anterior peripheral synechiae in primary glaucoma. Amer. J. Ophthalm. 8:433–449
71. Urech D: Hans Goldmanns Beitrag zur Glaukomforschung – seine Bedeutung für die Glaukomdiagnostik. Inaug. Diss. Zürich 1989
72. van Buskirk EM, Cioffi GA (1992) Glaucomatous optic neuropathy. Amer J Ophthalmology 113:447–452
73. Vogt A (1930) Lehrbuch und Atlas der Spaltlampenmikroskopie des lebenden Auges. II. Auflage. Erster Teil: Technik und Methodik, Hornhaut und Vorderkammer. Springer, Berlin, S. 2 ff
74. Vogt A (1931) Lehrbuch und Atlas der Spaltlampenmikroskopie des lebenden Auges. Band II J. Springer, Berlin
75. Vogt A (1942) Lehrbuch und Atlas der Spaltlampenmikroskopie des lebenden Auges. Band III Schweizer Verlagshaus, Zürich
76. Vossius A (1898) Lehrbuch der Augenheilkunde, Franz Deuticke Leipzig und Wien
77. Weber A (1877) Die Ursache des Glaucoms. Graefe's Archiv Ophthalm. 23:1–91

Lack of Knowledge About Glaucoma: A Possible Risk Factor for Blindness from the Disease

N. Pfeiffer

Introduction

Glaucomatous disease remains one of the veritable problem areas in ophthalmology. In spite of numerous advances in the field, the prevalence of blindness from the disease appears, remarkably, to be nearly the same now as many decades ago. There are several explanations for this: The relative longevity of the population has contributed to an increased proportion of the elderly in many countries. However, mechanisms of the development of glaucoma, mechanisms of the damage process and questionable success of the treatment available may also contribute to the rather slow advances in the prevention of blindness from glaucoma. Many of the areas are discussed in this volume. It is also surprising that glaucoma remains one of the leading causes of irreversible blindness, not only in so-called developing but also in industrialized countries. A major problem appears to be that the disease often is only detected after a major proportion of visul function, as measured by perimetry, has already been lost. In fact, studies from various countries suggest that in most cases glaucoma is detected only after late stages of the disease have been reached (Leydhecker 1973). Thies review suggested that in 6.4 % of patients glaucoma was only detected after complete blindness had occurred in at least one eye. A recent population-based study, the Baltimore Eye Survey, revealed that even in an urban population with good access to medical care, 50 % of glaucoma patients were undetected (Telsch et al. 1991). What could be the reasons for this unfavourable proportion of detected and undetected glaucomas?

At present, there appears to be an uncertainty as to the proper definition of glaucoma. While optic nerve damage and visual field defects are part of the definition, there is an ongoing argument whether or not increased intraocular pressure should be part of the definition. This is puzzling, as elevated intraocular pressure (IOP) is a substantial part of the definition of both ocular hypertension, on the one hand, and of all secondary glaucomas, on the other. As long as there is no clearcut definition of the disease, there will be deficits in its detection. Also, screening methods either are ineffective, or too complicated, and/or too expensive. An IOP cut-off point of 18 mm Hg would render a sensitivity and specificity of 65 % for the detection of glaucoma (Tielsch and Katz 1991). Standard clinical perimetry, such as the Goldmann method, renders positive results only after apparently 30 %–40 % of optic nerve fibers have already been lost (Quigley 1982). Electrophysiological testing would improve the diagnostic yield but is impractical for a large population group (Pfeiffer et al. 1993). However, some risk factors have been identified, such as higher age, a first degree relative with glaucoma, myopia and being of African heritage. It appears reasonable that patients will only present themselves for adequate screening if there is an awareness for this almost asymptomatic disease and if they know that they may have additional risk factors for the development of glaucoma.

What Do Patients Know About Glaucoma?

When patients present upon first diagnosis of the disease, the treating ophthalmologist is frequently confronted with the same pattern: (1) The diagnosis was made "by chance", for example, upon prescription of reading glasses. (2) The patient did not note any symptoms. (3) The patient had not heard of glaucoma. (4) The patient is not aware that he or she might have been at risk. (5) The patient does not know whether or not close blood relatives might have glaucoma. (6) If the patient has information on the disease it might be grossly false.

In fact a recent study suggested that patient knowledge of glaucoma is rather poor. After patients attending glaucoma clinics received a questionaire, they were randomized into two groups. One group was only followed up, while the other group underwent an education program using brochures and a video. Knowledge delivered through brochures and videos was reassessed after 2 weeks and 6 months. While at 2 weeks the educated group performed better than the group without education the effect had completely worn off upon reexamination after 6 months (Kim et al. 1997). In this study knowledge of patients was tested who already had the disease for various periods of time. Their knowledge should be better than that of the healthy population. Further education in addition to and beyond what they had already learned from their treating physician by personal research did not necessarily last for very long. However, if one aims to diagnose new glaucoma patients, it is also of interest to establish what undiagnosed glaucoma patients know about glaucoma.

What Does the General Population Know about Glaucoma?

In a survey from our own group, we investigated the knowledge of the undiagnosed general population about glaucoma (Pfeiffer et al. 1993). In the western part of Germany, a representative study of the German population was performed by means of fact to face interviews conducted with 2000 people. The purpose of the study was to assess the knowledge of the general population with respect to glaucomatous disease, its signs and symptoms, possible treatment and the source of information.

1. **Knowledge of the term glaucoma:** When asked which eye diseases were known, 47 % named glaucoma as an answer. There was an apparent correlation with age. While glaucoma was mentioned by only 37 % of persons age 34 and younger, it was mentioned by 57 % of persons 55 and older. Among persons who had not yet had contact with an eye health care provider, only 29 % (all age groups) mentioned glaucoma.

2. **Understanding of glaucoma:** When given a list of possible effects of glaucoma, 28 % selected the danger of blindness, 21 % increased intraocular pressure and 10 % visual field defects. Again, there was a positive correlation with age.

3. **Glaucoma as an asymptomatic disease:** It is important that there is an understanding that glaucoma is a relatively asymptomatic disease. However, most people expect reading difficulties, red eyes or other apparent symptoms. Only a small proportion of the general population (12 % overall, 10 % of the group aged 34 and younger, 14 % of the group aged 55 and older) could imagine that symptoms might be rare.

4. **Risk factors for glaucoma:** When a selection of possible risk factors was offered, high age (60 years and older) was selected by 31 %, while the age group of 40–59 years was not thought to be at risk (12 %). A blood relative with glaucoma (21 %) was considered to be a much higher risk factor than myopia (4 %).

5. **Treatment options:** We assumed that people will only present for screening if treatment is available and not too invasive. When asked about the expectations concerning treatment modalities, only 22 % knew about topical application of eye drops. Some 27 % had heard of laser treatment and 60 % knew about surgery. Some 11 % believed that no treatment whatsoever was available.

6. **Source of information:** The major source of information about glaucoma appears to be from friends (28 %), print media (23 %) or television/radio (12 %). Ophthalmologists are a relatively small source of information (9 %). A surprisingly large group knew somebody who suffered from glaucoma (14 %).

References

Leydhecker W (1973) Glaukom. Ein Handbuch, 2. Aufl. Springer, Berlin, Heidelberg, New York

Tielsch JM, Sommer A, Katz J, Royall RM, Quigley HA, Javitt J (1991) Racial variations in the prevalence of primary open-angle glaucoma: The Baltimore eye survey. JAMA 266:369–374

Tielsch JM, Katz J, Singh K et al. (1991) A population-based evaluation of glaucoma screening: the Baltimore Eye Survey. Am J Epidemiol 134:1102–1110

Quigley HA, Addicks EM, Green WR (1982) Optic nerve damage in human glaucoma. III Quantitative correlation of nerve fiber loss and visual field defect in glaucoma, ischemic neuropathy, disc edema, and toxic neuropathy. Arch Opthalmol 100:135–146

Pfeiffer N, Bach M, Tilmon B (1993) Predictive value of the Pattern-Electroretinogram. Invest. Opthalmol Vis Sci 34 (Nr. 5); 1710–1715

Kim S, Stewart JF, Emond MJ, Reynolds AC, Leen MM, Mills RP (1997) The effect of a brief education program on glaucoma patients. J Glaucoma 6:146–151

Pfeiffer N, Krieglstein GK (1993) Knowledge about glaucoma in the population. Invest Ophthalmol Vis Sci 34: 1798

Livingstone PM, Lee SE, De Paola C, Carson CA, Guest CS, Taylor HR (1995) Knowledge of glaucoma, and its relationship to self-care practice, in a population sample. Aust N Z J Ophthalmol 23:37–41

CHAPTER 4

Compliance with Medical Therapy in Chronic Glaucoma

I. Goldberg

Definition of Compliance

"The extent to which patients' behaviour (in terms of taking medications, following diets, or executing other life-style changes) coincides with the clinical prescription" is Sackett's definition of compliance [1]. Encompassing a spectrum from occasional forgetfulness to never following the recommended schedule [2], non-compliance can be regarded as the intentional or accidental failure to comply with a physician's expressed or implied directions in the self-administration of any medication [3].

Compliance encompasses an individual's active participation in his/her own health care: seeking medical advice, keeping appointments and following implicit and overt recommendations.

As physicians, we consider in great detail the indications and contra-indications for surgical procedures and, with even greater interest, the means by which each step in an operation can be made safer and more effective. We have tended to avoid the same attention to medical management. Although much time, effort and expense is devoted to developing and testing new drugs, and into incorporating them into management strategies, we do not assess whether or not our patients are taking them effectively and as advised, nor how to recognise or to minimise non-compliance. The latest medical advances are to no avail if the patient is not acting to get the agents to the receptors.

Importance of Compliance

Over 10 % of visual loss from glaucoma has been estimated to be caused by non-compliance [4–6].

Defaulting can be associated with progressive visual loss in a patient whose intra-ocular pressures (IOPs) at the times of consultations are measured as "safe" – because use of eye drops increases on the days before and after seeing the doctor [7]. Told that "your pressures are good", the patient's non-compliant behaviour between visits can be reinforced inadvertently. Alternative clinical possibilities include intra-cranial pathology or normal tension glaucoma, and so, if non-compliance is not suspected, expensive and possibly invasive investigations can be employed or the already partly ignored medical therapy accelerated, thereby increasing the chances of systemic and local side effects.

Table 1. Techniques for measuring compliance

Patient self-report:
  Questionnaire
  Diary or daily record
  Interview "post-hoc"
Health professional "guesstimate"
Therapeutic result
Metabolic consequences of the drug(s)
Calculation of:
  Tablet number used
  Volume of liquid used
  Weight of liquid used
  Number of prescriptions filled
Measurement of medication, metabolite, or marker in blood, urine, salvia, faeces.
Medication monitor

Technique for Measuring Compliance

Ideally, techniques for measuring compliance should be objective, unobtrusive (i.e., not affect the very behaviour being assessed), accurate, practical and inexpensive. None of the current methods satisfies all these criteria (Table 1).

Because it is relatively inexpensive and easy to perform, patient interview is appealing. However, patients may complain "how can you honestly expect me to remember what I have forgotten?" And there can be a wide divergence between compliance rates as reported by patients and those measured more objectively. One spectacular example involved children prescribed oral penicillin for streptococcal pharyngitis [8]. Although 83 % of the parents reported continued administration of the drug after 9 days of therapy, 82 % of the children had no penicillin detectable in their urine. In another example, of glaucoma patients supposedly instilling pilocarpine drops four times daily, 99 % claimed in interview to have instilled their drops at least 75 % of the time, whereas a medication monitor hidden within the bottle detected that only 66 % of the patients were at least this regular, 15 % of patients instilling pilocarpine less than 50 % of the time, and 25 % of patients missing their medication altogether more than 1 day per month [9].

Perhaps this finding is not as startling as it might seem. In one study [10], even if patients were asked, 69 % would not admit to problems with their medications; in another [11], 40 % of defaulting patients said that they had never had any intention of following their doctor's advice. "Patients who admit defaulting are usually telling the truth; patients who report that they are following the prescription may or many not be" [12].

Dyscompliance

Not only must patients self-administer drops at the correct times and in the correct amounts, but they must also master a technique to do so. Table 2 summarises the actions required.

Elderly patients with arthritis and/or tremor can find this procedure beyond them. In one survey [13], 27 % of glaucoma patients failed to place the drop into the con-

Table 2. Actions required for successful eye drop self-administration

Break steril seal.
Shake if necessary.
Remove lid.
Hyperextend neck if sitting or standing.
Raise arm above shoulder.
Grasp bottle with thumb and index finger.
Invert bottle over eye.
Hold bottle over eye so that tip does not contact lids or lashes.
Hold eye open.
Hold lower eyelid everted to "catch" the drop.
Squeeze bottle to eject one drop.
Instil drop into conjunctival sac.
Close eye gently while lowering arm and replacing bottle lid.
Avoid blinking and keep eyelids closed for at least two minutes.
Simultaneously, press over lacrimal sac with pulp of index finger for at least two minutes.
Wipe excess drop(s) off skin of eyelids.
Repeat for second eye, or combine technique so that both eyes treated simultaneously.

junctival sac, and of these, 25 % were unaware that they had missed the eye. Those patients taught instillation techniques did better than those not tutored, particularly if the instructions were repeated periodically.

Prevalence of Non-compliance

Overall, clinicians should assume that at least one-third of patients will default from prescribed medical therapy from occasionally to often, and that they will not be accurate necessarily in identifying those patients. In certain circumstances, this rate can be expected to be higher [14].

Factors Associated with Non-compliance

No single determinant of non-compliances has emerged. Most of the associated factors can be grouped under the following headings:

The Patient

Increased frequency of missed appointments, an unstable home or family situation, dissatisfaction with the treatment, and a poor understanding of the disease and its treatment all appear to be correlated with non-compliance.

Most patients who admitted to defaulting were unable to explain what disease they had, or what were the aims of treatment [15]. Of 62 patients in one glaucoma clinic who knew that glaucoma was associated with raised IOP, and that regular drop instillation could prevent blindness, two-thirds were compliant; of those who did not grasp these concepts, only one-third followed the regimen [16].

Perception of the "sick role" is a potent factor: lack of concern about one's health in general, and in particular, that the disease in question does not pose a threat to one's well-being, or that the prescribed treatment is not going to help, all contribute to defaulting [17].

Glaucome has been regarded as one of the most important areas in which the patient's viewpoint can alter significantly the therapeutic result [18].

Denial of the diagnosis and of the disease process are relevant [19]. Patients often do not understand and do not retain what they have been told by their doctor, particularly if detailed information is provided immediately after a threatening diagnosis has been made. Such a situation may engender a shock-like state during which very little if anything is absorbed and digested mentally or emotionally. For the medically uninitiated, material presented may be conceptually too complex, or the language may be too difficult.

The Disease

Diseases that produce severe symptoms or disability promote compliance [15]. As an asymptomatic, chronic disease requiring life-long, expensive treatment and supervision with no subjective improvement, glaucoma fosters non-compliance [20].

The Medical Regimen

Poor compliance correlates with increased regimen complexity; a greater number of drugs, required to be taken more frequently, with further life-style disruption. More side effects, particularly those which are alarming or unexpected, provoke defaulting.

Referring to pilocarpine-induced brow ache, fluctuating distance focus, and poor vision in dim illumination, a patient wrote passionately "(the) threat of a handicapped old age was always present, but use of miotics added to this a severe immediate disability, preventing the full use and enjoyment of eyes which ... were optically sound" [21].

An increased frequency of consumption of prescribed medications is associated with defaulting: in the treatment of epilepsy, 87 % of patients on once-daily tablets were compliant, compared with only 39 % on a four times a day program [22]. Long-term rates of compliance with anti-glaucoma medications are estimated at 95 % with timolol, 70 % with pilocarpine, 60 % with systemic carbonic anhydrase inhibitors, and 30 % with adrenaline [23].

Duration of therapy is also important: although patients may be willing to take drugs for a limited period, when therapy is extended indefinitely, defaulting becomes more common [2]. Once more, by its very nature as an incurable and life-long disease, glaucoma promotes non-compliance.

The Doctor-Patient Relationship

Just as poor communication between clinical and patient leads to more defaulting, so perception of the physician as warm, caring, friendly, accessible, active and thorough encourages compliance. Similarly, an increased waiting time to see the doctor, and a doctor's apparent lack of time or concern contributes directly to non-compliance. Being seen by a different clinician at each visit, and even long waiting times to be served at the pharmacy, also may enhance subsequent non-compliance [12].

One fact emerges clearly: no matter how well a clinician knows a patient, or how well that clinician feels able to predict compliant behaviour, physician's judgements are often no more accurate than chance [24].

Compliance is often assumed, the physician's often not-inconsiderable ego permitting little else. When defaulting becomes apparent, the patient is blamed, sometimes with anger and rejection. Rather, it should be recognised that the management situation is inadequate to meet than patient's needs [2].

Strategies to Enhance Compliance

Explain Glaucoma

As discussed above, patients who understand the relevant concepts of a disease and its treatment are more compliant with that therapy, and have more realistic expectations of both the clinician and the management strategies. Misconceptions and misunderstandings of the condition and its treatment are the rule among glaucoma patients, not the exception. In the long term, patient adherence with symptomatic, non-curative, costly medications cannot be expected without patient knowledge and understanding. Explanations, needing to be repeated periodically, must be simple and clear.

Minimise the Treatment Regimen

- Use the least number of drugs, at the lowest concentrations, the fewest number of times necessary.
- As IOP can fluctuate widely, a one-eyed therapeutic trial is needed at initiation and acceleration of therapy: record the time of applanation tonometry and of the last drug instillation; review after a pharmacologically appropriate period at the same time of day.
- Introduce one drug at a time, to one eye only if possible, and measure IOP changes to both eyes to gauge efficacy and side effects.
- Substitute before adding drugs.

Minimise Inconvenience

- Try to fit the dosage regimen into each patient's life-style, with their active involvement. Determine the patient's daily routine (e.g. times for waking, morning break, lunch, return from work, evening meal, bedtime) and link the appropriate milestones in the day with the desired instillation schedule.
- For working patients, one set of drops at work, and another at home might be useful (if cost is not an issue).

- For patients with memory problems, write out the schedule in large clear letters, labelling the bottles descriptively as well as by name (e.g., the lilac-top bottle).
- For those with poor sight, use large coloured squares to match the bottle tops.
- Allergies to medications actually may be to the preservative – if patients understand this they may be more willing to try alternatives

Teach Installation Techniques

Fraunfelder's technique [25] is recommended:
- Look up.
- Gently pull the lower eyelid away from the globe to form a "cup".
- By looking at it, position the inverted bottle or dropper directly over the eye without touching anything with the tip.
- Instil one drop (or more if the first is not felt – refrigerate the bottle if necessary to assist with this).
- Look down.
- Release the lower eyelid.
- Gently close the eye without blinking or squeezing the eyelids, and avoiding rolling the eye around.
- Press against the lacrimal sac with the tip of the index finger for at least 3 min.
- Reflex tearing can be minimised by avoiding the cilia, and by applying drops into the fornix rather than onto the cornea.

Once explained, check that the patient or a helper can perform these steps. Review the technique from time to time. Reinforce the need to wait at least 5 min between different drops to reduce "wash-out" of the first by the second.

In one study, 21 % of patients always relied on someone else to instill their eye drops, an additional 33 % had help sometimes, and 57 % had difficulties in self-administration [10]. These included problems with breaking the bottle top seal, raising their arms above their heads, titling their head backwards, holding and squeezing the bottle, directing the drop, fear of hitting the eye (leading to the bottle being held too high), involuntary blinking, and poor sighting of the bottle tip [10].

Severe physical difficulties were noted in 25 %–50 % of glaucoma patients – particularly in the elderly with arthritis and/or tremor. Increasing digit pressure on the bottle to expel a drop led to increased hand tremor, and 13 % could not expel a drop at all, let alone into the eye [16].

When a group of glaucoma patients was interviewed and then observed self-administering eye drops, 27 % separated two or more medications by less than 1 min, a mean of 2.4 drops was instilled into each eye each time, 45 % made contact between the bottle tip and ocular tissues, and 4 % placed the drop onto the skin of an eyelid and rolled their heads around till the drop spilled into the conjunctival sac [26, 27]. No patients closed their eyes after instillation, and none used lacrimal sac occlusion.

Measured by radio-immunoassay 1 h after drop instillation, nasolacrimal duct occlusion reduced the timolol concentration in plasma by 67 %; eyelid closure reduced it by 65 % [28]. After conjunctival instillation of fluorescein, nasolacrimal duct occlusion increased its peak anterior chamber concentration by 69 % (by 46 %

with eyelid closure), and its duration of detection in the anterior chamber by 100 % (by 33 % with eyelid closure) [28].

Predict Likely Side Effects

Nothing reinforces patient confidence in the clinician as much as accurate prediction of effects and side effects. Patients are usually grateful to be made aware in advance of what to expect. This knowledge also protects them from fear and panic, and the physician from avoidable late night and weekend calls when anticipated side effects occur.

Use Compliance Aids

Try to encourage open communication with your glaucoma patients, minimising guilt about difficulties with their treatment program. Make them aware of compliance aids such as instillation frames and some eye drop bottles with numbers on the caps, both of which have been shown to enhance compliance.

Communicate with Relevant Medical Colleagues

Ensure that all medical practitioners involved in a patient's overall care are fully aware of the anti-glaucoma regimen. If need be, educate your colleagues about the potential systemic side effects and drug interactions of topical therapies. Be sure those colleagues are happy with what you are prescribing. Remind patients to tell all other doctors they consult about their glaucoma and their eye drops.

Who has the Time?

All these suggestions require additional time, which many if not most busy ophthalmologists do not have. Trained staff can assist, especially if the patient perceives the effort as one co-ordinated by a concerned and involved clinician. Aids such as user-friendly information pamphlets and booklets, audio- and video-tapes extend this kind of reinforcement. Expect to have to repeat much of the advice from to time as the years of treatment unfold.

Community support groups are important. Several organisations produce regular newsletters, run support group meetings, provide educational material and special information sheets for glaucoma patients and their families. Find one near you which can reiterate your messages to your patients in clear, easy-to-understand language.

These strategies are summarised in Table 3.

Table 3. Strategies to improve compliance

Educate the patient about the disease and the treatment.
Teach the patient how and when to apply eye drops.
Fit the medications into that patient's daily routine.
Use the minimal number of drugs, frequency of daily drops and tablets, and concentrations/
strength of drugs.
Measure the response in a controlled fashion (therapeutic trial).
Measure the duration of the response.
Discuss potential systemic and local side effects with the patient and other involved doctors.
Take measures to minimise or to eliminate medication side effects.
Maintain open and empathetic communication with the patient.
Train staff to support patients and to reinforce your efforts.
Use aids (literature, tapes, videos, devices).
Encourage access to a community support group.

Conclusions

Our primary goal in glaucoma management is to preserve our patient's sight and to maintain their quality of life. Cure is not yet within our reach. Even when considerable sight has been lost, we can provide appreciated support and reassurance.

While "every patient is a potential defaulter...(and) compliance can never be assumed" [29], let us do whatever we can to minimise defaulting, thus making our medical treatment safer and more effective. In so doing, we are elevating our science to the noblest art of medicine.

References

1. Sackett DA, Haynes RB (eds) (1976) Compliance with therapeutic regimes, Baltimore, Johns Hopkins University Press
2. Davidson SI, Akingbehin T (1980) Compliance in Ophthalmology, Trans Ophthalmol UK, 100:286
3. Boyd JR et al (1974) Drug defaulting. I Determinants of compliance patterns. Am J Hosp Pharm 31:362
4. Ashburn FS Jr, Goldberg I, Kass MA (1980) Compliance with ocular therapy. Surv Ophthalmol 24:237
5. Spaeth GL (1971) Pathogenesis of visual loss in patients with glaucoma. Trans Am Acad Ophthalmol Otolaryngol 75:296
6. Van Buskirk EM (1986) The compliance factor. (editional) Am J Ophthalmol 101:609
7. Kass MA (1987) Compliance with topical pilocarpine therapy. Am J Ophthalmol 101:515
8. Bergman AB, Werner RJ (1963) Failure of children to receive penicillin by mouth. N Engl J Med 268:1334
9. Kass MA, et al. (1986) Compliance with topical pilocarpine therapy. Am J Ophthalmol 101:515
10. Winfield AJ et al. (1990) A study of the causes of non-compliance by patients prescribed eye drops. Br J Ophthalmol 74:477
11. Linn LS, Davis MS (1973) Occupational orientation and overt behavior – the pharmacist as drug advisor to patients. Am J Public Health 63:502
12. Kass MA, Meltzer DW, Gordon MO (1984) The Compliance Factor. In Drance SM, Neufeld AH: Glaucoma: applied pharmacology in medical treatment. Grune & Stratton, New York
13. Brown MM, Brown GC, Spaeth GL (1984) Improper topical self-administration of ocular medication among patients with glaucoma. Can J Ophthalmol 19:2
14. Goldberg I (1996) Compliance. In: Ritch R, Shields MB, Krupin T (eds) The Glaucomas. St Louis, Mosby, p1375
15. Spaeth GL (1970) Visual loss in a glaucoma clinic. I Sociological considerations. Invest Ophthalmol 9:73

16. Vincent PA (1970) Patients' viewpoint of glaucoma therapy. Sight Sav Rev 42:213
17. Kass MA (1978) Non-compliance to ocular therapy: glaucoma report. Ann Ophthalmol 10:1244
18. Riffenburgh RS (1966) Doctor-patient relationship in glaucoma therapy. Arch Ophthalmol 75:204
19. Bloch S et al. (1977) Patient compliance in glaucoma. Br J Ophthalmol 61:531
20. Zimmermann TJ, Zalta AH (1983) Facilitating patient compliance in glaucoma therapy. Surv Ophthalmol 28:252
21. Anonymous (1964) The Miotic Life. Br J Ophthalmol 48:354
22. Cramer J et al. (1989) How often is medication taken as prescribed? A novel assessment technique. JAMA 261:3273
23. Worthern DM (1976) Patient compliance and the „usefulness product" of timolol. Surv Ophthalmol 23:403
24. Caron HS, Roth HP (1968) Patients's co-operation with a medical regimen. Diffuculties in identifying the non-co-operator. JAMA 203:922
25. Fraunfelder FT (1976) Extra-ocular fluid dynamics: how best to apply topical ocular medication. Trans Am Ophthalmol Soc 74:457
26. Kass MA et al. (1982) Patient administration of eye drops. Part I. Interview: Ann Ophthalmol 14:775
27. Kass MA et al. (1982) Patient administration of eye drops. Part II Observation. Ann Ophthalmol 14:889
28. Zimmerman TJ et al. (1984) Improving the therapeutic index of topically applied ocular drugs. Arch Ophthalmol 102:551
29. Porter AWM (1969) Drug defaulting in general practice. Br Med J 1:218

CHAPTER 5

Mechanisms of Glaucoma Development in Pseudoexfoliation Syndrome

U. Schlötzer-Schrehardt, M. Küchle, and G.O.H. Naumann

Introduction

Pseudoexfoliation (PEX) syndrome is a common, age-related, clinically relevant, but still underestimated disorder, which is characterized by the multifocal production and progressive accumulation of an abnormal fibrillar extracellular material in many intra- and extraocular tissues including skin and connective tissue portions of various visceral organs (Schlötzer-Schrehardt et al. 1992; Streeten et al. 1992). It is now recognized as a systemic disorder, the clinical significance of which still has to be defined.

Patients with PEX syndrome are at an approximately ten fold increased risk for the development of a rather aggressive type of secondary open-angle glaucoma, also termed capsular glaucoma (Vogt 1926), but also for the development of secondary angle-closure glaucomas (Bartholomew 1981). The PEX-associated, chronic open-angle glaucoma, which develops in approximately 50 % of patients, differs from primary open-angle glaucoma (POAG) by a more serious clinical course and worse prognosis and is presently the most common recognizable cause of open-angle glaucomas worldwide (Ritch 1994). Accordingly, the frequency of PEX among chronic glaucoma patients is ususally high, e.g. 60 % of glaucoma patients in the "Middle-Norway-Eye-Screening Study" (Ringvold et al. 1991), 87 % of glaucoma patients requiring trabeculectomy in Northern Greece (Konstas and Allen 1989), and about 40 % of glaucoma patients undergoing filtering surgery in our institution. These figures reflect the enormous distribution of the disorder and underscore its significance as one of the most frequent causes of vision deterioration in older people.

Apart from being a major cause of glaucoma, PEX causes a wide spectrum of intraocular complications comprising phakodonesis and spontaneous lens (sub)luxation due to zonular instability (Fig. 1A), blood-aqueous barrier impairment and pseudouveitis, melanin dispersion, formation of posterior synechiae, nuclear cataract formation, early corneal endothelial decompensation, and a significantly higher rate of intra- and postoperative complications in cataract surgery, such as inadequate pupillary dilation, zonular ruptures, vitreous loss, postoperative inflammatory responses and fibrin reaction, secondary cataract formation, and postoperative decentration of the intraocular lens (Fig. 1B) (Naumann et al. 1998). All of these complications can be explained by active involvement of all anterior segment tissues in the basic pathological matrix process, which also causes increased intraocular pressure (IOP) by active involvement of the outflow tissues (Schlötzer-Schrehardt and Naumann 1997).

Fig. 1A,B. Complications in eyes with PEX syndrome. A Spontaneous dislocation of the lens with adhering zonular remnants and PEX material. B Spontaneous luxation of a posterior chamber lens 5 years after cataract surgery

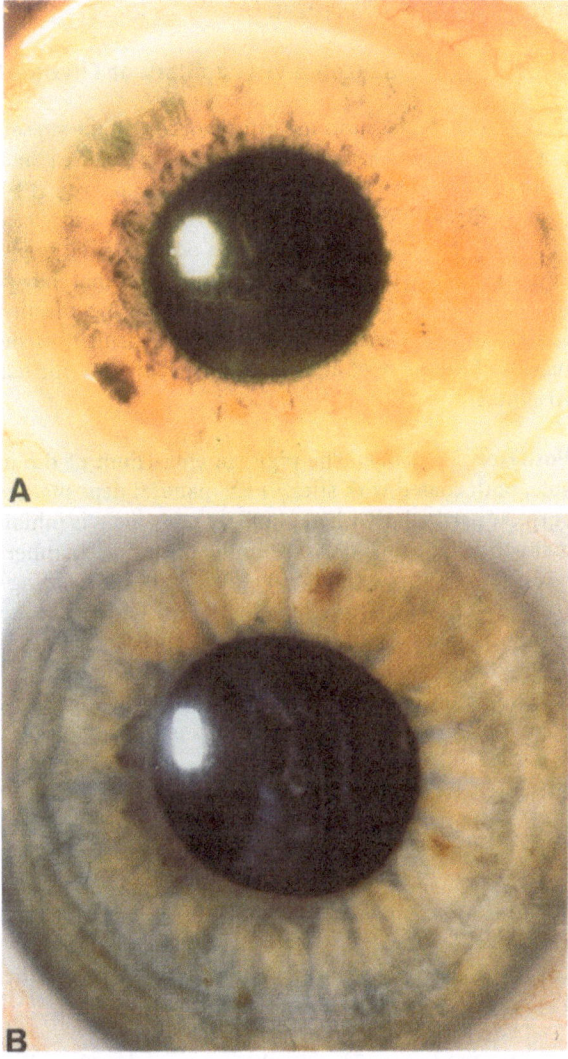

Despite many new findings and insights in recent years, the etiology of PEX syndrome remains obscure and the pathogenesis of chronic pressure elevation remains controversial. The purpose of this review is to present an overview of various pathogenetic factors and mechanisms that may contribute to glaucoma development in patients with PEX syndrome.

Angle-Closure Glaucoma

Angle-Closure Glaucoma via Pupillary or Ciliary Block

Glaucoma in PEX syndrome usually occurs in the presence of an open chamber angle, but an association between PEX and angle-closure glaucoma via *pupillary block* is not rare either. Ritch (1994) found clinically apparent PEX syndrome or PEX material deposits in conjunctival biopsies in 28.3 % of consecutive patients with angle-closure glaucoma. Moreover, narrow angles occur in a large proportion of patients (Gross et al. 1994). Characteristic features of PEX eyes that may predispose to the development of pupillary block angle-closure glaucoma include the formation of posterior synechiae, an increased iris rigidity, an impairment of the blood-aqueous barrier and increased viscosity of aqueous humor, and anterior lens subluxation due to zonular weakness.

Posterior Synechiae. The pigment epithelium of the iris and the anterior lens capsule, both coated with sticky PEX material deposits, tend to adhere before and after surgery, particularly when pupillary movement is inhibited by miotic therapy. In such a situation, aqueous pressure in the posterior chamber causes the iris to bulge at its weakest and thinnest point, the iris root, thus occluding the angle by apposition of the iris to the trabecular meshwork. The existence of broad circular posterior synechiae in miosis may hide the diagnosis of such an iridocapsular block ("masked PEX"). Therefore, in eyes with spontaneous or miotic-induced circular posterior synechiae, a PEX syndrome should be ruled out, e.g. by high-resolution ultrasound biomicroscopy, which may detect PEX deposits on the zonules (Fig. 2) (Naumann et al. 1998).

Increased Iris Rigidity. Reduction of iris elasticity by accumulating PEX material within the iris stroma and dilator and sphincter muscles may contribute to poor pupillary motility and advance pupillary block (Fig. 3) (Asano et al. 1995).

Blood-Aqueous Barrier Impairment. Marked breakdown of the blood-aqueous barrier in eyes with PEX syndrome results in a significant increase in aqueous protein concentration and viscosity of aqueous humor further facilitating pupillary block (Table 1) (Küchle et al. 1992, 1994, 1995).

Zonular Weakness. The zonules are severely affected early in the course of PEX syndrome and reveal an impaired anchorage both on the anterior lens capsule and in the ciliary epithelium explaining the clinically observed zonular instability (Fig. 4) (Schlötzer-Schrehardt and Naumann 1994). Weakening of the zonular support and subsequent laxity of the lens many cause a slight anterior displacement of the lens predisposing to the development of a pupillary block. This tendency of the lens to phakodonesis and anterior movement is consistent with a reduced anterior chamber volume in eyes of PEX patients (Gharagozloo et al. 1992).

In extreme and rather rare cases, anterior subluxation of the lens may be so pronounced due to marked zonular weakness that a *ciliary block* angle-closure glaucoma ("malignant glaucoma") is induced by contraction of the ciliary muscle, where aque-

Fig. 2A,B. Masked PEX.
A Circular posterior syn-
echiae firmly adherent to
the anterior lens surface
after pharmacologic dila-
tion. B High-resolution
anterior segment ultra-
sound biomicrograph
showing PEX deposits
(*arrows*) on the anterior
zonular insertion to the
lens surface hidden behind
dense posterior synechiae

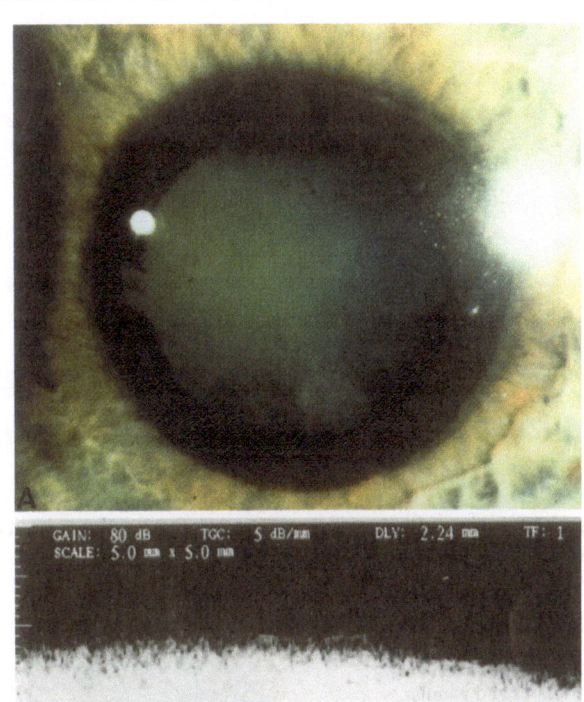

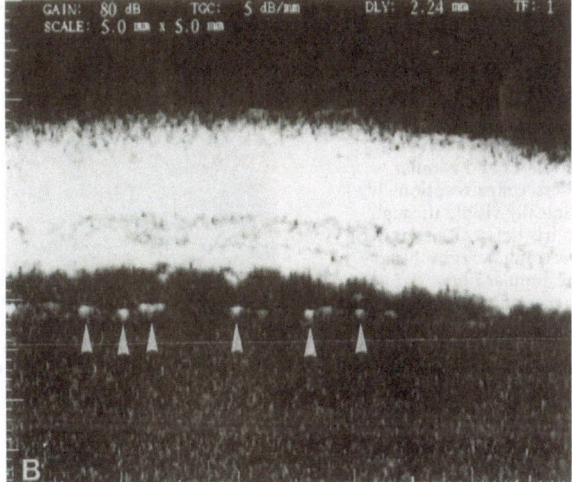

Table 1. Aqueous flare values (photon counts/ms) in normal controls, pseudoexfoliation (PEX) without and with secondary open-angle glaucoma (SOAG) and primary open-angle glaucoma (POAG)

Group	Eyes (n)	Flare values (mean ± SD)	Range	Significance (p value)
Normal controls	164	4.6 ± 1.1	2.0– 7.2	
POAG eyes	100	4.7 ± 1.6	2.0– 7.4	0.1
All PEX eyes	90	14.3 ± 9.2	6.0–43.2	< 0.000
PEX with SOAG	40	14.5 ± 9.8	7.4–43.2	
PEX without SOAG	50	14.1 ± 7.9	6.0–42.0	0.5

From Küchle et al. (1995).
Statistic: Mann-Whitney test.

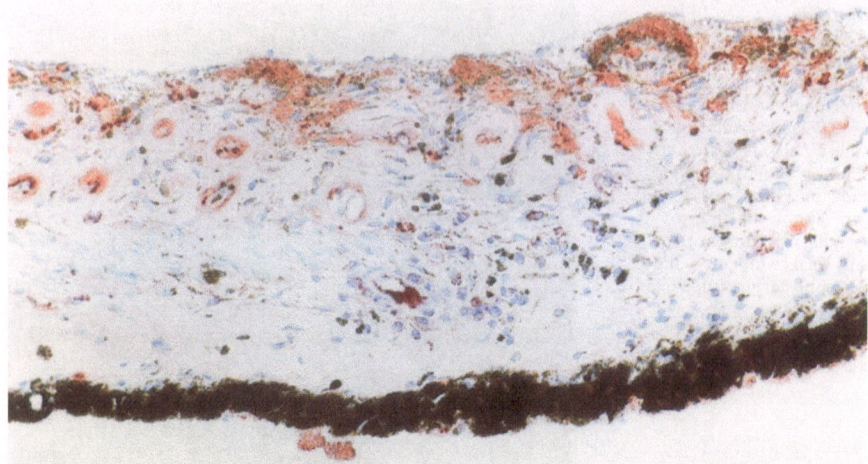

Fig. 3. Massive accumulation of PEX material within the iris stroma as demonstrated by a specific immunohistochemical stain (*red color*) 200x

Fig. 4A,B. Zonular involvement in PEX syndrome. **A** PEX deposits on ciliary processes and zonular fibers, only exceptionally clinically visible through an iris defect. **B** Scanning electron micrograph showing zonular fibers encrusted with PEX material

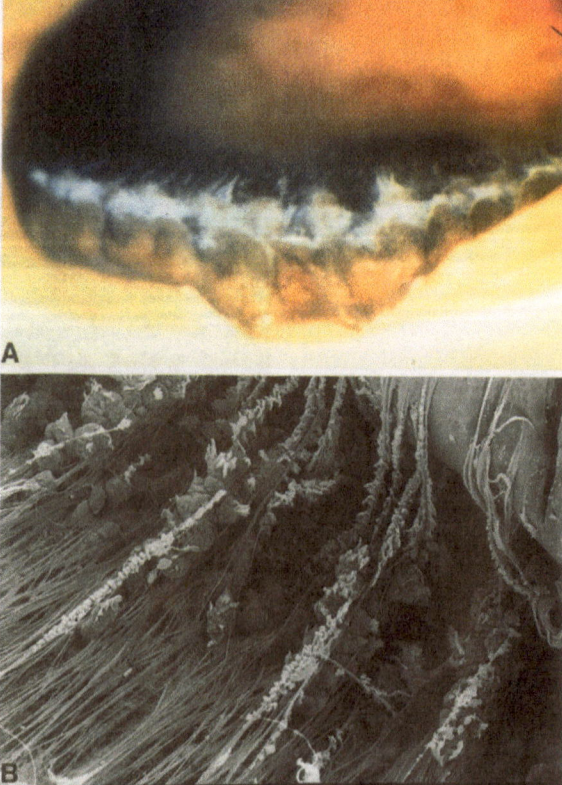

ous humor pressure causes the whole lens to move forward and block the angle (Von der Lippe et al. 1993; Naumann and von der Lippe 1995).

Miotics may aggravate both pupillary and ciliary block in eyes with PEX.

Secondary Angle-Closure Following Central Retinal Vein Occlusion with Rubeosis Iridis

Branch or central retinal vein occlusions appear to be more common in patients with PEX syndrome (Fig. 5). In a retrospective study, 6.0% of patients with branch and 6.9% of patients with central retinal vein thrombosis revealed PEX (Cursiefen et al. 1997). In another series, about 33% of all eyes enucleated for neovascular glaucoma caused by central retinal vein occlusion and rubeosis iridis had coexistent PEX syndrome (Karjalainen et al. 1987). Pathogenetically, the high IOP values could be causative for the venous thrombosis. Iris neovascularization (rubeosis iridis) often follow-

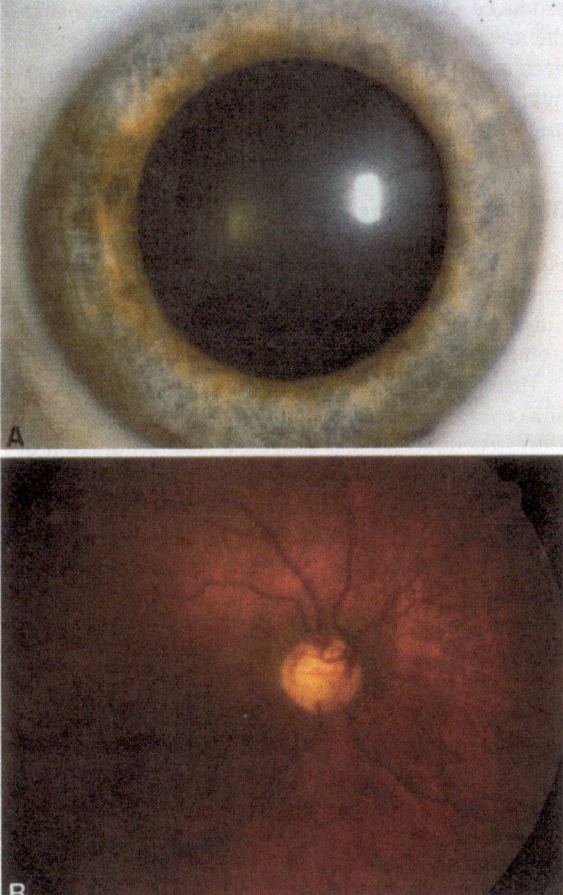

Fig. 5A,B. Central retinal vein occlusion in an eye with PEX sydrome

ing retinal vein occlusion can cause secondary angle-closure glaucoma by newly formed vessels and connective tissue elements proliferating on the surface of the trabecular meshwork or by formation of anterior synechiae closing the chamber angle.

Open-Angle Glaucoma

Chronic open-angle glaucomas caused by PEX syndrome are hypertensive glaucomas associated with an increase in aqueous outflow resistance (Johnson and Brubaker 1982; Gharagozloo et al. 1992).

Although the pathogenetic mechanisms of chronic pressure elevation has been a matter of much debate, one widely accepted view is that capsular glaucoma is a secondary open-angle glaucoma resulting from obstruction of the outflow pathways either by PEX material or melanin granules or both. However, the pathogenetic mechanism of glaucoma development may involve several factors. Potential mechanisms include obstruction of the meshwork by PEX material, either endogenously produced ("endotrabecular") or passively deposited ("exotrabecular"), blockage of the meshwork by melanin granules liberated from the iris pigment epithelium, trabecular cell dysfunction and degenerative changes, an increased viscosity of aqueous humor and accumulation of aqueous proteins in the meshwork structures, and migration of damaged corneal endothelial cells over the chamber angle.

Obstruction of the Trabecular Meshwork by PEX Material

Flakes of PEX material can be occassionally seen in the chamber angle during gonioscopy and obstruction of the meshwork by PEX material is generally considered the most likely cause of elevated IOP in PEX eyes. This idea has been supported by electron microscopic observations and morphometric studies:

Histopathologically, most PEX deposits can be found in the juxtacanalicular tissue adjacent to Schlemm's canal and also in the uveal part of the meshwork (Fig. 6A,C). Ultrastructural findings suggest a local production of PEX fibers by the juxtacanalicular connective tissue cells and the endothelial cells lining Schlemm's canal (Fig. 6D), resulting in a progressive accumulation of PEX material in the subendothelial area. In early cases, subendothelial PEX material ocurred in isolated clumps, but in more advanced cases, it frequently formed a continuous layer beneath the inner wall of Schlemm's canal, thus limiting aqueous access to Schlemm's canal and impairing drainage of aqueous humor (Fig. 6A,C). In further advanced stages, the accumulating PEX masses may cause a considerable disorganization of the normal tissue architecture, including narrowing and focal collapse of the canal lumen, disruption of its endothelial lining, and splitting into smaller channels (Fig. 6B) (Schlötzer-Schrehardt and Naumann 1995).

Furthermore, a statistically significant positive correlation has been observed between the amount of PEX material in the trabecular meshwork and the presence or absence of glaucoma (Schlötzer-Schrehardt and Naumann 1995) and even with the extent of glaucomatous optiv nerve damage (Gottanka et al. 1997) substantiating the hypothesis of obstruction of outflow channels.

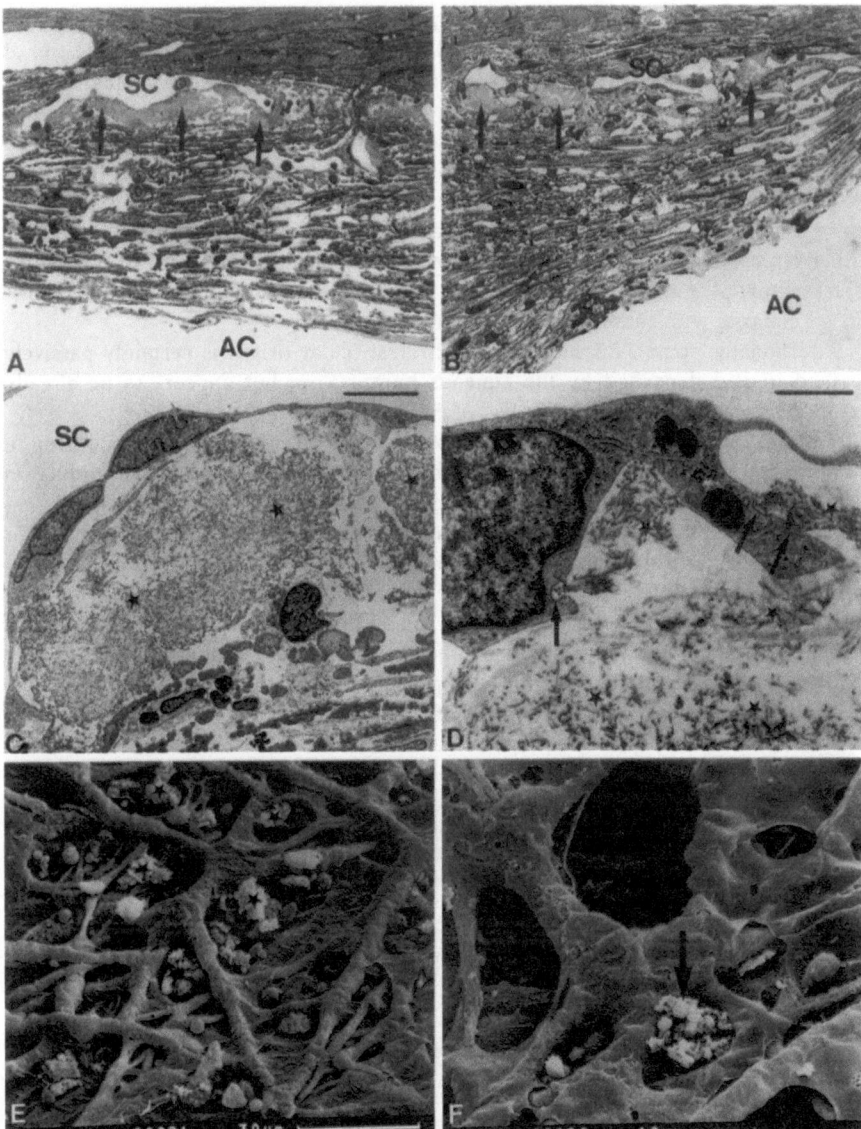

Fig. 6A–F. Obstruction of the trabecular meshwork by PEX material. **A** Light micrograph showing accumulation of PEX material in the juxtacanalicular meshwork (*arrows*) adjacent to Schlemm's canal (SC) (AC anterior chamber; 360x). **B** Light micrograph showing disorganization of Schlemm's canal (SC) area by PEX accumulations in the juxtacanalicular tissue (*arrows*) (300x). **C** Transmission electron micrograph showing accumulation of PEX material (*) beneath the inner wall of Schlemm's canal (SC) (*bar* = 5 μm). **D** Apparent production (*arrows*) of PEX fibers (*) by a trabecular cell with phagocytosed melanin granules (bar = 1μm). **E, F** Scanning electron micrographs of the inner meshwork surface showing PEX deposits (arrow, *) in the uveal pores

Thus, the main pathologic alterations appear to involve local production and sub-endothelial accumulation of PEX material in the juxtacanalicular region, the site of greatest resistance to aqueous outflow, and subsequent degenerative changes in this delicate and decisive portion of the meshwork impairing drainage of aqueous humor into Schlemm's canal. This means that the meshwork cannot be simply considered as a sieve, the pores of which are mechanically clogged by PEX clumps, but the meshwork cells are actively involved in the generalized pathologic matrix process affecting many other intra- and extraocular tissues as well. This degenerative fibrillopathy may either represent an overproduction of an abnormal fibrillar extracellular material or a lack of turnover and breakdown leading to a progressive buildup of the locally produced material with subsequent degenerative changes.

Additionally, some PEX material of extratrabecular origin is certainly passively washed in and deposited by the aqueous humor flow, but appears to be already trapped between the uveal cords (Fig. 6E,F).

Thus, the PEX material within the trabecular meshwork appears to result from a combination of passive deposition in the inner portions and active local production in the outer portions, both contributing to increased outflow resistance (Fig. 7).

Nevertheless, the question remains as to why some eyes with PEX appear to never develop glaucoma, although mean IOP levels in PEX eyes are generally higher than in unaffected control eyes. Possible causative factors for this phenomenon may be simply the amount of PEX material present in the outflow structures, interindividual differences in managing the metabolic disturbance and load of abnormal matrix material, the presence or absence of additional predisposing factors, or interindividual differences in the susceptibility to damage of the optic nerve or retinal ganglion cells.

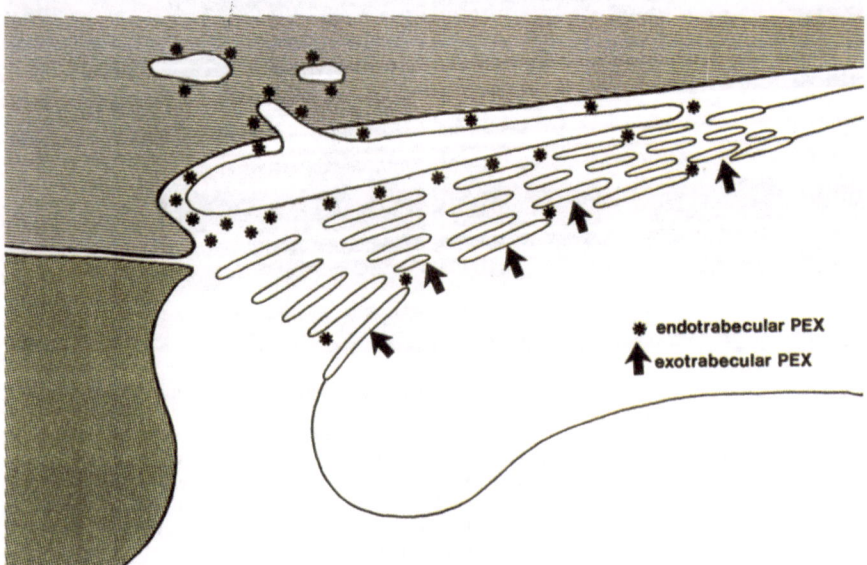

Fig. 7. Schematic representation of the trabecular meshwork in PEX syndrome showing the localization of PEX deposits of presumed endotrabecular and exotrabecular origin

Dispersion of Melanin Granules

Whether PEX material alone is responsible for IOP elevation or whether melanin dispersion plays a crucial role, remains debatable.

Increased pigmentation of the trabecular meshwork region in the chamber angle, particularly in the inferior portion and more pronounced in the affected than in the non-affected fellow eye, represents a chatacteristic clinical sign and an early diagnostic finding in PEX eyes. Asymmetry of trabecular pigmentation without other cause should alert to the diagnosis of PEX in early stages. Unlike primary melanin dispersion syndrome, the melanin distribution in the chamber angle of PEX eyes tends to be rather uneven and splotchy (Fig. 8A). Melanin dispersion is caused by abrasive movements of the pupillary iris against the irregular lens capsule surface during pupillary action and rupture of the degenerative iris pigment epithelial cells with liberation of melanin granules (Fig. 8B). Loss of melanin and its dispersion through the anterior chamber are reflected by transillumination defects at the pupillary margin

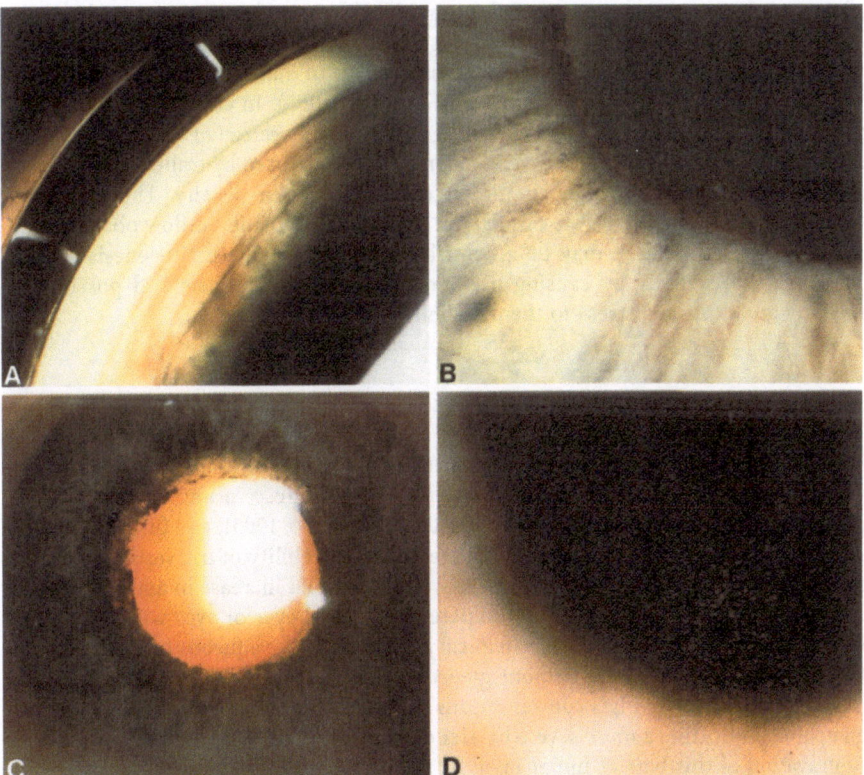

Fig. 8A–D. Dispersion of melanin granules in PEX syndrome. A Iridocorneal angle pigmentation. B Dispersion of melanin granules from the iris pigment epithelium following mydriasis and deposition of melanin granules on the iris surface. C Atrophy of the peripupillary pigment epithelium. D Deposition of melanin granules inferiorly on the corneal endothelium

(Fig. 8C), and pigment deposition on anterior segment structures, e.g. on the iris surface (Fig. 8B), on the corneal endothelium (Fig. 8D), and along Schwalbe's line and the trabecular meshwork.

Dispersion of melanin granules and PEX material in the anterior chamber is common after diagnostic or therapeutic pupillary dilation and may lead to marked transient IOP rises, sometimes causing an acute open-angle glaucoma. This melanin dispersion can be quantified by laser tyndallometry. Together with an early corneal endothelial decompensation and diffuse corneal edema, such pressure peaks can mimic an acute pupillary block inspite of an open angle. Krause et al. (1973) noted a positive correlation between the degree of pressure rise and the amount of pigment liberation, which both reach a maximum after 2 h following mydriasis.

Melanin dispersion after diagnostic mydriasis or after surgery can be so pronounced that heterochromia iridum is produced.

Apart from acute and transient IOP rises due to melanin showers provoked by mydriasis, the role of melanin dispersion in chronic pressure elevation is controversial. Although glaucoma is usually more common in the eye with the more heavily pigmented meshwork (Puska 1995), the degree of pigmentation does not always correlate with IOP and the severity of glaucoma (Tarkkanen 1962; Konstas et al. 1993).

Moreover, no significant correlation was found between the number of intratrabecular melanin granules and the presence or absence of glaucoma in a histomorphometrical study (Schlötzer-Schrehardt and Naumann 1995). In contrast to classic pigmentary glaucoma, the melanin granules were mostly restricted to the innermost uveal portions of the meshwork, were generally phagocytosed by trabecular endothelial cells, and showed a high circumferential variation in density. These findings speak against a significant role of melanin granules in causing outflow obstruction.

Nevertheless, melanin may be a contributing factor in the pathogenesis of PEX glaucoma, particularly by causing pressure peaks after mydriasis and possibly by exerting an additional stress to the metabolically damaged cells.

Increased Viscosity of Aqueous Humor

Evidence of blood-aqueous barrier impairment in PEX eyes both with and without glaucoma has been demonstrated by studies using fluorescein angiography, fluorophotometry, laser tyndallometry (Küchle et al. 1992, 1994, 1995), and histologic tracer studies (Küchle et al. 1996) indicating increased permeability of iris vasculature. This compromised barrier function leads to a two to three fold increase in aqueous protein concentrations and flare values as compared to normal eyes or eyes with cataract or POAG, thereby altering the physiochemical properties of the aqueous humor (Table 1). Whereas in eyes with PEX without glaucoma only the albumin concentration was increased, albumin and IgG concentrations were significantly higher in PEX eyes with glaucoma, indicating a more severe barrier defect (Moreno-Montanes and Blesa 1995). Aggravation of this barrier impairment by miotic therapy should be kept in mind.

Increased amounts of albumin have been detected immunohistochemically also in the trabecular meshwork of PEX eyes (Küchle et al. 1996). The PEX material accumulating in the meshwork may serve as a nidus for accumulation of serum proteins and thereby further decrease outflow facility (Fig. 9).

Fig. 9. Tranmission electron micrograph showing immunogold labelling for albumin: accumulation of albumin within PEX deposits (*) beneath the inner wall of Schlemm's canal (SC) (*bar* = 1μm)

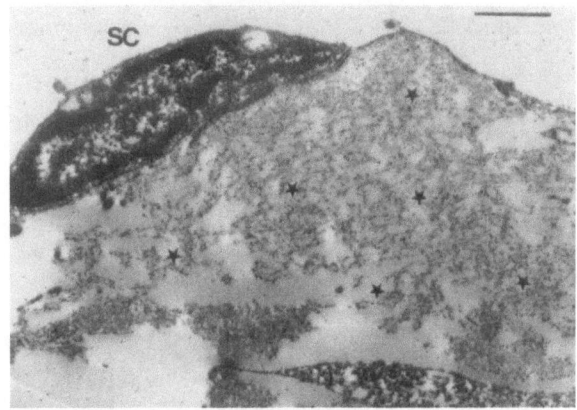

Migration of Corneal Endothelial Cells Over the Chamber Angle

Evidence of a damaged corneal endothelium (corneal endotheliopathy) in PEX eyes with and without glaucoma has been shown in specular microscopic, clinical, and histopathologic studies (Knorr et al. 1991; Schlötzer-Schrehardt et al. 1993; Seitz et al. 1995; Naumann and Schlötzer-Schrehardt 1994; Naumann 1995).

Occasionally, proliferating corneal endothelial cells may migrate beyond Schwalbe's line over the chamber angle, producing a pretrabecular connective tissue sheet including PEX and other extracellular components covering the inner surface of the meshwork (Fig. 10A–C) (Schlötzer-Schrehardt et al. 1993; Morrison and Green 1988). Although this appears to be a sporadic phenomenon, possibly depending on the elimination of contact inhibition between corneal and trabecular endothelial cell populations by PEX clumps along Schwalbe's line (Fig. 10D), it may contribute to pressure rise in some patients with PEX syndrome.

The characteristic anterior chamber hypoxia measured in PEX eyes (Helbig et al. 1994) may be of significance for the abnormal behavior of corneal endothelial cells. This is consistent with the observations by Zagorski et al. (1989) that a decreased oxygen level increases corneal endothelial cell proliferation in tissue culture.

Conclusion

Pseudoexfoliation syndrome, producing increased IOP by a series of pathologic events, has to be acknowledged as a specific cause of glaucomas. The underlying disease in the abnormality responsible for the production and deposition of the pathognomonic PEX material in many intra- and extraocular tissues including the trabecular meshwork. Unique features, such as the obvious production of PEX fibers in the juxtacanalicular tissue, and rather non-specific pathogenetic factors, such as melanin dispersion, may cooperate in glaucoma development.

Despite many new insights in recent years, PEX syndrome still remains greatly underdiagnosed leading to unexpected problems in clinical management and sur-

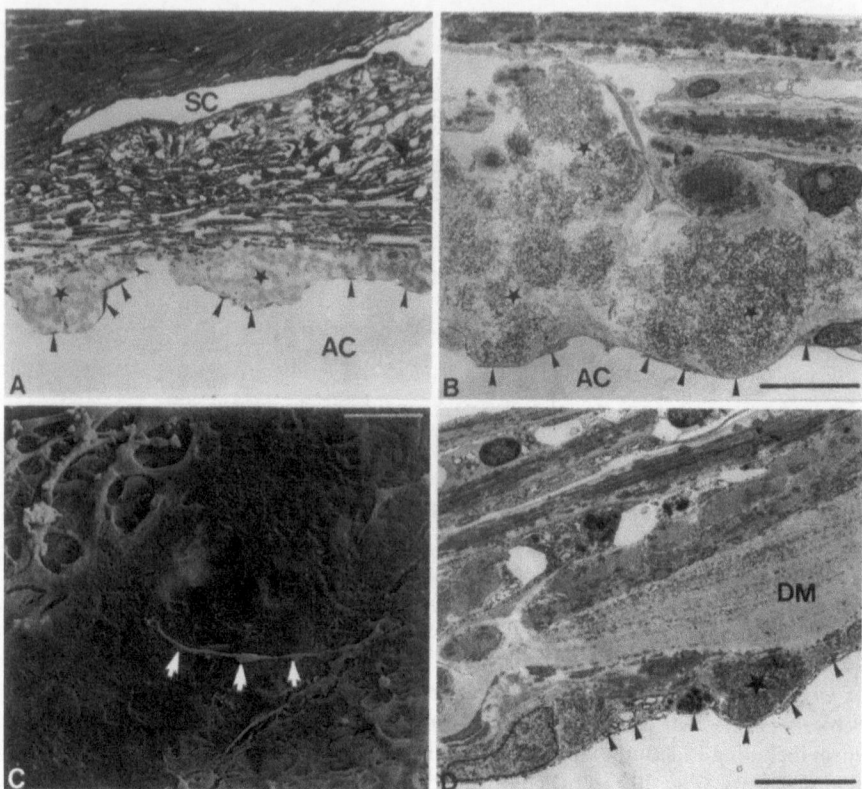

Fig. 10A–D. Migration of corneal endothelial cells over the chamber angle in PEX syndrome. **A** Light micrograph showing a pretrabecular sheet of PEX material (*) produced by migrating corneal endothelial cells (*arrowheads*) (*AC*, anterior chamber; *SC* Schlemm's canal; 340x). **B** Pretrabecular sheet of PEX material (*) surrounded by migrating corneal endothelial cells (*arrowheads*) by transmission electron microscopy (*bar* = 10 μm). **C** Scanning electron micrograph showing a fibroblastic corneal endothelial cell (*arrows*) migrating towards the trabecular meshwork (*bar* = 30 μm). **D** PEX clump (*) deposited along the transition zone between cornea and trabecular meshwork, possibly facilitating corneal endothelial migration (*arrowheads*) beyond Schwalbe's line (*DM*, Decement's membrane; *bar* = 10 μm)

gery. Reasons for frequent failure in making an accurate diagnosis of PEX syndrome include the asumption that the associated glaucoma should be treated identically to POAG and that it is, therefore, unimportant to differentiate it. Many cases which are treated initially as POAG disclose intraocular PEX material later on.

PEX glaucoma is, however, clearly differentiated from POAG both clinically and histopathologically and has a specific pathophysiologic cause. Clinically, eyes with PEX glaucoma have higher mean IOP values, greater diurnal fluctuations in IOP, a greater amount of melanin dispersion and acute pressure peaks, worse optic disc damage, and a more rapid loss of visual field, a poorer response to medical treatment, and therefore a more frequent necessity of surgical intervention (Konstas et al. 1993).

In addition, histomorphometric data indicate fundamental differences in nature: whereas a significant increase in juxtacanalicular plaque material and a decrease in trabecular meshwork cellularity have been reported in POAG (Rohen 1983; Alvarado et al. 1984), no differences in plaque concentrations and cellularity from normal eyes have been found in PEX glaucoma (Lütjen-Drecoll et al. 1986; Schlötzer-Schrehardt and Naumann 1995). These histopathologic differences might help to explain the different response to medical therapy, the different responsiveness to steroids, and the more severe clinical course and management as compared to POAG. But alterations in the composition of the extracellular matrix of the lamina cribrosa (Netland et al. 1995) and vascular factors (Mitchell et al. 1997) also have to be considered.

Although sufficient evidence now suggests differing pathomechanisms of glaucoma development and two separate entities, treatment modalities of PEX glaucoma and POAG are classically still similar or even identical. Instead of merely attempting to lower IOP, the final common pathway of a number of different diseases, therapeutic measures should take into account the unique features and specific pathomechanism as far as known (Naumann et al. 1998). Modern methods of cell and molecular biology will hopefully advance our knowledge of the pathophysiology of PEX syndrome and lead to more specific treatment approaches intervening at initial steps in the series of events before glaucomatous damage occurs.

Eyes with PEX syndrome and PEX glaucoma deserve special attention and concern, and increased awareness and accurate diagnosis of this common condition is not only important in the early detection and management of a specific and frequent type of glaucoma, but also in the management of many additional risks before, during, and after surgery.

References

1. Asano N, Schlötzer-Schrehardt U, Naumann GOH (1995) A histopathologic study of iris changes in pseudoexfoliation syndrome. Ophthalmology 102:1279–1290
2. Alvarado J, Murphy C, Juster R (1984) Trabecular meshwork cellularity in primary open-angle glaucoma and non-glaucomatous normals. Ophthalmology 91:564–579
3. Bartholomew RS (1981) Pseudoexfoliation and angle-closure glaucoma. Glaucoma 3:213–216
4. Cursiefen C, Händel A, Schönherr U, Naumann GOH (1997) Das Pseudoexfoliationssyndrom bei Patienten mit retinalem Venenast- und Zentralvenenverschluß. Klin Mbl Augenheilkd 211:17–21
5. Gharagozloo NZ, Baker RH, Brubaker RF (1992) Aqueous dynamics in exfoliation syndrome. Am J Ophthalmol 114:473–478
6. Gottanka J, Flügel-Koch C, Martus P, Johnson DH, Lütjen-Drecoll E (1997) Correlation of pseudoexfoliative material and optic nerve damage in pseudoexfoliation syndrome. Invest Ophthalmol Vis Sci 38:2435–2446
7. Gross FJ, Tingey D, Epstein DL (1994) Increased prevalence of occludable angles and angle-closure glaucoma in patients with pseudoexfoliation. Am J Ophthalmol 117:333–336
8. Helbig H, Schlötzer-Schrehardt U, Noske W, Kellner U, Foerster MH, Naumann GOH (1994) Anterior-chamber hypoxia and iris vasculopathy in pseudoexfoliation syndrome. German J Ophthalmol 3:148–153
9. Johnson DH, Brubaker RF (1982) Dynamics of aqueous humor in the syndrome of exfoliation with glaucoma. Am J Ophthalmol 93:629–634
10. Karjalainen K, Tarkkanen A, Merenmies L (1987) Exfoliation syndrome in enucleated haemorrhagic and absolute glaucoma. Acta Ophthalmol 65:320–322
11. Knorr HLJ, Jünemann A, Händel A, Naumann GOH (1991) Morphometrische und qualitative Veränderungen des Hornhautendothels bei Pseudoexfoliationssyndrom. Fortschr Ophthalmol 88:786–789
12. Konstas AG, Allan D (1989) Pseudoexfoliation glaucoma in Greece. Eye 3:747–753
13. Konstas AGP, Jay JL, Marshall GE, Lee WR (1993) Prevalence, diagnostic features, and response to trabeculectomy in exfoliation glaucoma. Ophthalmology 100:619–627

14. Krause U, Helve J, Forsius H (1973) Pseudoexfoliation of the lens capsule and liberation of iris pigment. Acta Ophthalmol 51:39–46
15. Küchle M, Nguyen NX, Horn F, Naumann GOH (1997) Quantitative assessment of aqueous flare and aqueous "cells" in pseudoexfoliation syndrome. Acta Ophthalmol 70:201–208
16. Küchle M, Ho TS, Nguyen NX, Hannappel E, Naumann GOH (1994) Protein quantification and electrophoresis in aqueous humor of pseudoexfoliation eyes. Invest Ophthalmol Vis Sci 36:748–752
17. Küchle M, Nguyen N, Hannappel E, Naumann GOH (1995) The blood-aqueous barrier in eyes with pseudoexfoliation syndrome. Ophthalmic Res 27 Suppl 1:136–142
18. Küchle M, Vinores SA, Mahlow J, Green WR (1996) Blood-Aqueous barrier in pseudoexfoliation syndrome: evaluation by immunohistochemical staining of endogenous albumin. Graefes Arch Clin Exp Ophthalmol 234:12–18
19. Lütjen-Drecoll E, Shimizu T, Rohrbach M, Rohen JW (1986) Quantitative analysis of "plaque material" in the inner and outer wall of Schlemm's canal in normal and glaucomatous eyes. Exp Eye Res 42:443–455
20. Mitchell P, Wang JJ, Smith W (1997) Association of pseudoexfoliation syndrome with increased vascular risk. Am J Ophthalmol 124:685–687
21. Moreno-Montanes J, Blesa JL (1995) IgG, albumin and total IgG index in the aqueous humor of eyes with pseudoexfoliation syndrome. Acta Ophthalmol Scand 73:249–251
22. Morrison JC, Green WR (1988) Light microscopy of the exfoliation syndrome. Acta Ophthalmol 66 (Suppl):5–27
23. Naumann GOH, Schlötzer-Schrehardt U (1994) Corneal endotheliopathy in pseudoexfoliation syndrome (Letter). Arch Ophthalmol 112:297–298
24. Naumann GOH (1995) Corneal Transplantation in Anterior Segment Diseases. The 56. Bowman Lecture 1994. Eye 9:395–421
25. Naumann GOH, von der Lippe I (1995) Increased prevalence of occludable angles and angle-closure glaucoma in patients with pseudoexfoliation syndrome (Letter). Am J Ophthalmol 1995; 119:526
26. Naumann GOH, Schlötzer-Schrehardt U, Küchle M (1998) Pseudoexfoliation syndrome for the comprehensive ophthalmologist. Intraocular and systemic manifestations. Ophthalmology 105:951–968
27. Netland PA, Ye H, Streeten BW, Hernandez MR (1995) Elastosis of the lamina cribosa in pseudo-exfoliation syndrome with glaucoma. Ophthalmology 102:878–886
28. Puska P (1995) The amount of lens exfoliation and chamber-angle pigmentation in exfoliation syndrome with or without glaucoma. Acta Ophthalmol Scand 73:226–232
29. Ringvold A, Blika S, Elsas T, Guldahl J, Brevik T, Hesstvedt P et al. (1991) The Middle-Norway eye-screening study. II. Prevalence of simple and capsular glaucoma. Acta Ophthalmol 69:273–280
30. Ritch R (1994) Exfoliation syndrome and occludable angles. Trans Am Ophthalmol Soc 92:845–944
31. Ritch R (1994) Exfoliation syndrome – the most common identifiable cause of open-angle glaucoma. J Glaucoma 1994; 3:176–178
32. Rohen JW (1993) Why is intraocular pressure elevated in chronic simple glaucoma? Anatomical considerations. Ophthalmology 90:758–765
33. Schlötzer-Schrehardt U, Koca MR, Naumann GOH, Volkholz H (1992) Pseudoexfoliation syndrome. Ocular manifestation of a systemic disorder? Arch Ophthalmol 110:1752–1756
34. Schlötzer-Schrehardt U, Dörfler S, Naumann GOH (1993) Corneal endothelial involvement in pseudoexfoliation syndrome. Arch Ophthalmol 111:666–674
35. Schlötzer-Schrehardt U, Naumann GOH (1994) A histopathologic study of zonular instability in pseudoexfoliation syndrome. Am J Ophthalmol 118:730–743
36. Schlötzer-Schrehardt U, Naumann GOH (1995) Trabecular meshwork in pseudoexfoliation syndrome with and without open-angle glaucoma. A morphometric, ultrastructural study. Invest Ophthalmol Vis Sci 36:1750–1764
37. Schlötzer-Schrehardt U, Naumann GOH (1997) Pseudoexfoliations-Syndrom: Morphologie und Komplikationen. In: Naumann GOH et al. Pathologie des Auges, vol II. Springer, Heidelberg, pp 1373–1422
38. Seitz B, Müller EE, Langenbucher A, Kus MM, Naumann GOH (1995) Endotheliale Keratopathie bei Pseudoexfoliationssyndrom: quantitative und qualitative Morphometrie mittels automatisier-ter Videobildanalyse. Klin Monatsbl Augenheilkd 207:167–175
39. Streeten BW, Li Z-Y, Wallace RN, Eagle RC, Keshgegian AA (1992) Pseudoexfoliative fibrillopathy in visceral organs of a patient with pseudoexfoliation syndrome. Arch Ophthalmol 110:1757–1762

40. Tarkkanen A (1962) Pseudoexfoliation of the lens capsule: A clinical study of 418 patients with special reference to glaucoma, cataract, and changes of the vitreous. Acta Ophthalmol 71 Suppl:1–98
41. Vogt A (1926) Ein neues Spaltlampenbild: Abschilferung der Linsenvorderkapsel als wahrscheinliche Ursache von senilem chronischem Glaukom. Schweiz med Wschr 56:413
42. von der Lippe I, Küchle M, Naumann GOH (1993) Pseudoexfoliation syndrome as a risk factor for acute ciliary block angle closure glaucoma. Acta Ophthalmol 71:277–279
43. Zagórski Z, Gossler B, Naumann GOH (1989) Effect of low oxygen tension on the growth of bovine corneal endothelial cells in vitro. Ophthalmic Res 21:440–442

Wound Healing and Scarring of the Developing Filtering Bleb – A Major Challenge in Glaucoma Surgery

F. Grehn, G. Picht, U. Welge Lüssen, and E. Lütjen-Drecoll

Introduction

Trabeculectomy has become the standard surgical procedure for primary open-angle glaucoma (POAG) during the last few decades. Modifications of the technique and preoperative assessment of risk factors have constantly reduced the rate of acute postoperative complications. The main challenge that remains is, however, the lack of predictability of postoperative wound healing and scar formation at the filtering site [1–3]. The basic mechanisms of wound healing in glaucoma filtering surgery are still poorly understood [4–6]. Antimetabolites such as Mitomycin C and 5-fluorouracil (5FU) are now routinely used to reduce scar formation in high risk cases, but their mechanisms of action are not specific [5, 7–9].

The following report summarizes the main clinical aspects to be considered that may lead to increased success rate of filtering surgery and outlines some new aspects of research of post-trabeculectomy wound healing.

The Importance of a Classification of the Developing Filtering Bleb

Filtering blebs develop in various forms during the postoperative period [10–13]. The slit-lamp morphology of filtering blebs is a strong indicator of the prognosis of the function of the bleb. Misconceptions are frequently encountered that possibly prevent adequate postoperative treatment of the filtering bleb:
1. In contrast to common belief, the postoperative level of intraocular pressure (IOP) has little predictive value of the long-term outcome and functionality of the filtering bleb. This holds true especially during the first 2–3 weeks after surgery.
2. The initial site of scarring is rarely the scleral flap, but much more frequently the subconjunctival connective tissue. If the scleral flap obliterates, this occurs mostly secondary to scarring of the subconjunctival tissue.
3. Treatment with local antiglaucoma drugs for postoperative IOP elevation during the first 3–4 weeks may trigger additional scarring via the following mechanisms:
   (a) Decrease of flow through the filtering bleb due to aqueous suppressive drugs, hence the filtering site is not sufficiently held open by flow of aqueous
   (b) Opening of the blood-aqueous and blood-tissue barriers when parasympathomimetics and epinephrine are used [14–17]
   (c) Increase of inflammatory mechanisms of wound healing by most of the antiglaucoma drugs [14–17]

4. The modulation of wound healing (i.e. postoperative 5FU injections) at the filtering site is ineffective if started too late.

The major turning point for postoperative decision making is the period of the second and third week. In many cases, if the IOP goes up again, the increase occurs during this period. It is then important to correctly interpret the mechanism of IOP elevation. The following causes are common: (a) beginning of scar formation, (b)
increase of IOP induced by postoperative steroid treatment (c) IOP elevation due to
still incomplete drainage through subconjuctival lymph vessels and veins.

According to the mechanism that is present, the following measures have to be
taken into consideration: Beginning of scar formation needs intervention such as 5FU
injections, needling of the filtering bleb, or both. In case of steroid-induced IOP elevation, the steroids should be simply reduced or discontinued. In this case, the IOP
will return to normal values within a few days unless other causes of IOP elevation
are present. If incomplete drainage vessel development without scar formation is present during the first 3 weeks, one can simply follow the bleb development and should
not reduce aqueous flow with antiglaucoma drugs.

Adequate decision on the above mentioned causes can best be done by slit-lamp
biomicroscopy of the filtering bleb.

There are a few simple signs that allow the decision between favourable and unfavourable development of the filtering bleb in the postoperative period [12,13]. These
are the following:

1. The state of vascularization determines future wound healing properties: Little or
   no vascularization is typically a favourable sign of bleb function (Fig. 1). Strong
   vascularization is a sign of impending scar formation (Fig. 2).
2. The appeerence of "cork screw" vessels is a sign of active fibril contraction during
   connective tissue formation (Fig. 3).
3. Presence of microcysts signify favourable filtering bleb development (Fig. 4).
   These microcysts probably are a morphological equivalent of free access of aqueous to lymphatic vessels. They can best be seen with regredient light from a narrow beam of the slit-lamp.

Fig. 1. Little conjunctival
vessel formation of the
filtering bleb and diffuse
transition of bleb borders as
a sign of favourable bleb
development

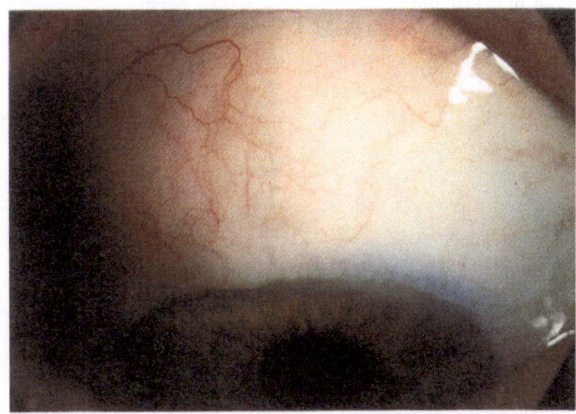

Fig. 2. Strong vascularization of the filtering bleb and
the surrounding conjunctiva
as a sign of unfavourable
bleb development. Demarca-
tion of bleb borders

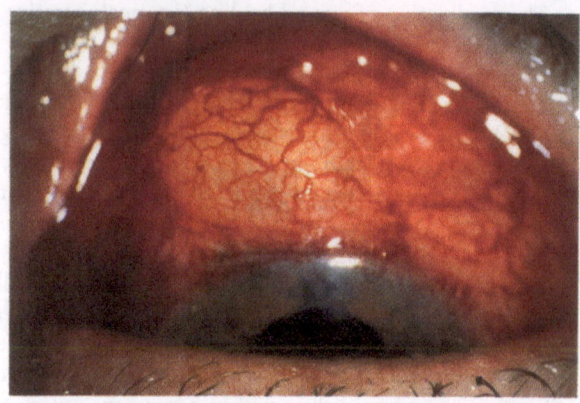

Fig. 3. Cork screw vessels
on the filtering bleb as a
sign of impending active
scar formation during the
development of the filtering
bleb

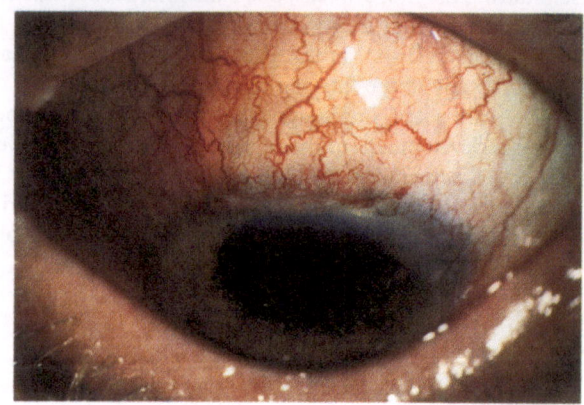

Fig. 4. Conjunctival microcysts of the filtering bleb

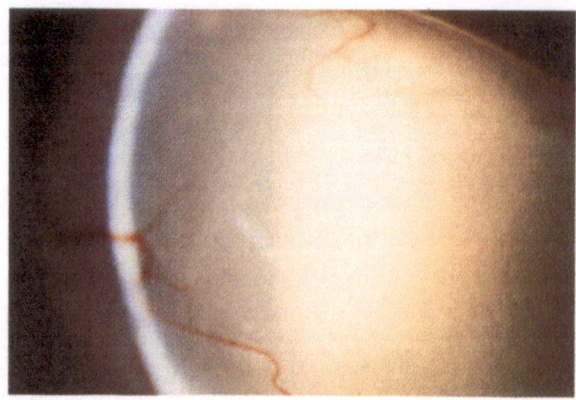

Fig. 5. Encapsulated, dome-shaped filtering bleb

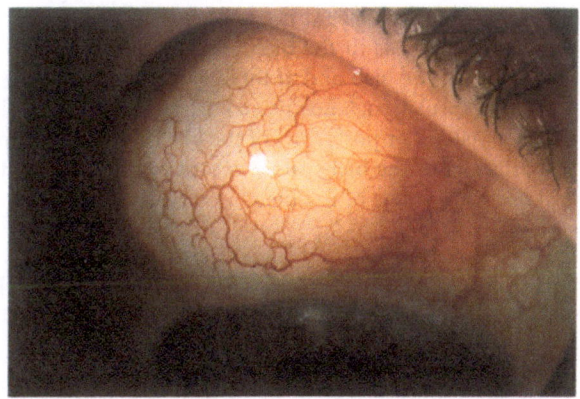

4. Bleb borders give important information on the activity of the wound healing process: If sharp borders are present, an encapsulated bleb may develop and scar formation will increase (see Fig. 2).
5. Monocystic appearance ("encapsulated bleb") is an unfavourable sign of bleb function (Fig. 5). The dome-shaped bleb consists of a dense capsule of connective tissue. The aqueous humor flows freely though the scleral flap area but is not resorbed from the episcleral lake. As an additional morphologic sign for cystic encapsulation, the superficial conjunctiva can be moved with a glass spatula and glides on the dense connective capsule tissue.

Grading System of Filtering Blebs

We currently use a grading system of filtering blebs for documentation (Table 1).

For vascularization, 0 means no or less vessels compared to the conjunctiva adjacent to the filtering bleb (see Fig. 1), 1 means equal vascularization compared to the adjacent conjunctiva, 2 means stronger vascularization compared to the adjacent conjunctiva, and 3 means heavy vascularization (see Fig. 2).

For cork screw vessels, 0 means absence of cork screw vessels, 1 means presence of a fewer number of cork screw vessels than of other vessels, 2 means an equal number of cork screw vessels compared to other vessels, 3 means a preponderance of cork screw vessels compared to other vessels.

Table 1. Semiquantitative grading system for filtering blebs

Vascularization	0	1	2	3
Cork screw vessels	0	1	2	3
Microcysts	0	1	2	3
Encapsulation	0	1	2	3
Movableness of superficial bleb conjunctiva	Yes			No
Height of the bleb	As estimated in corneal thickness equivalents (slit beam)			

For microcysts, 0 means no microcysts, 1 means microcysts at the area of the bleb, 2 means microcysts in the bleb and at two sides adjacent to the bleb, and 3 means microcysts in the bleb and at three sides adjacent to the bleb.

For encapsulation, 0 means no encapsulation of the bleb, 1 means encapsulation at one side (lateral or posterior) of the bleb, 2 means encapsulation at two sides (lateral or posterior) of the bleb, and 3 means encapsulation at all three sides (both lateral and posterior sides) of the bleb.

Outcome of Filtering Procedures Using Intensified Postoperative Treatment

In a retrospective study [11], 113 eyes of 113 patients were followed after trabeculec-tomy. The above described criteria for bleb classifications were used for therapeutic decisions during the first few weeks after operation and during 6 months postopera-tively. Success of filtering surgery was defined as intraocular pressure (IOP) < 21 mm Hg including IOP reduction of at least 20% of the initial IOP without antiglaucoma-tous treatment.

The success rate using these IOP criteria was 88.5% after 6 months. This favour-able success rate was achieved by using an intensified postoperative regimen for post-operative treatment. In 47.6% of the operated eyes, signs of scar formation of the fil-tering bleb were suspected. 38.9% of eyes had a modification or intensification of their topical steroid or cycloplegic treatment. Subconjunctival 5-FU injections were given in 28.5%, the combination of needling and 5-FU injections was performed in 14.2% and laser suturolysis was made in 6.2% of the 113 eyes.

Although follow-up period was only 6 months in this study, a prerequisite for a long-term functioning filtering bleb is the adequate development of the bleb during the various stages of wound healing. Hence, the assessment of the morphological signs of the development filtering bleb is crucial for further treatment decisions.

The Role of Aqueous Humor Transforming Growth Factor β-2 in the Development of the Filtering Bleb

A number of growth factors are involved in wound healing after glaucoma surgery. Khaw [18] found TGFβ-2 to be a major modulator of wound healing after experimen-tal glaucoma surgery. Tripathi et al. [19] and Picht et al. [20] found TGFβ-2 increased in glaucoma eyes. In contrast to primary open angle glaucoma, TGFβ-2 was normal in pseudoexfoliation glaucoma [20].

We were interested in the role of TGFβ-2 concerning the development of filtering blebs after filtration surgery.

A comparison of the outcome of filtration surgery and TGFβ-2 values taken during surgery is, of course, difficult to establish. Usually, surgeons make numerous attempts to overcome bleb obliteration when a risk for scarring of the filtering site is antici-pated. As a consequence, antimetabolites are sometimes given during surgery (mito-mycin C or 5-FU) and/or after surgery (5-FU) and may lead to favourable outcome despite a preoperatively high-risk situation. In addition, secondary procedures, like

Fig. 6. TGFβ-2 values in POAG classified according to clinical filtering bleb appearance. Eyes whose blebs developed signs of scarring after trabeculectomy showed higher average preoperative TGFβ-2 values than eyes that developed favourable blebs after trabeculectomy

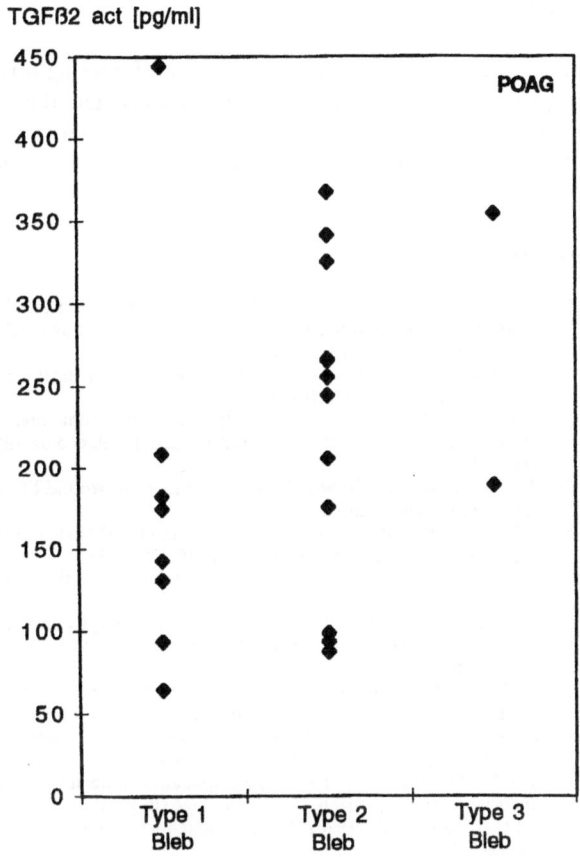

needling and 5-FU injection of varying doses, are applied taking into account the postoperative development of the filtering bleb and the postoperative IOP.

When we compared TGFβ-2 values and clinical outcome, we tried to define simple clinical outcome criteria: (a) IOP decrease in percentage of preoperative values, (b) classification of filtering bleb according to slit-lampe criteria into favourable (type 1 bleb), intermediate (type 2 bleb), and unfavourable (type 3 bleb) appearance, as described above [12, 13], (c) absence or need of further intervention (post-operative subconjunctival 5-FU injections and/or needling, surgical revision after surgery).

POAG eyes with favourable bleb development (type 1 bleb) had lower TFGβ-2 values than eyes with less favourable (type 2 bleb) or unfavourable bleb (type 3 bleb, Fig. 6).

The POAG eyes that had undergone previous laser surgery showed a tendency of higher activated TGFβ-2 values than those that had no previous laser surgery.

Hence it seems likely that TGFβ-2 is one of the factors that influence bleb development after glaucoma surgery also in humans. The possibility to influence TGFβ-2 activity by injecting anti-TGFβ-2 has recently suggested by Khaw et al. [18].

Conclusions

The major problem for long-term success of filtering surgery is wound healing. Glaucoma surgeons should: (1) preoperatively evaluate the risks for scarring in the individual situation and (2) use intensified post-operative treatment when the first signs of bleb scarring appear in the early post-operative period.

References

1. Schwartz AL, Van Veldhausen PC, Gaasterland DE, Ederer F, Sullivan EK, Cyrlin MN, Agis Investigators (1999): The advanced glaucoma intervention study (AGIS): 5. Encapsulated bleb after initial trabeculectomy. Am J Ophthalmol 127:8–19
2. Oh Y, Katz LJ, Spaeth GL, Wilson P (1994) Risk factors for the development of encapsulated filtering blebs. Ophthalmology 101:629–634
3. Shingelton BJ (1996) Management of the failing glaucoma filter. Ophthalmic Surg Rev 27:445–451
4. Skuta GL, Parrish RK (1987) Wound healing in glaucoma filtering surgery. Surv Ophthalmol 32:149–170
5. Khaw PT, Migdal CS (1996) Current techniques in wound healing modulation in glaucoma surgery. Curr Op Ophthalmol 7:24–33
6. Addicks EM, Quigley HA, Green R, Robin AL (1983) Histological characteristics of filtering blebs in glaucomatous eyes. Arch Ophthalmol 101:795–798
7. Fluorouracil Study Group (1996) Five-year follow-up of the fluorouracil filtering study group. Am J Ophthalmol 121:349–366
8. Mietz H, Arnold G, Kirchhof B, Diestelhorst M, Krieglstein GK (1996) Histopathology of episcleral fibrosis after trabeculectomy with and without mitomycin C. Graefes Arch Clin Exp Ophthalmol 234:364–368
9. Hutchinson AK, Grossniklaus HE, Brown RH, McManus PE, Bradley CK (1994) Clinicopathologic features of excised mitomycin filtering blebs. Arch Ophthalmol 112:74–79
10. Hitchings RA, Grierson I (1983) Clinico pathologic correlation in eyes with failed fistulizing surgery. Trans Ophthal Soc UK 1983; 103:84–88
11. Picht G, Mutsch Y, Grehn F (1999) Komplikationen nach Glaukomoperation – Häufigkeit und therapeutische Konsequenzen. Ophthalmologe (in press)
12. Picht G, Grehn F (1998) Sickerkissenentwicklung nach Trabekulektomie. Ophthalmologe 95:380–387
13. Picht G, Grehn F (1998) Classification of filtering blebs in trabeculectomy: biomicroscopy and functionality. Curr Op Ophthalmol 9,II, 2–8
14. Broadway DC, Grierson I, Hitchings RA (1993) Adverse effects of topical antiglaucomatous medications of the conjunctiva. Br J Ophthalmol 77:790–796
15. Broadway DC, Grierson I, O'Brian C, Hitchings RA (1994) Adverse effects of topical antiglaucoma medication I: The conjunctival cell profile. Arch Ophthalmol 112:1437–1445
16. Sherwood MB, Grierson I, Millar L, Hitchings RA (1989) Longterm morphological effects of antiglaucoma drugs on the conjunctiva and Tenon's capsule in glaucomatous eyes. Ophthalmology 98:327–335
17. Broadway DC, Grierson I, Stürmer J, Hitchings RA (1996) Reversal of topical antiglaucoma medication effects on the conjunctiva. Arch Ophthalmol 114:262–267
18. Khaw PT, Cordeiro MF (1998) Neutralizing effects of new recombinant human TGF-β2 monoclonal antibody on in vitro human conjunctival fibroblast-mediated scarring response [ARVO Abstract]. Invest Ophthalmol Vis Sci 39(4):S1107. Abstract No. 5115
19. Tripathi RC (1994) Aqueous humor in glaucomatous eyes contains an increased level of TGFβ-2. Exp Eye Res 59:723–727
20. Picht G, Welge-Luessen U, Grehn F, Luetjen-Drecoll E. TGFβ-2 levels in the aqueous humor in different types of glaucoma and the relation of filtering bleb development. J Glaucoma (submitted)

CHAPTER 7

Neurotransmitter Receptors as Potential Targets of Glaucoma Pathogens

C.-M. Becker

Amino Acid Neurotransmitter in the Retina

Visual signal transduction in the retina essentially depends on a limited number of amino acids which serve as excitatory or inhibitory mediators of synpatic neurotransmission (Brandstätter et al. 1998). Comparable to the situation in the mammalian CNS, glutamate is the principal excitatory neurotransmitter while γ-aminobutyric acid (GABA) and glycine primarily serve as inhibitory mediators. Analysis of these neurotransmitter systems reveals that the retina displays a distinct chemical architecture of synaptic transmission: Vertical transmission, mediated by glutamate, primarily confers excitatory synaptic signals generated by photoreceptors to ganglion cells via bipolar cells. In contrast, GABA and glycine serve as mediators of horizontal transmission by the horizontal and amacrine cells (Fig. 1). Fast neurotransmission by amino acids depends on ligand-gated ion channels including glycine, $GABA_A$, $GABA_C$, and two principal classes of glutamate receptors, the AMPA/kainate and the NMDA-responsive subtype (Enz et al. 1996; Brandstätter et al. 1998).

Fig. 1. Functional architecture of amino acid neurotransmitters prevailing in the retina. (From Brandstätter et al. 1998; Wässle et al. 1998)

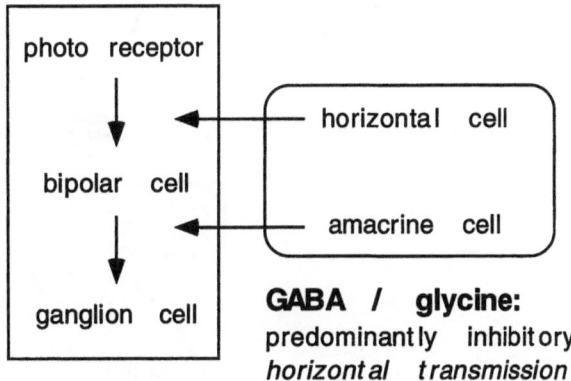

glutamate:
predominantly   excitatory
vertical   transmission

photo receptor

bipolar cell

ganglion cell

horizontal   cell

amacrine   cell

GABA / glycine:
predominantly   inhibitory
horizontal   transmission

As exemplified for NMDA and glycine receptors, receptor dysfunction has been identified as an underlying molecular mechanism of various neurological disorders. In particular, NMDA receptors have not only been associated with neuronal plasticity under physiological conditions, e.g., long-term potentiation and depression, but also with pathological conditions characterized by excitation-mediated neuronal damage. Excessive activation of NMDA receptors by sudden increases in free glutamate levels has been observed following brain trauma and cerebral ischemia. These conditions are thought to elicit massive increases in intracellular calcium concentrations, resulting in neuronal damage and cell death. In a similar way, AMPA/kainate receptors are believed to be involved in some models of ischemic neuronal cell damage. In contrast, mutations of glycine receptor genes cause hypertonic motor disorders in the human and in mutant mouse models. By analogy, alterations in synaptic receptor function should therefore be expected to represent a potential mechanism of retinal pathology in glaucoma and other conditions resulting in a pronounced loss of vision.

Pharmacology, Structure, and Genetics of the NMDA Receptor

NMDA receptors are ligand-gated cation channels widely expressed in mammalian CNS, e.g. hippocampus, cerebral cortex, and retina. They form a subpopulation of ionotropic glutamate receptors which is characterized by high calcium permeability and selectivity for the synthetic agonist N-methyl-D-aspartate. The NMDA receptor complex (Fig. 2) carries distinct functional domains which are distinguishable by

Fig. 2. Ligand topology of the NMDA receptor complex

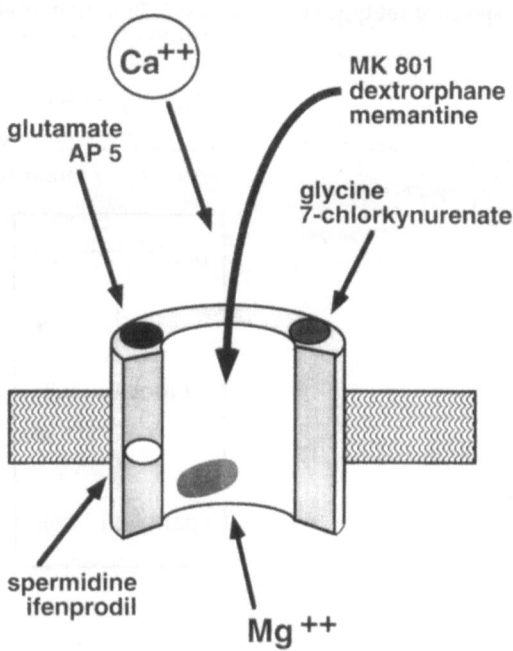

radioligand binding and subject to pharmacological modulation (Monagham et al. 1989):

1. While the agonist binding domain is recognized by [³H]glutamate, applicability of this ligand for binding studies is restricted by its low affinity ($K_D \approx 3$ μmM). In contrast, the antagonistic aminophosphonic acid [³H]CGP-39653 serves as a high affinity NMDA receptor marker.

2. At the NMDA receptor, glycine acts as an essential co-agonist. Gating of the instrinsic cation pore by glutamate binding essentially depends on the occupation of a high affinity glycine binding site ($K_D \approx 100$ nM). Glycine binding to the NMDA receptor is insensitive to strychnine.

3. The cation pore is sensitive to blockage by non-competitive antagonists including MK 801 (dicozilpine), memantine, and ketamine. [³H]MK 801 is a high affinity radioligand ($K_D = 2$ nM) that serves as a valuable tool for analysis of NMDA receptors. In contrast, memantine and ketamine are in clinical use for symptomatic therapy of Parkinson's disease and intravenous anesthesia, respectively.

4. Further binding sites have been characterized for magnesium (Mg^{2+}), zinc (Zn^{2+}), and biogenic polyamines (spermine, spermidine).

NMDA receptors exist as protein isoforms assembled from various subunits. According to a widely accepted topological model, these polypeptides cross the postsynaptic membrane three times (segments A, B, C), while a hairpin inserted between transmembrane segments A, and B is assumed to delineate the cation pore (Hollmann and Heinemann 1994). All of these NMDA receptor oligomers comprise an obligatory subunit NR1 that exists in several splice variants (Sugihara et al. 1992; Durant et al. 1993). The corresponding human gene GRIN1 (glutamate receptor, ionotropic, N-methyl-aspartate 1) comprises 21 exons which are distributed over about 31 kb. By fluorescence in situ hybridization, it has been localized to the chromosomal region 9q34.3-qter (Zimmer et al. 1995).

In addition to NR1, NMDA receptor protein complexes contain at least one of the other NMDA receptor subunits, NR2A–D, as demonstrated by recombinant expression experiments (Laurie and Seeburg 1994). While heterogeneity of NR1 subunit variants is generated by alternative splicing (Lo et al. 1998), the various NR2 polypeptides are encoded by individual genes, termed GRIN2A–D (Table 1). The efficient formation of NMDA receptor channels depends on the coexpression of both NR1 and NR2 subunit cDNAs (Monyer et al. 1992; Ishii et al. 1993). In rodent CNS, the NR2

Table 1. Homology of human and murine NMDA receptor subunit genes

Human Subunit	Gene	Chromosome	Murine Subunit	Gene	Chromosome
NR1	GRIN1	9q34.3	ζ (zeta)	Grin1	2 (12.0 cM)
NR2A	GRIN2A	16p13	ε1 (epsilon 1)	Grin2A	16 (3.4 cM)
NR2B	GRIN2B	12p12	ε2 (epsilon 2)	Grin2B	6 (64.5 cM)
NR2C	GRIN2C	17p25	ε3 (epsilon 3)	Grin2C	11 (78.0 cM)
NR2D	GRIN2D	19q13.1-qter	ε4 (epsilon 4)	Grin2D	7 (23.5 cM)

Subunit designation gene symbol, and chromosomal localization are given for a particular human NMDA receptor subunit and its murine homologue (Online Mendelian Inheritance in Man, 1999). For murine chromosomal loci, the relative position is given in centiMorgan (cM) as listed in the Mouse Genome Database (1999).

subunit variants A–D display characteristic regional and developmental expression patterns, while the NR1 subunit appears to be widely distributed throughout the brain (Monyer et al. 1992; Gass et al. 1993; Mülhardt et al. 1994). These observations have led to the proposal that the different splice variants of NR1 assemble with distinct members of the NR2 subunit types, differing in gating kinetics (Ishii et al. 1992), sensitivity to blockage by Mg^{2+}, and responsiveness to the coagonist glycine (Kleckner and Dingledine 1992). Although the exact stoichiometry of NMDA receptor subunit composition still remains elusive, both tetra- and pentameric models have been proposed (Herkert et al. 1998).

Developmental studies have shown that two major receptor isoforms prevail during maturation of rodent cerebral cortex. Apparently, preexisting assemblies of NR1 and NR2B polypeptides are continuously replaced by oligomeric receptors containing the NR2A subunit. This conclusion is based on several lines of evidence: (1) During the first postnatal week, developmental onset of NR2A expression succeeds NR2B expression (Sheng et al. 1994); (2) expression of the NR2A subunit coincides with the appearence of a low affinity ifenprodil binding site in rat brain (Williams et al. 1993); (3) in immunoprecipitation experiments, NR1 antigen solubilized from rat brain is preferentially co-precipitated with NR2A rather than with NR2B polypeptide by NR1-specific antibodies (Blahos and Wenthold 1996). In rat CNS neurons, NR2B antigen undergoes a pronounced redistribution during maturation. In immature neurons, NR2B antigen accumulates in axonal growth cones and variscosities, while a punctated distribution pattern with redistribution to somato-dendritic spheres is seen in mature cells (Herkert et al. 1998). The association of NR2B with axonal growth cones and processes of immature neurons suggests a role of NMDA receptors in neurite outgrowth and pattern formation (Fig. 3).

There is increasing knowledge about the cellular distribution of NMDA receptor isoforms in mammalian retina, most of these observations relying on in situ hybridization studies. These data indicate that the NMDA receptor subunits NR1 and NR2A–D are expressed in the retina, in addition to several of the structurally related AMPA/kainate receptor subunits (Watanabe et al. 1994; Brandstätter et al. 1994; Wenzel et al. 1997). Immunohistology has led to the identification of the NR2A subunit in

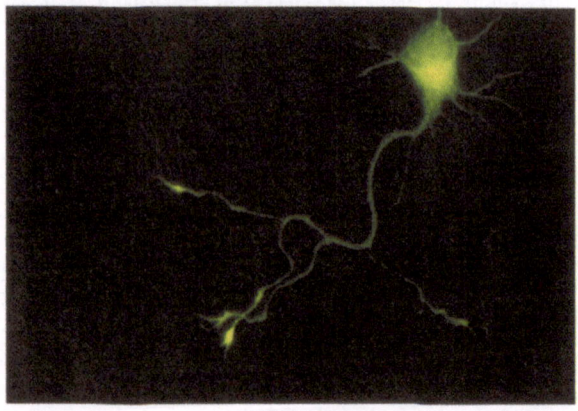

Fig. 3. Distribution of NR2B antigen in cultured hippocampal neurons (2.5 days in culture). Note branching of the prominent axon and enhanced immunoreactivity in growth cones. (From Herkert et al. 1998)

retinae of several mammalian species (Hartveit et al. 1994). NR2A antigen was found throughout the retina, in particular in the outer segments or red/green and blue cone photoreceptors, B-type horizontal cells, several types of amacrine cells, Müller cells and the majority of cells in the ganglion cell layer (Goebel et al. 1998). Functional ionotropic glutamate receptors, including the NMDA subtype, have been characterized in detail on retinal ganglion cells (Sucher et al. 1997; Brandstätter et al. 1998). Thus, it may be a safe assumption that genetic disorders affecting NMDA receptor genes (Table 1) would also interfere with glutamatergic transmission in the retina.

Glycine Receptor Structure and Genetics

Initially, glycine was identified as the principal inhibitory neurotransmitter in spinal cord and brainstem. After vesicular release from presynaptic terminals, a depressant action on neuronal activity is exerted by binding to postsynaptic receptors that exist in various isoforms. Glycine-mediated inhibition underlies the segmental regulation of spinal mononeurons by small interneurons including the Renshaw cells, but is also present in other CNS areas. The inhibitory action of glycine is distinct from its modulatory function as a co-agonist to glutamate at the NMDA receptor (Becker et al. 1994; Becker 1995).

Strychnine-sensitive glycine receptors (GlyRs) represent a family of ligand-gated chloride channels that exist as pentameric protein complexes. The GlyR isoform prevailing in brainstem and spinal cord of adult mammals is an assembly of ligand-binding α1 and structural β subunits (Becker 1995; Becker and Langosch 1998). In addition, α2, α3, and α4 subunit genes have been identified in human and rodents (Becker and Langosch 1998; Nikolic et al. 1998). Mature GlyR subunits are thought to cross the postsynaptic membrane four times, with transmembrane segment M2 delineating the inner wall of the anion pore. Determinants of ligand-binding have been assigned to the large extracellular NH_2-terminal domain of the α subunit variants. Glycinergic agonist responses also depend on amino acid residues situated within the extracellular loop linking segments M2 and M3 (Becker and Langosch 1998). The chromosomal localizations of the human genes encoding the α1 (GLRA1), α2 (GLRA2), α3 (GLRA3), and β subunits (GLRB) have been identified (Table 2).

Disturbances of glycinergic transmission play a role in strychnine intoxication as well as in genetic alterations. Glycine binding is efficiently antagonized by the plant

Table 2. Homology of human and murine glycine receptor subunit genes

GlyR Subunit	Human Gene	Chromosome	Murine Gene	Chromosome
α1	GLRA1	5q31.2	Glra1	11 (30.0 cM)
α2	GLRA2	Xp21.2-p21.3	Glra2	X (72.0 cM)
α3	GLRA3	4q33-q34	Glra3	8 (26.0 cM)
α4	GLRA4	[Xq21-q22?]	Glra4	X (56.0 cM)
β	GLRAB	4q31.3	Glrb	3 (36.0 cM)

The human chromosomal representation of the glycine receptor α4 subunit is not known. Rather, the position in brackets denotes the human chromosomal region linked by synteny homology to the murine Glra4 locus.

alkaloid strychnine which produces both increases in muscle tone and exaggerated startle responses to external stimuli (Becker 1995). Symptoms of the human neurological disorder, hyperekplexia (startle disease, stiff baby syndrome, STHE, MIM#149400), are reminiscent of strychnine-induced GlyR dysfunction. Affected infants display exaggerated startle responses and severe muscle stiffness which may result in fatal apnea. During the first year of life, muscle tone returns to normal while excessive startling, which may culminate in immediate, unprotected falling, persists into adulthood (Brune et al. 1996). Dominant traits of hyperekplexia were found to correlate with GLRA1 missense mutations affecting segment M2 and the extracellular M2–M3 loop (Becker and Langosch 1998). In two recessive traits, amino acid exchanges have been identified within segment M1 (Becker and Langosch 1998). Moreover, homozygosity for a null allele demonstrated that the complete loss of GLRA1 gene function may be tolerated in the human (Brune et al. 1996). Homologous phenotypes shown by mouse lines carrying GlyR α1 and β mutant alleles further support the causative role of GlyR alterations in hypertonic motor disorders (Mülhardt et al. 1994; Saul et al. 1994; Kling et al. 1997). Taken together, the pathogenesis of motor disorders may serve as a paradigm for alterations of neuronal circuits, including those underlying signal processing in the retina (Pinto et al. 1994; Wässle et al. 1998).

Targets of Glaucoma Pathogens?

The concept of excitotoxic cell death predicts that ischemia, trauma, and other neuronal lesions produce an excessive increase in intracellular calcium concentrations, thus triggering cell death (Beal 1992). As ligand-gated calcium channels, NMDA receptors are thought to be mediators of excitotoxicity (Fig. 4). Consistent with this hypothesis, antagonists of NMDA receptor function exert neuroprotective effects (Becker et al. 1995; Storch-Hagenlocher et al. 1996). Glaucoma is characterized by a chronic loss of ret-

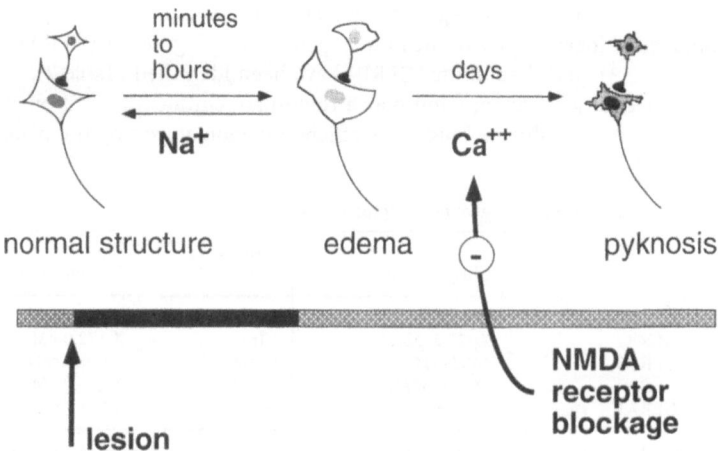

Fig. 4. Stages of neuronal excitotoxicity. (See Beal 1992)

inal ganglion cells, the cause of which is unknown. As potential glaucoma pathogens, direct lesions induced by increased intraocular pressure have been proposed to generate shear forces at the lamina cribrosa. In contrast, damage of retinal ganglion cells may as well be secondary to an accumulation of toxic factors induced by glaucoma, including the excitotoxic amino acid glutamate. It may be speculated that the relese of glutamate reflects ischemic conditions induced by a nutritive deficit due to increases of intraocular pressure during glaucoma. Experimental ischemia indeed induces enhanced release of transmitters, such as GABA, in the rabbit retina (Osborne et al. 1995).

This hypothesis is consistent with amino acid analyses performed on the vitreous body from patients undergoing cataract extraction. In this particular study, glutamate levels were found to be elevated twofold in patients with glaucoma as compared with patients suffering from cataracts only (Dreyer et al. 1996). Similar observations were made in dogs with breed-related primary glaucoma, in which animals with primary glaucoma had significantly elevated vitreal glutamate concentrations (Brooks et al. 1997). Therefore, the loss of ganglion cells occurring in open-angle glaucoma may, at least in part, be attributed to pathological increases in intraocular glutamate (Dreyer and Grosskreutz 1997). As analyzed in retinal explants, glutamate and related receptor agonists effectively induce retinal neurodegeneration (Romano et al. 1995). These studies have confirmed that the neurotoxic actions of glutamate include mediation by Ca^{2+} (Sucher et al. 1997) as well as by nitric oxide (Adachi et al. 1998). Formation of endogenous endotoxins may represent another pathogenic mechanism. Inflammation results in the release of the metabolite of tryptophane, quinolinic acid, which acts as an NMDA-like agonist (Stone 1993).

Conversely, neuroprotective strategies, such as application of NMDA receptor antagonists, prevented the loss of retinal ganglion cells in the experimental paradigms used (Lombardi et al. 1994; Weber et al. 1995; Sucher et al. 1997). Effective drugs included NMDA antagonists such as the channel blockers MK-801 (Chaudhary et al. 1998) and memantine (Lagreze et al. 1998), as well as the non-opioid analgesic flupirtine (Osborne et al. 1998). While these findings offer intriguing promises for an effective treatment of glaucomatous ganglion cell loss, a note of caution may be warranted. The experimental paradigms used hardly reflect the chronic course of this blinding disease. Moreover, some researchers failed to correlate the distribution of glutamate receptor subunits NR1 and GluR2 in the retina of macaques with neurons vulnerable to experimental glaucoma (Hof et al. 1998). Still, therapies protecting neurons against glutamate toxic effects may finally prove to be useful in the management of glaucoma.

As additional players, other members of the ligand-gated ion channel superfamily should be taken into account. In the mature nervous system, glycine receptors mediate inhibitory currents, due to a negative equilibrium potential for chloride ions generated by K^+ / Cl^- cotransporter KCC2 (Rivera et al. 1999). Following mechanical trauma, however, ligand-gated chloride channels revert to excitatory action (van den Pol et al. 1996), potentially exaggerating excitotoxic lesions inflicted upon a neuron. This hypothesis would imply that glycine receptors, in addition to their role in motor disorders, may also contribute to the pathogenesis of neuronal cell loss in glaucoma. Given the high therapeutic potential of ligand-gated neurotransmitter receptors, further analysis of these proteins in the pathogenesis of glaucoma may finally result in new protective therapies.

Acknowledgements. Helpful discussions with Dr. Matthias Herkert are gratefully acknowledged. This work was supported by the Bundesministerium für Bildung und Forschung and the Deutsche Forschungsgemeinschaft (SFB 539, Glaukome einschließlich Pseudoexfoliations-Syndrom).

References

Adachi K, Kashii S, Masai H, Ueda M, Morizane C, Kaneda K, Kume T, Akaike A, Honda Y (1998) Mechanism of the pathogenesis of glutamate neurotoxicity in retinal ischemia. Graefes Arch Clin Exp Ophthalmol 236:766–774

Beal FM (1992) Mechanism of excitotoxicity in neurologic disease. FASEB J 6:3338–3344

Becker CM (1995) Glycine receptors: Molecular heterogeneity and implications for disease. The Neuroscientist 1:130–141

Becker CM, Langosch D (1998) The inhibitory glycine receptor. In: Stephenson FA, Turner AJ (eds) Amino acid neurotransmission. Portland, London, pp 93–112

Becker CM, Hoch W, Schramm M, Wolters I, Betz H (1994) Influence of NMDA receptor antagonists on glycine isoform expression in spinal cord cultures. In: Hartmann A, Yatsu F, Kuschinsky W (eds) Cerebral ischemia and basic mechanisms. Springer, Berlin pp 180–189

Blahos J, Wenthold RJ (1996) Relationship between N-methyl-D-aspartate receptor NR1 splice variants and NR2B subunits. J Biol Chem 271:15669–15674

Brandstätter JH, Hartveit E, Sassoe-Pronetto M, Wässle H (1994) Expression of NMDA and high-affinity kainate receptor subunit mRNAs in the adult rat retina. Eur J Neurosci 6:1100–1112

Brandstätter JH, Koulen P, Wässle H (1998) Diversity of glutamate receptors in the mammalian retina. Vision Res 38:1385–1397

Brooks DE, Garcia GA, Dreyer EB, Zurakowski D, Franco-Bourland RE (1997) Vitreous body glutamate concentration in dogs with glaucoma. Am J Vet Res 58:864–867

Brune W, Weber RG, Saul B, von Knebel-Döberitz M, Grond-Ginsbach K, Kellermann K, Meinck HM, Becker CM (1996) A GLRA1 null mutation in recessive hyperekplexia challenges functional role of glycine receptors. Am J Hum Gen 58:989–997

Chaudhary P, Ahmed F, Sharma SC (1998) MK801 – a neuroprotectant in rat hypertensive eyes. Brain Res 792:154–158

Dreyer EB, Grosskreutz CL (1997) Excitatory mechanisms in retinal ganglion cell death in primary open angle glaucoma (POAG). Clin Neurosci 4:270–273

Dreyer EB, Zurakowski D, Schumer RA, Podos SM, Lipton SA (1996) Elevated glutamate levels in the vitreous body of humans and monkeys with glaucoma. Arch Ophthalmol 114:299–305

Durand GM, Bennett MV, Zukin RZ (1993) Splice variants of the N-methyl-D-aspartate receptor NR1 identify domains involved in regulation by polyamines and protein kinase C. Proc Natl Acad Sci 90:6731–6735

Enz R, Brandstätter JH, Wässle H, Bormann J (1996) Immunocytochemical localization of the GABAc receptor rho subunits in the mammalian retina. J Neurosci 15:4479–4490

Gass P, Mülhardt C, Sommer C, Becker CM, Kiessling M (1993) NMDA and glycine receptor mRNA expression following transient global ischemia in the gerbil brain. J Cerebr Blood Flow Metab 13:337–341

Goebel DJ, Aurelia JL, Tai Q, Jojich L, Poosch MS (1998) Immunocytochemical localization of the NMDA-R2A receptor subunit in the cat retina. Brain Res 808:141–154

Hartveit E, Brandstätter JH, Sassoe-Pronetto M, Laurie DJ, Seeburg PH, Wässle H (1994) Localization and developmental expression of the NMDA receptor subunit NR2A in the mammalian retina. J Comp Neurol 348:570–582

Herkert M, Röttger S, Becker CM (1998) The NMDA receptor subunit NR2B of neonatal brain: Complex formation and enrichment in axonal growth cones. Eur J Neurosci 10:1553–1562

Hollmann M, Heinemann S (1994) Cloned glutamate receptors. Annu Rev Neurosci 17:31–108

Hof PR, Lee PY, Yeung G, Wang RF, Podos SM, Morrison JH (1998) Glutamate receptor subunit GluR2 and NMDAR1 immunoreactivity in the retina of macaque monkeys with experimental glaucoma does not identify vulnerable neurons. Exp Neurol 153:234–241

Ishii T, Moriyoshi K, Sugihara H, Sakurada K, Kadotani H, Yokoi M, Akazawa C, Shigemoto R, Mizuno N, Masu M, Nakanishi S (1992) Molecular characterization of the family of the N-methyl-D-aspartate receptor subunits. J Biol Chem 268:2836–2843

Kleckner NW, Dingledine R (1991) Regulation of hippocampal NMDA receptors by magnesium and glycine during development. Mol Brain Res 11:151–159

Kling C, Koch M, Saul B, Becker CM (1997) The frameshift mutation oscillator (Glra1^{spdot}) produces a complete loss of glycine receptor α1 polypeptide in mouse central nervous system. Neuroscience 78:411–417

Lagreze WA, Knorle R, Bach M, Feuerstein TJ (1998) Memantine is neuroprotective in a rat model of pressure-induced retinal ischemia. Invest Ophthalmol Vis Sci 39:1063–1066

Laurie DJ, Seeburg PH (1994) Regional and developmental heterogeneity in splicing of the rat NMDAR1 mRNA. Eur J Pharmacol 268:335–345

Lo W, Molloy R, Hughes TE (1998) Ionotropic glutamate receptors in the retina: moving from molecules to circuits. Vision Res 38:1399–1410

Lombardi G, Moroni F, Moroni F (1994) Glutamate receptor antagonists protect against ischemia-induced retinal damage. Eur J Pharmacol 271:489–495

Monaghan DT, Bridges RJ, Cotman CW (1989) The exitatory amino acid receptors: Their classes, pharmacology, and distinct properties in the function of the central nervous system. Annu Rev Pharmacol Toxicol 29:365–402

Monyer H, Sprengel R, Schoepfer R, Herb A, Higuchi M, Lomeli H, Burnashev N, Sakmann B, Seeburg PH (1992) Heteromeric NMDA receptors: molecular and functional distinction of subtypes. Science 256:1217–1221

Mouse Genome Database (MGD), Mouse Genome Informatics, The Jackson Laboratory, Bar Harbor, Maine, 1999. World Wide Web URL: http://www.informatics.jax.org/)

Mülhardt C, Fischer M, Gass P, Simon-Chazottes D, Guénet JL, Kuhse J, Betz H, Becker CM (1994) The spastic mouse: Aberrant splicing of glycine receptor β-subunit mRNA caused by intronic insertion of L1 element. Neuron 13:1003–1015

Online Mendelian Inheritance in Man, OMIM (TM). Center for Medical Genetics, Johns Hopkins University (Baltimore, MD) and National Center for Biotechnology Information, National Library of Medicine (Bethesda, MD) 1999, World Wide Web (URL:http://www.ncbi.nlm.nih.gov/omim/)

Osborne NN, Wood J, Muller A (1995) The influence of experimental ischaemia on protein kinase C and the GABAergic system in the rabbit retina. Neuropharmacology 34:1279–1288

Osborne NN, Cazevieille C, Wood JP, Nash MS, Pergande G, Block F, Kosinski C, Schwarz M (1998) Flupirtine, a nonopioid centrally acting analgesic, acts as an NMDA antagonist. Gen Pharmacol 30:255–263

Pinto LH, Grünert U, Studholm K, Yazulla S, Kirsch J, Becker CM (1994) Glycine receptors in the retinas of normal and spastic mutant mice. Invest Ophthalmol Vis Sci 35:3633–3639

Rivera C, Voipio J, Payne JA, Ruusuvuori E, Lahtinen H, Lamsa K, Pirvola U, Saarma M, Kaila K (1999) The K$^+$/Cl$^-$ co-transporter KCC2 renders GABA hyperpolarizing during neuronal maturation. Nature 397:251–255

Romano C, Price MT, Olney JW (1995) Delayed excitotoxic neurodegeneration induced by excitatory amino acids agonists in isolated retina. J Neurochem 65:59–67

Saul B, Schmieden V, Mülhardt C, Gass P, Kuhse J, Becker CM (1994) Point mutation of glycine receptor α1 subunit in the spasmodic mouse affects agonist responses. FEBS Lett 350:71–76

Sheng M, Cummings J, Roldan LA, Jan YN, Jan LY (1994) Changing subunit composition of heteromeric NMDA receptors during development of rat cortex. Nature 368:144–147

Stone TW (1993) Neuropharmacology of quinolinic and kynurenic acids. Pharmacological reviews 45:309–379

Storch-Hagenlocher B, Becker CM, Hacke W (1996) Calciumantagonisten bei neurologischen Erkrankungen. In: Kübler W, Tritthart HA (eds) Calciumantagonisten: Forschung und Klinik, Vergangenheit, Gegenwart und Zukunft. Steinkopf, Darmstadt, pp 273–284

Sucher NJ, Lipton SA, Dreyer EB (1997) Molecular basis of glutamate toxicity in retinal ganglion cells. Vision Res 37:3483–3493

Sugihara H, Moriyoshi K, Ishii T, Masu M, Nakanishi S (1992) Structures and properties of seven isoforms of the NMDA receptor generated by alternative splicing. Biochem Biophys Res Commun 185:826–832

van den Pol AN, Obrietan K, Chen G (1996) Excitatory actions of GABA after neuronal trauma. J Neurosci 16:283–292

Wässle H, Koulen P, Brandstätter JH, Fletcher EL, Becker CM (1998) Glycine and GABA receptors in the mammalian retina. Vis Res 38:1411–1430

Watanabe M, Mishina M, Inoue Y (1994) Diffential distribution of the NMDA receptor channel subunit mRNAs in the mouse retina. Brain Res 634:328–332

Weber M, Bonaventure N, Sahel JA (1995) Protective role of excitatory amino acid antagonists in experimental retinal ischemia. Graefes Arch Clin Exp Ophthalmol 233:360–365

Wenzel A, Benke D, Möhler H, Fritschy JM (1997) N-methyl-D-aspartate receptors containing the NR2D subunit in the retina are selectively expressed in rod bipolar cells. Neuroscience 78:1105–1112

Williams K, Russel S, Shen YM, Molinoff PB (1993) Developmental switch in the expression of NMDA receptors occurs in vivo and in vitro. Neuron 10:267–278

Zimmer M, Fink TM, Franke Y, Lichter P, Spiess J (1995) Cloning and structure of the gene encoding the human N-methyl-D-aspartate receptor (NMDAR1). Gene 159:219–223

CHAPTER 8

Genetic Risk Factors for Glaucoma

J. Hetherington

Introduction

The most common forms of glaucoma are essentially insidious and require the help of risk factors, or predictors, which aid in providing a diagnosis as early as possible. Finding a reliable test could reduce the incidence of visual loss, require fewer exams for low risk patients, identify individuals requiring more attention and reduce the cost of care. Early literature describes the use of nicotine, cold water immersion, head-down position, carotid compression and immune globulin typing as examples of researchers' attempt toward glaucoma detection. A classic example of the effort to find risk factors included the well known, 12 year Glaucoma Collaborative Study. Unfortunately testing that included tonography, tonometry with water provocative testing, along with other methods, did not prove fruitful in spite of their anticipated merit. However, the study did provide evidence that elevated pressures do not necessarily produce damage in many patients.

Ophthalmologists have already established a moderately useful set of glaucoma risk factors after several years and numerous population studies. Not all studies agree but there is a consensus on risks to be considered in managing our glaucoma cases. These risks include: family history, elevated intraocular pressure, race, age, myopia, diabetes and hypertension. Other factors that might be considered predictors include, for example: presence of exfoliation, pigment dispersion, appearance of the optic nerve, inflammation, narrow angles, history of trauma and steroid response.

The past 50 years of the science age and advances in genetics have provided an entire new and creative potential for predicting glaucoma. Benefits also include the possibility of better understanding the disease, predicting outcomes, and curing or controlling glaucoma. At this meeting it is useful to review genetic advances in glaucoma, its clinical usefulness, and to give some expectation for the future. The level of presentation will be directed toward the clinician rather than the geneticist, therefore information of methods, techniques used and detailed discussion will be disregarded.

Juvenile Open-Angle Glaucoma

Juvenile open-angle glaucoma, an area of intensive genetic investigation, is logically the most fruitful place to search because of the early onset (ages 15–35) of high introcular pressure, visual field defects and optic nerve damage with a poor response to medications. The pattern of inheritance is easier to define.

Diagnostic clues for the clinician are derived from an awareness that most cases are autosomal dominant with a 50-50 chance of inheriting this form of glaucoma, fortunately a rare condition. Early detection is now possible via discovery of the TIGR (trabecular meshwork inducibe glucocorticoid response) gene and its linkage to glaucoma. The gene was cloned from the steroid-induction studies of trabecular meshwork cells (Nguyen and Polansky 1993, 1998) and localized in chromosome 1, at the boundary of 1q23–24 (Nguyen et al. 1998), which is within the genetic GLC1A locus originally demonstrated to have a link to JOAG pedigrees (Sheffield et al. 1993) and to COAG pedigrees (Stone et al. 1997). The gene was cloned independently by Kubota et al. in 1997, and its genetic product was termed myocilin due to its homology to myosin protein and its expression in photoreceptor cilia.

Juvenile open-angle will likely be the first form of glaucoma to be completely mapped, with other loci defined in the near future. A GLC1A gene defects is detectable in 70 %–80 % of juvenile glaucoma patients.

Chronic Open-Angle Glaucoma

Genetic analysis would be far simpler of chronic open-angle glaucoma demonstrated a typical mendelian pattern of inheritance. The inheritance of chronic open-angle glaucoma (COAG) determined by pedigree varies from autosomal dominant to no clear pattern, suggesting a multi-factorial mode of inheritance. This variability and the fact that COAG is a disease of late onset makes the task of finding the gene difficult. Pedigree studies reportedly show a risk of 4 %–16 % for relatives with COAG (Leske 1983).

Several mutations, clustered at the 3' end of the TIGR gene, were shown to associate with glaucoma. These mutations account for 3 %–5 % of COAG cases and some mutations seem to correlate with the severity of the disease making them useful markers. For example, the Gln368Stop mutation was found in late onset COAG (Stone et al. 1998); the Tyr437His mutation was found in juvenile onset cases, but not in the adult onset form and the Pro370Leu mutation represents cases of severe juvenile glaucoma (Shirato et al. 1998). Current studies suggesting that mutations which potentially affect the rate of expression of the TIGR gene (accounting for an increased amount of TIGR protein being made) could produce a much higher incidence of glaucoma. This concept is further supported by studies that showed over 50 % of trabecular meshwork tissues from glaucoma patients had larger amounts of TIGR protein compared to the tissues from normal individuals (Lutjen-Drecoll et al. 1998). The observation appears to agree with a potential role of the TIGR protein and its high homology to a mucous protein, olfactomedin (Yokoe and Anholt, 1993), in obstructing the outflow pathway due to its association with pathways of secretion and high viscosity (Polansky et al. 1997). The identification of the TIGR gene as a risk factor was suggested in a study of middle age glaucoma patients which showed a linkage of the GLC1A locus in patients with optic nerve and visual field damage, but not to those without damage although with the same pressures (Brezin et al. 1997).

It is important to know that the TIGR gene was also found to be in tissues other than the trabecular meshwork including photo receptor, iris, ciliary body, sclera and choroid (Ortega et al. 1997). The genetic heterogeneity of adult onset glaucoma is evident from the multiplicity of chromosomal loci associated with the disease. In addition to GLC1A several other loci have been identified that segregate with COAG, suggesting the heterogeneous nature of glaucoma.

The importance of extracellular molecules on glaucoma pathogenesis received further support from isolation of the PCOLCE2 candidate gene for COAG. The PCOLCE2 is a type-1 procollagen COOH-terminal proteinase enhancer protein and is a member of a gene family that plays a role in regulating the levels of type 1 collagen and other fibrinous proteins. The gene was identified by expression in the trabecular meshwork cells (Wirtz et al. 1997). Based on the gene localization within the inclusion of the GLC1C locus (3q21–24) and its potential role in collagen synthesis. PCOLCE2 was proposed as a candidate gene for COAG. If mutations are confirmed, identification of the PCOLCE2 gene suggest a role of the meshwork collagen beam in glaucoma pathogenesis.

Heterogeneity is revealed, with data linking cases of adult open angle glaucoma to 2cen-q13 (GLC1B) (Stoilova et al. 1996). This particular family showed no defects to the TIGR (GLC1A) gene. Patients in this group of this different phenotype presented with a milder form of glaucoma and only a moderate pressure elevation. Within this group of adult COAG, some patients did not show linkage to the GLC1B gene. Polygenic heterogeneity is also supported by the finding of a family with linkage to two genes in the 3q21-region (GLC1C) (Wirtz et al. 1997). Lichter's (Lichter et al. 1997) group found no mutations in the TIGR gene in a Panamanian family but they may be linked to other loci. A large number of cases from a French Canadian family were classified as autosomal dominant and phenotypically variable, and mapped to TIGR, GLC1B and IRIDI gene loci (Vincent 1997). The clinical characteristics are similar to the previously described GLC1B group, again supporting the heterogeneous nature of glaucoma. To date there are six gene loci (GLC1A to GLC1F) identified for different subtypes of COAG.

Pigmentary Glaucoma

The definition between pigment dispersion syndrome and pigmentary glaucoma and COAG is unclear, and thus difficult to evaluate genetically. Gramer et al. (1998) determined that family history and myopia are risk factors for the development of pigmentary glaucoma. Theories suggest that pigmentary glaucoma is basically an abnormality in the development of the angle, mechanical contact of the iris to the lens, an abnormality of the iris pigment layer, or only a form of COAG. These conditions follow an autosomal dominant inheritance pattern, similar to COAG. (Wiggs et al. 1997) discovered a locus at the telomere of chromosome 7 (7q35-36) in four families that is linked to pigment dispersion syndrome, and although pigmentary glaucoma is often found in families of diagnosed COAG, there was no linkage to the GLC1A locus.

Normal Tension Glaucoma

Recent screening programs revealed a higher incidence of low tension glaucoma than estimated with variations among populations. Very little is known about low tension glaucoma to the extent that only recently, in 1998, intraocular pressure was proven to be a risk factor (personal communication, Glaucoma Research Foundation). Optic nerve damage occurs when the pressure is lower than expected compared to other forms of glaucoma. This leads to theories of connective tissue abnormalities. Additionally, clinicians can only arbitrarily agree on a gray area of pressure levels that poorly define normal tension glaucoma, and many experts considers this condition a part of the COAG spectrum rather than a separate disease. The inability to define and categorize a disease makes genetic analysis difficult.

Genetic studies of normal tension glaucoma, aided by a family, show an autosomal dominant pattern of inheritance. In this pedigree, eight members of a family of five generations are affected (Bennett et al. 1989). Sarfarazi et al. (1998) mapped normal tension glaucoma in a British family to the 10q15–q14 region, locus GLC1E.

Congenital Glaucoma

Primary congenital glaucoma allows a moderately clear opportunity for analysis. An early onset with obvious symptoms of tearing, cloudy cornea and an enlarged eye bring patients to an ophthalmologist for diagnosis, in contrast to COAG that is insidious and often undiagnosed. Therefore pedigrees are easier to obtain. Linkage analysis, gene mapping, positional cloning and candidate genes have helped identify genes associated with glaucoma and developmental defects of the anterior segment.

Primary congenital glaucoma is, for the most part, autosomal recessive with linkage to the 2q21 GLC3A locus, with mutations in the CYP1B1 gene (Sarfarazi et al. 1995; Stoilova et al. 1997). This gene encodes the P450, a hepatic enzyme gene which is an interesting finding. Defects in the P450 (CYP1B1) gene are detectable in 70 %–80 % of congenital glaucoma cases making it a major genetic marker for this disease. It suggests an important relationship of metabolic pathways and regulation of eye development. Although not verified in all families, the 2p21 region appears to be a major locus in different ethnic groups and in a very high percentage of patients.

Another gene, FKHL7 (forkhead) recently identified, is related to the 6p25 locus for congenital glaucoma. FKHL7 may be related to other developmental glaucomas (Nishimura and Sheffield 1998).

A second, apparently less important locus, for primary congenital glaucoma links to 1p36 (GLC3B), an area that contains many oncogenes known to be associated with tumors (Akarasu et al. 1996). Graff et al. (1997) reported linkage of autosomal dominant congenital glaucoma to 1p36 and 2p21 and Mears et al. (1996) added chromosome 6p25 as a region responsible for iridogoniodysgenesis and primary congenital glaucoma.

Riegers Syndrome and Iris Hypoplasia

Riegers' syndrome is an autosomal dominant condition and involves marked abnormalities of the anterior segment, which maps to 4q25, accompanied by dental and facial defects that have been linked to the 4q25 RIEG1 gene locus (Heon et al. 1995a). Findings such as these differ, however, with those of other investigators due perhaps to variations in phenotypes. Phillips et al. (1996) mapped another locus, REIG2 to 13q14 region. Graff et al. (1997) mapped the developmental defect of the anterior chamber, termed iridogoniodysgenesis, to IGDA 6q25tel.

Marfan Syndrome

As an autosomal dominant connective tissue disease, Marfan syndrome involves a variety of organs including the cardiovascular and skeletal system, and the anterior segment of the eye. Dietz et al. (1991) found linkage to fibrillin-1 gene (locus 15p-21). Fibrillin is classified as a microfibrillar glycoprotein component of the extracellular tissues including the eye but not found in trabecular meshwork.

Weill-Marchesani Syndrome

Short stature, absence of zonules with spherophakia and glaucoma comprise the Weill-Marchesani syndrome, which shows an autosomal dominant inheritance pattern (Wirtz et al. 1997). As suspected, the organ abormalities involve connective tissues that also map a fibrillin protein found at 15q21. This finding points out the similarities to Marfan syndrome.

Posterior Polymorphous Dystrophy

Posterior polymorphous dystrophy (PPMD), also an autosomal dominant condition, involves the anterior segment, primarily the cornea, and is associated with glaucoma in approximately 20%–40% of patients. Linkage analysis maps PPMD to 20q11 segment of chromosome 20 (Heon et al. 1995). The condition is rare and likely will require larger groups of these patients to confirm these findings.

Nail Patella Syndrome

Lichter et al. (1997) first described a locus at 9q34 that is associated with COAG in patients with nail patella syndrome (NPS), a rare condition. A gene PBX3 mapped to this locus was found to have mutations associated with NPS (Dreyer et al. 1998). This finding could add information to the puzzle that would help solve the genetics of COAG, a far more common problem.

Summary

It is evident that genetics have become a very important strategy in the clinical approach to the care of glaucoma patients. The research activity is exciting and moving rapidly. Although in its present state genetic testing is of limited value in determining risk factor, its promise for the future is obvious.

Using risk factors, such as mutations in the TIGR gene, are at this stage limited when a family history is unavailable. However if a TIGR gene defect is known to be present in family members, a finding of the TIGR mutation in an individual would be a considered risk factor for glaucoma. There is a major interest in investigating possibilities of the TIGR gene for screening. It is also likely there will soon be a genetic test

Table 1. Genes and loci identified for glaucoma

Locus/year	cM/markers	Candidate gene/year	Authors	Glaucoma types
1q21-31 (1993) GLC1A	10 (D13665-D1S218)	TIGR (1993) (MYOC/CBS-670 GLC1A) (1997)	Nguyen, Polansky, Stone, Sheffield, Shimizu, Coca-Prados, Stone	JOAG, COAG
1p36 (1996) GLC3B	D1S2834-D1S402	N/D	Sarfarazi M	Primary Congenital
2cen-q13 (1997) GLC1B	(D2S2161-D2S1897) 11.2 (D2S2161-D2S176)	N/D N/D	Richards J Sarfarazi M	Middle-Age COAG Late 40s COAG LTF
2p21 (1996) GLC3A	10 (D13665-D1S218)	P450 (1997) (CYP1B1)	Sarfarazi M	Congenital
3p21-24 (1997) GLC1C	11 (D3S3637-D3S1744)	PCOLCE2 (1998)	Wirtz M	High pressure COAG
4q25-q27 (1996)	10 (D13554-D1S218)	RIEG (1996) Biocoid related	Murray	Rieger syndrome
6p25 (1997)	6.4 (D6S1600-D61617) 6per-D&S1617)	FKHL7 forkhead (1998) NQOS/BAC(1998) unknown RIEG N/D	Sheffield V Mears Murray Raymond V	Congenital IGDA Rieger syndrome Develp.
7q35-q36(1997)	5 (D7S2546-D7S550)	N/D	Wiggs J	Pigmentary glaucoma
8q23 (1998) GLC1D	6.3 (D81930-D8S592)	N/D	Sarfarazi M	COAG
9q34 (1997) GLC1F	Not known to us	PBX3 (LMX1B)	Lichter, P Wirtz M Dreyer S (1998) Richards J (1998)	Petella syndrome
10p14-p15 (1998) GLC1E	2.1 (D10S1729-D10S1644)	N/D	Sarfarazi M	Normal tension
11p13 (1998)	Not known to us	N/D	Richards J	Nanophthalmos
13q14 (1996) (second Rieger locus)	Not known to us	N/D	Philips J	Rieger syndrome-glaucoma
15p21.1 (1996)	Fibrillin region	Fibrillin-1	Wirtz M Wheathley HM	Weill-Marchesani-glaucoma Marfan syndrome-glaucoma
20q11 (1995)	30cM(D20S98-D20S108)	N/D	Heone and Stone	PPMD

Data established by J Heterhington and TD Nguyen.

This table descibes progress made in glaucoma research in the last few years. Fifteen loci that link to pedigrees with glaucoma were identified. Among these, six of them belong to primary open-angle glaucoma, two belong to primary congenitcal glaucoma and the rest are secondary congenital glaucoma. Seven candidate genes were identified (in italies and rhe genes are subjects for mutation and functonal studies to help identify risk population for glaucoma as well as understand glaucoma pathogenesis.

Note: Glaucoma research is a fast moving field. The author presents published data available to them at the moment of this writing and wish to apologize for incomplete information or lack of knowledge on findings of other laboratories. For oncenience, loci are listed by the order of chromosomes. Nomenclature for glaucoma: GLC1, open-angle glaucoma; GLC2, closed-angle glaucoma; GLC3, congenital glaucoma; A,B,C,D,E,F...gene number.

kit for congenital glaucoma using the CYP1B1 gene. Unfortunately numerous candidate genes have not demonstrated a direct association to COAG. Linkage to specific genes found by analysis in less common forms of glaucoma with good pedigrees, such as Riegers' syndrome, hopefully will provide clues to more common forms of glaucoma such as adult COAG. Other genetic factors such as promoter function, gene deletion, combination of genes and external factors may play a role in causing glaucoma. Genetic research in the future should also include, if possible, a more intense investigation of genes related to neuronal, vascular and connective tissue function. There is evidence that these factors, rather than pressure, may play an important part of some forms of glaucoma.

Genetic testing does provide useful information but care must be taken in its interpretation with guarded counseling of patients. Genetic testing is likely to become the most important determinant of risk factor for glaucoma within the next 5 years (Table 1).

References

Akarsu AN, Hossain A, Stoilo I, Turacli ME, Aktan SG, Barsoum-Homsy, Chevrette L, Sarfarazi M (1996) Mapping a major locus for primary congenital glaucoma (buphthalmos) to 2q21 and evidence for genetic heterogeneity. IOVS, 37(3), ARVO Abs#2075

Bennett SR, Alward WLM, Folberg R (1989) An autosomal dominant form of lowtension glaucoma. Am J Ophth 108:238–244

Brezin AP, Bechetoille A, Hamard P, Valtot F, Berkani M, Belmouden A, Adam MF, Dupont de Dinechin S, Bach JF and Garchon HJ (1997) Genetic heterogeneity of primary open angle glaucoma and ocular hypertension: linkage to GLC1A associated with an increased risk of severe glaucomatous optic neuropathy. J Med Genet 34:546–552

Dietz HG, Cutting GK, Pigritz RE et al. Marfans syndrome caused by de novo missense mutation in the Fibrillin gene. Nature 352:337–339

Dreyer SD, Zhou G, Baldini A, Winterpacht A, Zabel B, Cole W, Johnson RL, Lee B (1998) Mutations in LMX1B cause abnormal skeletal patterning and renal dysplasia in nail patella syndrome. Nature Gen, 19 (1):47–50

Graff C, Jerndal T, Wadelius C (1997) Fine mapping of the gene for autosomal dominant juvenile-onset glaucoma with iridogoniodysgenesis in 6p25-Tel. Hum Genet 101, 130–134

Gramer E, Thiele H, Ritch R (1998) Family history of glaucoma and risk factors in pigmentary glaucoma. A clinical study. Klin Monatsbl Augenheilk 212:454–464

Heon E, Sheth BP, Kalenak JW, Sunden SLF, Streb LM, Taylor CM, Alward WLM, Sheffield VC, Stone EM (1995a) Linkage of autosomal dominant iris hypoplasia to the region of the Rieger syndrome locus (4q25). Hum Mol Gen 4:1435–1439

Heon E, Mathers WD, Alward WLM, Weisenthal RW, Sunden SLF, Fishbaugh JA et al. (1995b) Linkage of posterior polymorphous corneal dystrophy to 20q11. Hum Mol Genet 4:485–488

Kubota R, Noda S, Wang Y, Minoshima S, Asakawa S, Kudoh J, Mashima Y, Oguchi Y and Shimizu N (1997) A Novel Myosin-like Protein (Myocilin) expressed in the connecting cilium of the photoreceptor: molecular cloning, tissue expression and chromosomal mapping, Genomics 41, 360–369

Kubota R, Noda S, Wang Y et al. (1997) A novel myosin-like protein (Myocillin) expressed in the conecting cilium of the photoreceptor: molecular cloning, tissue expression, and chromosomal mapping. Genomics 41:360–369

Kubota R, Noda S, Wang Y, Minoshima S, Asakawa S, Kudoh J, Mashima Y, Oguchi Y and Shimizu N (1997) A nobel Myosin-like protein (Myocilin) expressed in the connecting cilium of the photoreceptor: molecular cloning, tissue expression and chromosomal mapping. Genomics 41:360–369

Leske MC (1983) The epidemiology of open-angle glaucoma: a review. Am J Epidemiol 118:166–191

Lichter PR, Richards JE, Boehnke M, Ostman M, Camonon BD, Strigham HM, Downs CA, Lewis SB, Boyd BF (1997) Juvenile glaucoma linked to CLC1A gene on chromosome 1q in a Panamanian family. Amer J Ophthalmol 123:413–416

Lutjen-Drecoll E, May CA, Polansky JR, Johnson DH, Bloemendal H & Nguyen TD (1998) Localization of the stress proteins aB-crystallin and trabecular meshwork inducible glucocorticoid response in normal and glaucomatous trabecular meshwork. Invest Ophth Vis Sci 39:517–525

Mears AJ, Mirzayans R, Gould DB, Pearch WG, Walter MA (1996) Autosomal dominant iridogonidys-genesis anomaly maps to 6p25. Am J Hum Genet 59:1321–1327

Morissette J, Falardeau P, Dubois S, Bergeron J, Vonck P, Cote G, Anctil JL, Amyot M, Blondeau P, Bergeron E, Raymond V (1997) A common gene for development and familial open-angle glaucomas confined on chromosome 6p25 ASHG, 61(4). Abs# 1670

Mondette J, Falardeau P, Dubois S, Bergeron J, Vanck P, Cote G, Anctil JL, Amyot M, Blondeau P, Bergeron E et al. (1997) A common gene for development and familial open-angle glaucomas confined on chromone 6p25. Am J Hum Genet 61:A286

Nishimura DY, Swiderski RE, Alward WLM, Searby CC, Patil SR, Bennet SR, Kanis AB, Gastier JM, Stone EM, Sheffield VC (1998) The forkhead transcription factor gene FKHL7 is responsible for glaucoma phenotypes which map to 6p25. Nature Genetics 19:140–147

Nguyen TD, Huang W, Bloom E, Polansky JR (1993) Glucocorticoid (GC) effects on HTM cells: molecular biology approaches. In: Lutjen-Drecoll E (ed) Basis aspects of glaucoma research III. Shattauer, Stuttgart, New York, 331–343

Nguyen TD, Chen P, Chen H, Huang WD, Polansky JR (1999) Molecular biology and genetic studies of the major extracellular GC-induced glycoprotein cloned from HTM cells (abstract). Invest Ophthalmol Vis Sci (in press)

Nguyen TD, Chen P, Huang WD, Chen H, Johnson J, Polansky JR (1998) Gene structure and properties of TIGR, an olfactomedin-retaled glycoprotein cloned from glucocorticoid-induced trabecular meshwork cells. J. Biol. Chem. 273:6348–6350

Nguyen TD, Chen P, Chen H, Hetherington J, Lieberman M, Polansky JR (1997) Molecular biology and genetic studies of the putative gene, TIGR, for ourflow resistance in glaucoma, HGM '97 a47 (suppl)

Ortego J, Escribano J, Coca-Prados M (1997) Cloning and characterization of substrated cDNAs from a human ciliary body library encoding TIGR, a protein involved in juvenile open-angle glaucoma with homology to myosin and olfactomedin FEBS Lett 413:349–353

Phillips JC, DelBona EA, Haines JL, Praela AM, Cohen JS, Greff IJ, Wiggs JL (1996) A second locus for Rieger syndrome maps to chromosome 13q14. Am J Hum Genet 59:613–619

Sarfarazi M, Akersu AN, Hossain A, Turacli ME, Aktan SG, Barsoum-Homsy M, Chevrette L, Sayli BS (1995) Assignment of a locus (GLC3A) for primary congenital glaucoma (Buphthalmos) to 2p21 and evidence for genetic heterogeneity. Genomics 30:171–177

Sarfarazi M, Akarsu N, Hossain A, Turacli ME, Aktan SG, Barsoum-Homsy M et al. (1995) Assignment of a locus (GLC3A) for primary congenital glaucoma (buphthalmos) to 2p21 and evidence for genetic heterogeneity. Genomics 30:171–177

Sarfarazi M, Chico A, Stoilova D, Brice G, Desoit ??, Trifan OC, Poinoosawmy D, Crick KP (1998) GLC1E for adult onset chronic open angle glaucoma to the 10p15-14 region. Amer J Hum Gen 62:41–52

Sheffield VC, Stone EM, Alward WLM, Drack AV, Johnson AT, Streb LM, Nichols BE (1993) Genetic linkage of familial open angle glaucoma to chromosome 1q21-q31. Nature Genet 4:47–50

Sheffield VC, Stone EM, Alward WLM, Drack AV, Johnson AT, Streb LM, Nichols BE (1993) Genetic linkage of familial open angle glaucoma to chromosome 1q21-q31. Nature Genetics 4:47

Stoilova D, Child A, Trifan OC, Bradway D, Crick RP, Sarfarazi M (1996) A Search for chromosomal location of the Adult-Onset open angle glaucoma (GLC1B). Invest Ophthalmol Vis Sci 37(3), ARVO Abs#2073

Stoilova D, Child A, Trifan OC, Crick RP, Coakes RJ, Sarfarazi M (1996) Localization of a locus (GLC1B) for adult-onset primary open-angle glaucoma to the 2cen-q13 region. Genomics 36:142–150

Stone EM, Fingert JH, Alward WLW, Nguyen TD, Polanski JR, Sunden SLF, Nishimura D, Clark AF, Nystuen A, Nichols BE, Mackey DA, Rich R, Kalenak JW, Craven ER, Sheffield VC (1997) Identification of a gene that causes primary open angle glaucoma. Science 275:668–670

Stone EM, Fingert JH, Alward WLM, Nguyen TD, Polansky JR, Sunden SLF, Nishimura D, Clark AR, Nystuen A, Nichols BE, Mackey DA, Ritch R, Kalenak JW, Craven ER, Sheffield VC (1997) Identification of a gene that causes primary open angle glaucoma. Science 275:668–670

Suzuki Y, Shirato A, Tanaguchi F, O'Hara K, Nishimaki H, Ohta S (1987) Mutations in TIGR gene in familial open angle glaucoma in Japan. Amer J Hum Gen (1987) 61:1202–1204

Stoilov I, Akarsu AN, Sarfarazi M (1997) Identification of three different truncating mutations in cytochrome P4501B1 (CYP1B1) as the principal cause of primary congenital glaucoma (Buphthalmos) in families linked to the GLC3A locus on chromosome 2p21. Hum Mol Genet 6:641–647

Vincent R (1997) Molecular genetics of the glaucomas; mapping the first five "GLC" loci. Am J Hum Genet 60:272–277

Scheman JS, CG Mattox (1997) A gene responsible for the pigmentary dispersion syndrome maps to chromosome 7q35–36. Invest Ophthalmol Vis Sci 38(4), ARVO Abs#2678

Wirtz MK, Samples JR, Kramers PL, Rust K, Topinka JR (1997) Mapping a gene for adult-onset primary open angle glaucoma to chromosome 3q. Am J Hum Genet 60:296–304

Wirtz MD, Samples JR, Kramer PL, Rust K, Yount J, Ascott TS, Koler RD, Cisler J, Jahed A, Gorlin RJ, Godfrey M (1996) Weill-Marchesani syndrome – possible linkage of the autosomal dominant form to 15q21.1. Am J Med Gen 65:68–75

Yokoe H, Anholt RR (1993) Molecular cloning of olfactomedin, an extracellular matrix protein specific to olfactory neuroepithelium. Proc Natl Acad Sci USA, 90:4655–4659

CHAPTER 9

Molecular Genetics of Glaucoma*

H.-J. Garchon

Introduction

The past 2 years have seen considerable progress in the characterization of genetic factors that cause various forms of glaucoma [1–14]. These findings open the path to a better understanding of glaucoma pathogenesis. They also raise considerable hope for a better management of glaucoma patients. This is essentially because glaucomatous lesions of the optic nerve become rapidly irreversible, whereas they can be prevented by existing effective treatments. Prognosis therefore largely depends on an early diagnosis. Ideally, glaucoma patients should be identified at the preclinical stage, when optic nerve fibers are still minimally damaged. Genotyping provides an opportunity to characterize the constitutive predisposition of individuals to develop glaucoma, long before the onset of clinical disease. How this power will modify the management of glaucoma patients is still unclear. The aim of this review is to summarize these recent advances of glaucoma genetics, to describe their possible impact on clinical practice and to discuss our current approach in the search for additional genes that might predispose to glaucoma.

Mapped and Identified Glaucoma Genes: Recent findings

Several loci have been either identified molecularly or localized in the human genome. Besides the fact that the localization of a gene is an intermediate step toward its identification, there is a major qualitative difference between these two situations for a disease locus. For the first category of disease loci, the DNA sequence of the gene and its disease-causing alterations, also called mutations, could be defined. As a direct consequence of the knowledge of the gene sequence, its involvement can be assessed in isolated individuals. Regarding the second category of genes, the sole knowledge of their position in the genome, which is imprecise at the scale of the physical map of genes, is insufficient for testing their implication in disease occurrence in isolated patients. Comparison with affected relatives is necessary. In other words, a family study is required. This kind of analysis is called linkage analysis because it aims at determining whether markers closely linked to the suspected locus (whose exact position in the genome is unknown) actually cosegregate with the disease in the

* I am most indebted to my coworkers at INSERM Unit 25 and to Pr Alain Béchetoille, Dr. Françoise Valtot and Dr. Jean-Claude Dascotte for their fruitful collaboration.

Table 1. Identified glaucoma genes

Locus	Gene	Chromosomal location	Phenotype
GLC1A	TIGR/MYOC	1q24	Juvenile and adult-onset glaucoma
GLC3A	CYP1B1	2p21	Primitive congenital glaucoma
RIEG1,IH	PITX2	4q25	Rieger syndrome, iris hypoplasia
	FKHL7	6p25	Syndromic and primitive congenital glaucoma
NPS	LMX1B	9q34	Nail-patella syndrome and glaucoma

family, following a simple pattern of mendelian inheritance. Linkage analysis provides only a likelihood of the involvement of the locus in disease occurrence. A measure of this likelihood on a logarithmic scale, called lod-score (logarithm of the odds), is often given. A lod-score greater than 3 (odds are 1000 to 1 in favor of linkage, given the data) is considered as proof of linkage of the locus with the disease in the family. A lod-score below -2 makes unlikely a role for the genetic region under consideration. Between these two values, no conclusion can be reached. The power of this analysis depends on several parameters but critically on the number of affected persons available for testing. As a direct consequence, it is often difficult to draw firm conclusions from the study of small size families.

Tables 1 and 2 show the current lists of identified and mapped glaucoma genes respectively. Four of the identified genes (CYP1B1, PITX2, FKHL7, and LMXB1) determine rare forms of glaucoma associated with congenital and/or developmental anomalies [3-6]. In contrast, five of the mapped loci have been associated with adult-onset glaucoma [7-10]. Most of these localizations, however, rely on linkage analysis of few families, or even of one family. Their significance strongly depends on their future replication in independent studies. As explained above, the role of these loci currently cannot be assessed in patients with few affected relatives, not to mention in sporadic patients.

Taken together, these data confirm that the genetic control of glaucomatous disease is largely heterogeneous. It also appears that the genetic control of the commonest form of glaucoma, chronic open-angle glaucoma, remains to be characterized. These genetic findings are therefore of major significance for a better understanding of the pathogenesis of glaucoma but their relevance to the usual ophthalmology practice is still limited. A special case, however, should be made for the GLC1A gene. As

Table 2. Mapped glaucoma genes

Locus	Chromosomal localization	Phenotype
GLC1B	2qcen-q13	Adult-onset glaucoma
GLC1C	3q21	Adult-onset glaucoma
GLC1D	8q23	Adult-onset glaucoma
GLC1E	10q15	Adult-onset glaucoma
GLC1F	7q35	Adult-onset glaucoma
PDS1	7q36	Pigment dispersion
PDS2	18q11-q12	Pigment dispersion
GLC3B	1p36	Primitive congenital glaucoma
RIEG2	13q14	Rieger syndrome
IRID1	6p25	Iridogoniodysgenesis

discussed below, this gene is currently the only one to be implicated in a significant, even though minor, proportion of glaucomatous patients [1,15]:2 %-3 %, representing at least 100,000 patients in the European Union. In addition, the typing of GLC1A has a prognostic value: a comparative study of GLC1A-linked and GLC1A-unlinked families showed that the risk for the relatives of probands to develop glaucoma, as opposed to isolated ocular hypertension, and the risk to develop severe glaucomatous optic neuropathy were highly increased in GLC1A-linked families [16]. The GLC1A gene thus provides a unique ground for experimenting with the screening of mutation carriers at an already large scale and with genetic counseling of the healthy carriers who are at high risk of developing glaucoma.

The GLC1A/TIGR/Myocilin Gene

The GLC1A locus on chromosome 1q23-q24 was initially linked to a form of familial, juvenile-onset, open-angle glaucoma transmitted by an autosomal mode with high penetrance [17]. Subsequently, families with both juvenile- and adult-onset glaucoma were linked to this locus, which suggested that its expressivity was variable [18,19]. Molecular cloning of the GLC1A gene was achieved by combining positional cloning and candidate gene testing [1,2,20,21]. Most interestingly, this process disclosed a gene that had been independently discovered by Jon Polansky on the basis of its inducibility in cultured human trabecular meshwork cells upon glucocorticoid exposure, taken as a model of the steroid-induced glaucoma [22]. This gene, thus called TIGR (trabecular meshwork induced glucocorticoid response) or also myocilin, is of average size ($\sim$ 15 kilobases) and has a fairly simple genomic organization comprising three exons (Fig. 1). It encodes a 55 kDa protein (504 amino acids) whose function and subcellular localization are still a matter of investigation.

The protein sequence of TIGR shows a typical leucine zipper motif, which is usually found in dimerizing proteins, a N-terminal segment related to some myosins (25 % identical residues over 108 residues), hence the name of myocilin, and a C-terminal portion homologous (40 % identity) to olfactomedin, an abundant glycoprotein of the extracellular matrix of the olfactory neuroepithelium [23]. This latter

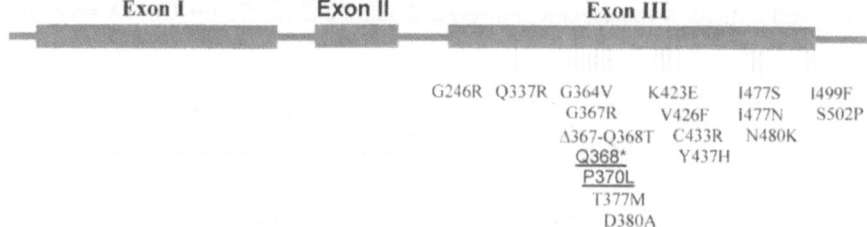

Fig. 1. Genomic organization of the TIGR gene and localization of the pathogenic mutations in the third exon. Mutations (under the exon III box) are designated by the position of the mutated amino acid, preceded by the wild-type amino acid and followed by the substituted amino acid. The one-letter amino acid coding convention has been used (A: alanine: C: cysteine; D: aspartic acid; E: glutamic acid; F: phenylalanine; G: glycine; H: histidine; I: isoleucine; K: lysine; L: leucine; M: methionine; N: asparagine; P: proline; Q: glutamine; R: arginine; S: serine; T: threonine; V: valine; Y: tyrosine; *: stop codon). The two underscored mutations are discussed in greater detail in the text.

region of 261 amino acids is exactly encoded by the third exon and is well conserved throughout evolution, from man to frog and worm. Remarkably, to this date, this olfactomedin-homology domain is the site of the 18 mutations proven to cause glaucoma (Fig. 1). It must therefore be critical for a normal function of the TIGR protein. Several additional but rare polymorphisms (coding or noncoding) have been described throughout the gene sequence [15]. Some of them have been suspected to cause glaucoma. However, as they have been identified in only one sporadic patient, even if they are absent from the control group, their unique observation cannot be statistically significant and their involvement in glaucoma pathogenesis remains to be firmly proven.

Most of the TIGR mutations causing glaucoma have been characterized in a single family, often of large size, or at most in a small number of families originating from a restricted geographical area. The two notable exceptions are the P370L (proline to leucine) and the Q368* (glutamine to stop) mutations. The first mutation, P370L, was identified in several pedigrees from France, Quebec, Japan, Germany and USA [2,24–27]. The two French pedigrees harboring this mutation were unrelated as shown by haplotype analysis. In the French Canadian family, the P370L mutation was shown to appear in one of the ancestors. It is also unlikely that the Japanese pedigree is related to the Caucasian families. This mutation therefore repeatedly occurred de novo.

The second mutation was found both in families and in sporadic patients, usually with middle-age or even late onset of disease. The penetrance of this mutation seems to be lower than that of other TIGR mutations as several healthy carriers were identified among patients' relatives. It has even been suggested that it was a neutral, non-pathogenic, polymorphism corresponding to a null allele (the Q368* mutation removes the 137 C-terminal amino acids of the TIGR protein). However, this mutation is by far the most recurrent of the TIGR mutations and account for approximately 2%-3% of all glaucoma cases whereas it remains very rare among several groups of unrelated healthy controls [1,2,15,25]. In addition and quite unexpectedly, French patients carrying this Q368* mutation appeared to have inherited their mutation from a unique ancestor (our unpublished data). Taken together, these data argue that this mutation is indeed pathogenic.

Phenotypic Variability

The phenotype associated with TIGR mutations typically comprises a normally open iridocorneal angle and an elevated intraocular pressure (IOP) that is rapidly associated with a severe alteration of the visual field if no treatment is undertaken. No other ocular or extraocular anomaly has been reported, which is important given that TIGR message expression is not restricted to the trabecular meshwork and the ciliary body [2,21]. This phenotype does not vary much qualitatively. In contrast, there is considerable quantitative variation regarding the age of diagnosis, the severity and the rate of progression of the disease. Thus, the P370L mutation consistently determines a juvenile onset of disease (median age in French patients, 11 years) with high IOP resisting to medical treatment and leading rapidly to severe alteration of the visual field in the absence of filtration surgery. With other mutations, however, the severity of the phenotype is more variable. Figure 2 shows the histograms of the distributions

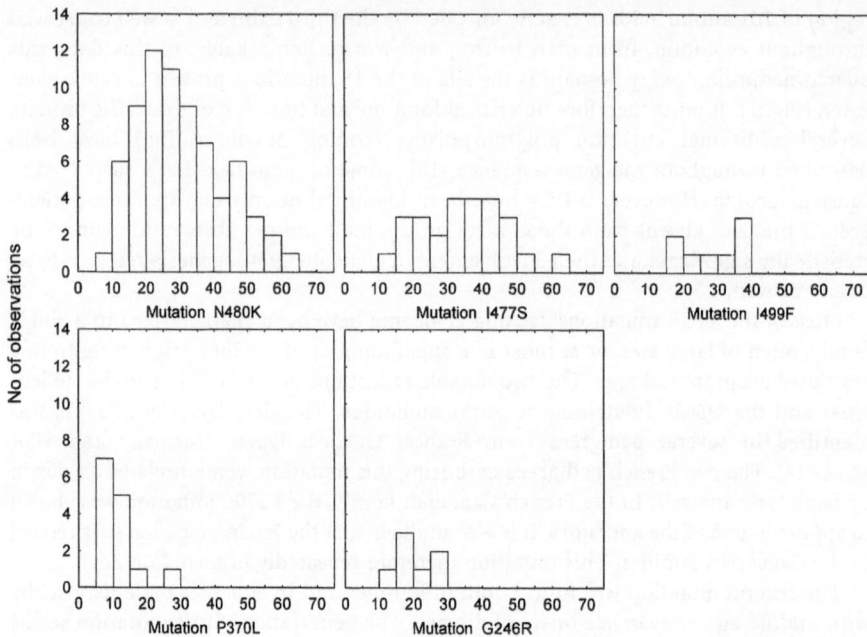

Fig. 2. Histograms of the distributions of ages at diagnosis for 5 mutations in French glaucoma families. The distribution were significantly different ($P < 1 \times 10^{-4}$, Kruskal-Wallis ANOVA test)

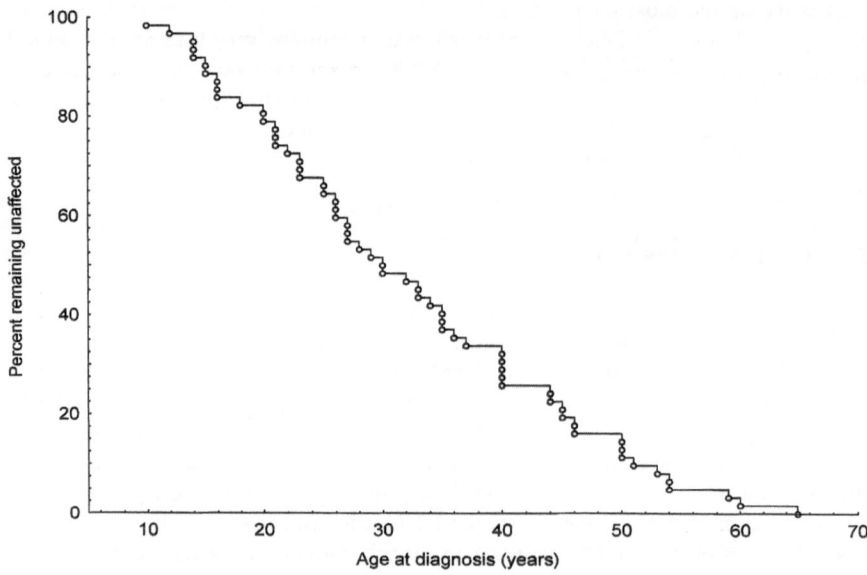

Fig. 3. Age-dependent penetrance of glaucoma in 86 persons carrying the N480K mutation inherited from the same ancestor. The proportion of remaining unaffected subjects has been plotted against the age at diagnosis

of the ages at diagnosis of glaucoma associated with five mutations in French families. Comparison using a nonparametric test indicated that these distributions for each mutation differed at a highly significant level ($P<10^{-4}$). Figure 3 shows the cumulated distribution of ages at diagnosis among 86 persons, belonging to six different pedigrees but all carrying the same mutation, N480K, that was in fact inherited from a unique ancestor [28]. The youngest patient was 10 years when his glaucoma was diagnosed. Conversely, a 46 year-old woman carrying the mutation was unaffected: her IOP curve was below 13 mm Hg and her visual field was repeatedly normal. This woman was the oldest of the 14 unaffected mutation carriers thus detected.

These observations indicate that the spectrum of phenotypes associated with TIGR mutations varies broadly from juvenile-onset glaucoma to nonpenetrance in adults. The nature of the mutation is just one of the factors of this variation. For a given mutation, the expressivity can also vary to a considerable extent. The factors that modify this expressivity are largely unknown. Still their knowledge would have important practical consequences. It would help anticipate the onset of disease and adjust the follow-up of at-risk mutation carriers.

A Search for Modifiers of TIGR Expressivity

Little is known about the factors that modify the expressivity of a gene. In principle, these factors can be genetic or environmental or both. Epidemiological surveys provided no strong evidence for specific environmental factors influencing glaucoma susceptibility, besides glucocorticoid exposure. In contrast, the search for modifying genetic factors appears as an open and very promising field of investigation, still in its infancy. A modifier locus can be defined as one that leads to qualitative or quantitative differences in the phenotype, including nonpenetrance of the major disease gene.

Ironically enough, the effect of a modifier locus in humans was discussed for the first time for the nail patella syndrome (NPS) by Renwick in 1957 (Table 3) [29]. This author observed a broad variability of the characteristic anomalies (of nails, knees and others) of this disease in several NPS pedigrees. There was a better correlation of disease severity between siblings than between parents and their children. Renwick's hypothesis was that the affected parent transmitted the main pathogenic allele of the disease gene to his/her children whereas a modifier allele at the same locus or close to it controlled the severity of disease and was received from the other normal parent. A similar observation was reported for the RP11 locus for retinitis pigmentosa [30]. These two diseases provide examples of allelic modifiers in trans of the major gene.

Table 3. Modifier loci

Position	Inheritance	Consequences	Examples
Allelic in trans	Dominant	Correlation among siblings	Nail-patella syndrome; Retinitis pigmentosa (RP11)
Pseudoallelic in cis	Dominant or recessive	Variation between families	R117H mutation in cystic fibrosis
Non allelic	Dominant	Variation between and within families	See Table 4

Table 4. Nonallelic modifiers in human diseases and traits

Disease or trait	Chromosomal location or gene	Strategy of identification
Familial hypertrophic cardiomyopathy	Angiotensin convertase	Candidate gene
Familial adenomatous polyposis	chr1p35-p36	Equivalent region suggested by a mouse model
Cystic fibrosis	chr19q13	Same as above
Persistence of fetal haemoglobin	chr6q23	Genome scan

An example of a pseudoallelic modifier in cis of the gene is found in the study of the R117H mutation of the CFTR gene causing fibrosis [31]. Depending on the haplotype on which this mutation occurs, the phenotype is more or less severe or even normal. Finally, the α^{LELY} polymorphism of the α-spectrin gene provides an example of a more complex allelic modifier of α-spectrin mutations that cause hereditary ellipsocytosis [32]. The LELY (low expression lyon) variant is frequent (25 %) and misses the nucleation site of α-spectrin that is encoded by exon 46 of the gene. Consequently, when the variant is in cis of the main disease-causing mutation, the mutated chain is less recruited and the disease is mild. Conversely, when the LELY variant is in trans, the normal chain is less recruited and the disease is severe.

Allelic or pseudoallelic modifiers are the easiest to assess. However, the most frequent situation is probably that of nonallelic modifiers. There are now several examples of modifier loci in mouse models. In humans, one can hope to identify such loci by testing candidate genes [33], by looking at genetic regions homologous to murine genetic regions shown to contain a modifier locus [34], or by scanning the genome systematically using dense maps of genetic markers [35], a formidable task despite continuing improvement of genotyping techniques. Table 4 summarizes these findings.

The observation of an important variation of disease severity within glaucoma families rules out a role for a pseudoallelic (in cis) modifier of TIGR mutation expressivity. From a preliminary analysis, there is no correlation between siblings that might reflect the existence of an allelic modifier in trans (our unpublished data). Putative modifier loci are therefore likely to be non-allelic to TIGR. The availability of large families grouping patients all carrying the same mutation inherited from a unique ancestor provides a valuable resource for an efficient search of such modifiers, following the examples just discussed. Finally, these modifiers could be implicated in other (unlinked to TIGR) forms of glaucoma.

TIGR Mutation Screening? Which Target Population?

The existence of effective treatments, provided that they are undertaken early enough, largely justifies the screening of TIGR mutation carriers. Their absolute frequency, over 100,000 persons in Western Europe, raises the question of the target population to be screened. Three levels of screening, each representing a target population of increasing size, can be viewed. The first level is that of the families of patients who carry an already identified TIGR mutation. In this simple situation of a known mutation, current techniques allow screening of numerous individuals efficiently. This level of screening focuses on a small population and is the most productive: the ratio of the number of newly identified carriers over the number of screened individuals is the highest. But eventually, few carriers are detected. Independently of the genetic screening, in our experience, the thorough investigation of pedigrees allowed recognition of already advanced glaucoma in patients unaware of their disease.

At the other end of the spectrum, the most extensive screening is that of the general population. Assuming a 1 % frequency for glaucoma patients in Western countries and a 2 % frequency for TIGR mutation carriers, one can expect to detect mutation carriers with a frequency of 2×10^{-4}. The cost of DNA collecting and genotyping on a very large scale may exceed by far the benefit resulting from disease prevention in healthy carriers. The throughput of current typing techniques is also too low to make feasible such an untargeted screening.

We therefore propose to investigate an intermediate level of screening corresponding to the population of glaucoma patients with first-degree relatives who would benefit from being identified as mutation carriers. Furthermore, as the Q368* mutation accounts for the vast majority of mutations, the screening could be limited to this mutation in a first step. In countries such as Germany or France, one can reasonably expect to identify 10,000–20,000 carriers of this mutation. The detailed characterization and the medical management of these persons and of their close relatives would already provide an invaluable experience for dealing with more complex gene screens when mutation detection techniques improve and when additional glaucoma genes are discovered.

References

1. Stone EM et al. (1997) Science 275:668–670
2. Adam MF et al. (1997) Hum Mol Genet 6:2091–2097
3. Stoilov I et al. (1997) Hum Mol Genet 6:641–647
4. Semina EV et al. (1996) Nature Genet 14:392–399
5. Bishimura DY et al. (1998) Nature Genet 19:140–147
6. Vollrath E et al. (1998) Hum Mol Genet 7:1091–1098
7. Stoilova D et al. (1996) Genomics 38:142–150
8. Wirtz MK et al. (1997) Am J Hum Genet 60:296–304
9. Trifan OC et al. (1998) Am J Ophthalmol 126:17–28
10. Sarfarazi M et al. (1998) Am J Hum Genet 62:641–652
11. Anderson J et al. (1997) Arch Ophthalmol 115:384–388
12. Akarsu AN et al. (1996) Hum Mol Genet 5:1199–1203
13. Phillips JC et al. (1996) Am J Hum Genet 59:613–619
14. Mears AJ et al. (1996) Am J Hum Genet 59:1321–1327
15. Alward WLM et al. (1998) New Engl J Med 338:1022–1027
16. Brézin AP et al. (1997) J Med Genet 34:546–552
17. Sheffield VC et al. (1993) Nature Genet 4:47–50
18. Morissette J et al. (1995) Am J Hum Genet 56:1431–1442
19. Meyer A et al. (1996) Hum Genet 98:567–571
20. Belmouden A et al. (1997) Genomics 39:348–358
21. Ortego J et al. (1997) FEBS lett. 413:349–353
22. Polansky J et al. (1997) Ophthalmologica 211:126–139
23. Yokoe H et al. (1993) Proc. Natl Acad Sci USA 90:4655–4659
24. Suzuki Y et al. (1997) Am J Hum Genet 61:1202–1204
25. Wiggs JL et al. (1998) Am J Hum Genet 63:1549–1552

26. Michels-Rautenstrauss KG et al. (1998) Hum Genet 102:103–106
27. Child A et al. (1998) J Med Genet, in press
28. Brézin AP et al. (1998) Am J Med Genet 76:438–445
29. Renwick JH (1957) Ann Hum Genet 21:159–169
30. McGee TL et al. (1997) Am J Hum Genet 61:1059–1066
31. Kiesewetter S et al. (1993) Nature Genet 5:274–278
32. Maillet P et al. (1996) Hum Mutat 8:97–107
33. Tesson F et al. (1997) J Mol Cell Cardiol 29:831–828
34. Dobbie Z et al. (1997) Hum Genet 99:653–657
35. Craig JE et al. (1996) Nature Genet 12:58–64

The TIGR Gene: Prospects for Understanding Glaucoma Mechanisms and Environmental/Genetic Interactions

J. R. Polansky, D. J. Fauss and C. C. Zimmerman

This paper focuses on conceptual and practical implications of the trabecular meshwork inducible glucocorticoid response (TIGR) gene in glaucoma research. We have recently reviewed advances that have led to the identification and cloning of a number of glaucoma genes, including TIGR (Polansky and Nguyen 1998). Here we extend the discussion of the TIGR gene research efforts into pathogenic mechanisms, including potential effects on protein procession pathways and environmental/genetic interactions. The current phase of research involves efforts by several major groups. Reports from the different approaches taken will require time to sort out. While interpretations of proposed findings must take place in a heuristic environment of give-and-take between the groups involved, this caution should not unduly limit our conceptual considerations. Since evaluations are moving at a rapid pace, with many reports concerning new discoveries relating to the TIGR gene and the expression of proposed defects anticipated in the literature this coming year, it is also useful to appreciate prior findings and their proposed implications to aid in this process.

The data presently available suggest that TIGR gene expression has a role steroid glaucoma, chronic open-angle glaucoma (COAG), and juvenile glaucoma - with potential effects that may also relate to exfoliation glaucoma and certain other secondary glaucomas. In this regard, it is important to emphasize that this gene was originally cloned and proposed to be a gene for primary open-angle glaucoma (POAG) as well as steroid glaucoma based on cell type-specific responses of our human trabecular meshwork (HTM) cell models for these entities. This has crucial implications for interpretation of the data and for providing a framework for follow-up research. It also suggests that further studies of the HTM cell models for glucocorticoid (e.g. dexamethasone) and oxidative (or phagocytic) 'stress' responses may uncover other important genes that act coordinately with TIGR in the glaucomatous process - as well as genes that may counteract the unwanted processes.

Originally, a key to the discovery of the TIGR gene was the observation of unusually large, progressive protein/glycoprotein inductions in HTM cells and meshwork tissues that matched the distinctive time course and dose-response defined for clinical (IOP) effects of corticosteroids. Experimental studies of HTM cultures (compared with a variety of other cell types) demonstrated the distinctive response of the cellular and extracellular 55 kDa gene products that led to the cloning of the TIGR gene. The demonstration that TIGR mRNA and protein expression were regulated by oxidative injury, phorbol ester treatment, and growth factor deprivation as well as corticosteroids provided additional information. The data led us to propose a relationship of the gene to other open-angle glaucomas (OAGs) in addition to steroid glaucoma.

The fact that the gene was induced by both glucocorticoids and oxidative (and other stress) treatments, suggested to us that TIGR gene expression could be of general relevance to pathogenic mechanisms in the different forms of glaucoma (Polansky et al. 1997).

At first our attention was mainly directed toward 'environmental' influences (including phagocytic, other unknown stress factors and other hormones in addition to glucocorticoids) rather than purely genetic ones. The current excitement over TIGR gene dects should not minimize the evidence suggesting a crucial influence on TIGR gene expression of environmental factors for understanding glaucoma pathogenic mechanisms. These concepts are outlined in Fig. 1 and 2, from our earlier work.

We had also predicted a role for genetic alterations in the TIGR gene, and this found support in evaluations of an extensive adult glaucoma pedigree showing restriction fragment length polymorphism changes using labeled TIGR cDNA that

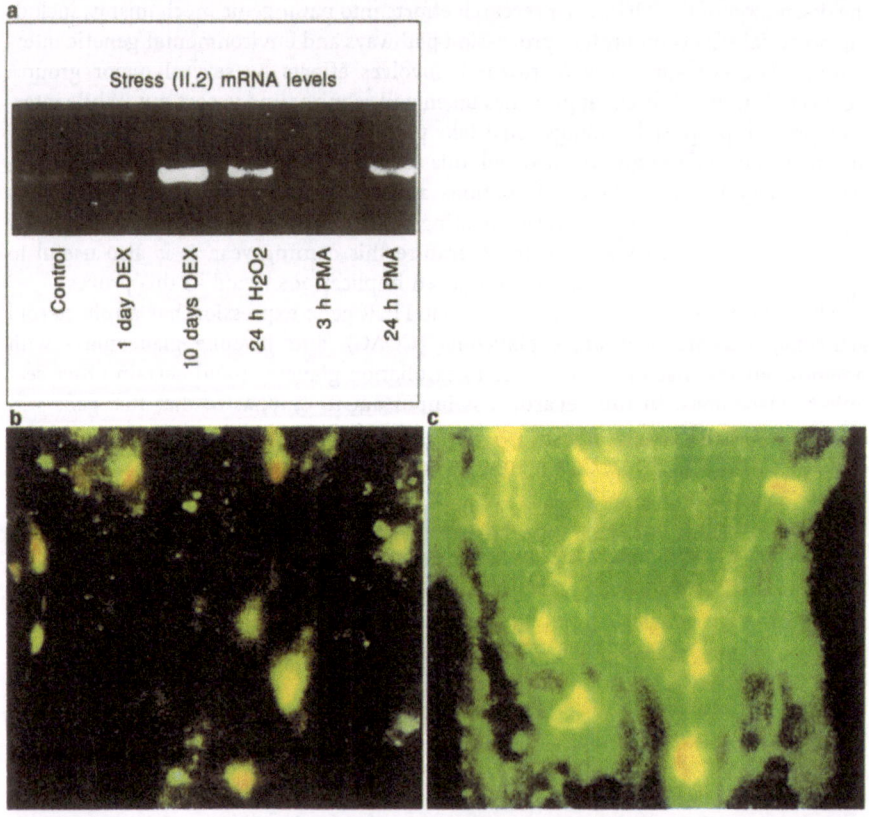

Fig. 1a-c. Modulation of TIGR expression by various inducers. **a** Example of PCR detecting changes in II.2 clone, 'TIGR'. **b, c** Effect of DEX induction of TIGR immunofluoresence after anterior segment tissues were maintained in perfusion culture for 20 days with (**c**) and without (**b**) DEX (550 nM). Frozen sections of unfixed tissue were then cut and treated with the TIGR antibody and visualized with an FITC secondary antibody (green). Nuclei were stained with propidium iodide and appear yellow-orange

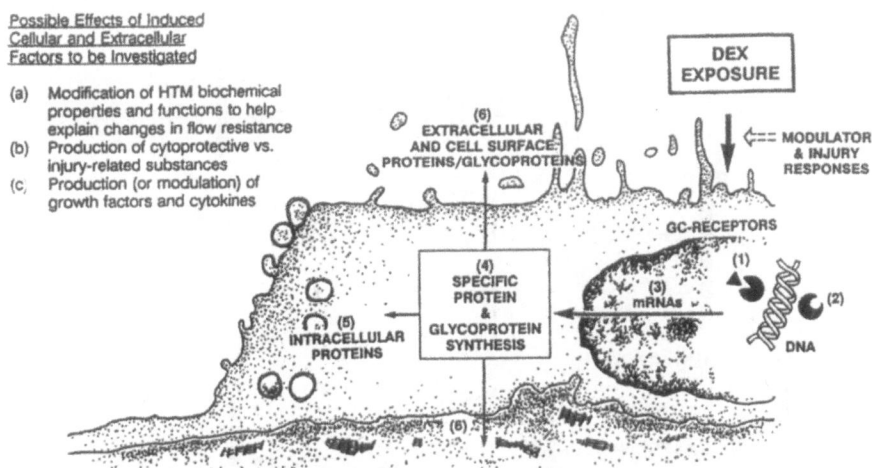

Possible Effects of Induced
Cellular and Extracellular
Factors to be Investigated

(a) Modification of HTM biochemical
     properties and functions to help
     explain changes in flow resistance
(b) Production of cytoprotective vs.
     injury-related substances
(c) Production (or modulation) of
     growth factors and cytokines

Fig. 2. HTM cell model for steroid and oxidative effects. From Polansky and Nguyen (1998)

associated with glaucoma (Nguyen et al., unpublishing findings). However, is was not until we found that the location of the TIGR gene was within the inclusion interval of the GLC1A locus for juvenile glaucoma families that the importance of parallel research being conducted using classic genetic approaches to juvenile glaucoma families was realized. The GLC1A locus for juvenile glaucoma has been narrowed from its original descriptions by classical genetic approaches by Sheffield, Stone, Alward, as well as Lichter and Richards, and Garchon; the studies also included the proposal by Raymond that the juvenile glaucoma gene could also be the same as one for COAG (see our 1998 review for references). The report that defined individual coding region defects in TIGR with random adult cases as well as many juvenile cases, by the Iowa group (Stone et al. 1997), had a substantial impact on the field. It led to the description of additional defects. This finding stimulated many different evaluations of the TIGR gene and its products and interest in potential genetic screening applications.

The initial proposals for genetic testing for TIGR gene defects were based on the Gln368Stop, a coding region defect associated primarily with adult OAG cases discovered by Stone et al. (1997). These may be justifiably questioned. However, the additional coding region defects being described, along with promoter sequence variants of potential functional significance, has added to the interest in TIGR gene studies for glaucoma diagnosis/prognosis. Since our review of the literature in 1998, the finding of several follow-up studies and findings from different groups have verified clinical implications of different disease-associated TIGR gene defects. Clinical correlates for specific TIGR coding region defects (e.g. the Tyr437His and the Pro370Leu mutations associated with severe, early-onset OAG; the Gln368stop with milder, adult-onset OAG) have found support in different populations and have provided a spectrum of ages to considered (and the possibility of 'protective' and/or 'susceptibility' genes that influence disease expression). The ability to apply this approach to a particular patient, and to provide information to aid in clinical decisions will improve as additional studies are performed sorting through disease mechanisms for the different defects.

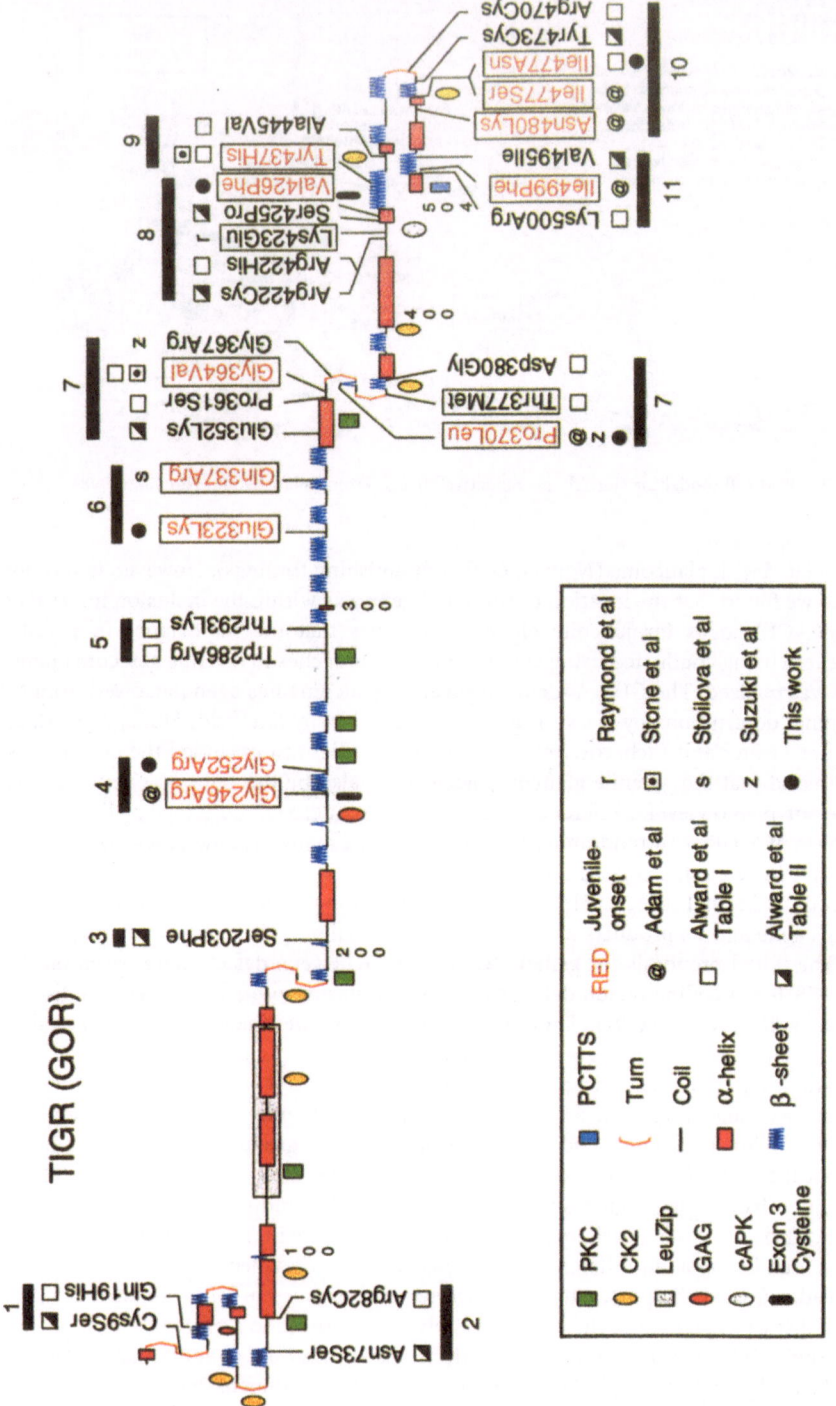

A relatively recent paper by Rozsa et al. (1998) demonstrated the clustering of coding region defects to restricted parts of TIGR (Fig. 3), especially in the gene's region of olfactomedin homology. The results have provided specific leads to evaluate functional changes in the abnormal TIGR proteins being generated. Olfactomedins (rather than myosin) show the greatest homology to TIGR (Nguyen et al. 1998). This is a family of proteins known to include other extracellular proteins/glycoproteins. Separate findings emphasize the importance of protein processing pathways, including different cellular and extracellular glycosylated forms. Recent findings in our laboratories show that certain stimuli better are stimulators of the glycosylated extracellular proteins compared with the cellular forms. Data suggest that glucococorticoids also stimulate some potentially important cellular forms of TIGR in addition to extracellular components (B. Yue, personal communication). An understanding of both of these 'normal' TIGR pathways could be relevant to understanding perturbations that could occur with the proposed TIGR mutations.

Protein processing studies using transfection with a biological marker such as green fluorescent protein (GFP) can be used to visualize TIGR pathways and protein targeting in HTM cells and other cell types. McKay and Stamer (personal communication) are actively investigating specific sites in the TIGR molecule for such targeting using this approach, which must still be confirmed by independent methods. An experiment we performed using a TIGR-GFP construct suggests the importance of the olfactomedin domain in targeting of the molecule, as presented in Fig. 4. As shown, deletion of the olfactomedin homology domain from TIGR produces an apparent massive increase in TIGR staining, potentially indicating defective targeting. More detailed HTM cell and cell-free evaluations of normal vs abnormal pathways for TIGR gene expression and protein biosynthesis offer exciting prospects to understand pathogenic mechanisms involved with specific TIGR gene defects at a basic biochemical and cellular level. We are particularly interested in evaluating the potential generation of abnormal forms of secretory and membrane proteins during processing, especially during the steps required for translocation or insertion into the endoplasmic reticulum (ER). These experiments are being done in collaborative studies with V. Lingappa's laboratory at our institution who has found ER processing defects relating to other clinical conditions. This approach has been found important in other genetic diseases and is providing clues to understanding the role of apo-B in artherosclerosis and defects in prion proteins in relation to neurodegenerative disorders. An application of similar approaches to evaluating important TIGR gene coding region defects is a promising area of current investigation. Interestingly, the region of TIGR's olfactomedin homology appears to correspond to a substantial 'pause' in protein processing (Lingappa, Zimmerman, and Polansky, unpublished observations) and to defects early on in this domain associated with glaucoma. Of importance is that these defects were not readily explained as affecting functional motifs identified by Rozsa et al. (1998). The possibility that a utilization of ER sorting functions which serve to eliminate abnormal forms of TIGR might activate stress pathways directly or indirectly needs to be considered, in addition to direct effects on the structural-functional properties of the TIGR protein/glycoprotein forms generated.

◄──

Fig. 3. TIGR gene structural analysis showing some of the coding region defects reported. (From Rozsa et al. 1998)

Fig. 4. TIGR constucts trasfected into confluente HTM cultures: affect of deletion of the olfactomedin homology domain (From Zimmermann and Polansky, unpublished data)

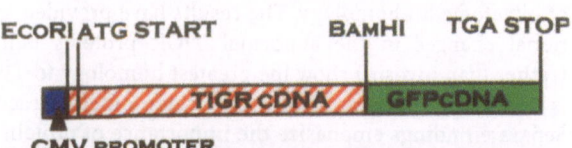

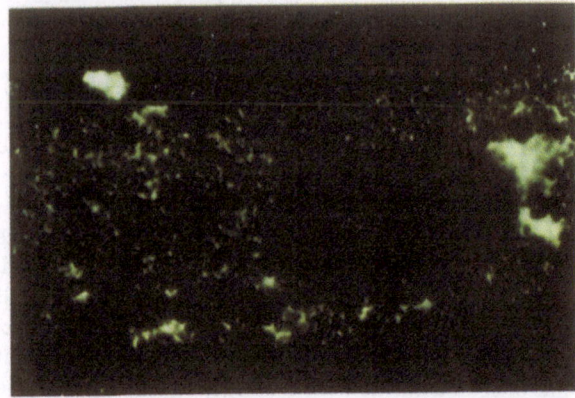

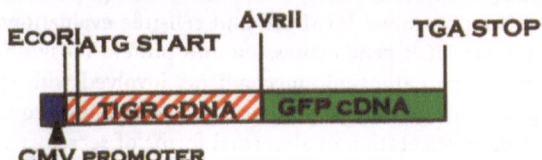

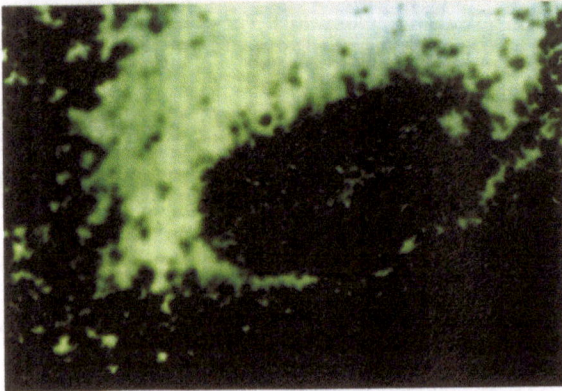

Sequence variants in TIGR's promoter that may have potential disease conse-quences are also being evaluated in addition to TIGR coding region defects. These proposed promoter 'defects' are being considered in relation to the development of glaucomatous visual field loss in ocular hypertension and possibly certain secondary glaucomas. Investigations by Nguyen et al. from our laboratories have supported putative roles for environmental factors and sequence variants that could influence the TIGR gene's promoter. These results may provide potentially valuable leads to help explain pathogenic mechanisms in chronic open-angle glaucoma and certain secondary glaucomas. Correlations of disease phenotypes with specific alterations in the TIGR gene, and genes that may directly or indirectly interact with TIGR, are cur-rently being investigated. In addition to the 4%–5% of random glaucoma cases that may be found with TIGR gene coding region defects, sequence variants in the gene's promoter may help define a significantly higher risk of developing the disease in spe-cific populations in a substantially higher percentage of adult glaucoma cases. Of par-ticular interest is the preliminary association of certain defects with more difficult to control glaucoma cases, which is being followed-up with clinical profile evaluations. The possibility that studies of other populations (e.g. ocular hypertensives, high ste-roid responders, exfoliation and pigment dispersion patients) may provide additional information about the value of such genetic 'susceptibility' or 'protection' effects involving genetic alterations is also being examined. Such evaluations are likely to generate the information we need to understand the value of genetic (possibly com-bined with environmental) tests in helping to make clinical decisions, including the level of scrutiny that might be justified for a glaucoma suspect, and provides indica-tions of the timing or method of therapy that could be helpful. Genetic testing offers potentially useful prospects for patients, physicians, and health management organi-zations. Genetic data also help to raise awareness of the need for glaucoma evaluation through the various nongenetic approaches available. This is crucial because of the limitations of IOP measurements for glaucoma screening. Increased patient aware-ness and improved knowledge of what may underlie the cause of glaucoma in differ-ent clinical settings suggests that the developing field of glaucoma genetics deserves attention.

The basic implications of TIGR gene research also include the search for potential interacting effects of different gene products, in addition to a reevaluation of some of the information obtained by early studies of corticosteroid responses and glaucoma genetics. Appropriate analyses of earlier data from clinical/experimental studies may have been confounded by a variety of influences that may soon be possible to sort out. Ongoing work will consider mechanisms by which alterations in the TIGR gene might produce their effects, as well as the discovery and definition of other hormones and factors that stimulate/regulate or interact with the gene. In addition to finding other genes that interact directly or indirectly with TIGR gene products (or pathways for their regulation), this concept has practical implications in potential future appli-cations of genetic testing and its interpretations.

In the coming years it will be important to take into account the spectrum of dif-ferent genetic and environmental influences, and to consider how different gene products could influence disease expression and the 'clinical profile' of an individual patient - rather than relying on an overly simplified genetic hypothesis. In this revised concept, genetic alterations in the structure of the gene can be modified by susceptibility and protective factors that still need to be defined, in addition to major influences involving putative changes in the gene's promoter and environmental/trans-acting factor influences on promoter function. The possibility of genetic factors in TIGR affecting other tissues, such as ciliary muscle, and other cell types that could contribute to visual field loss in glaucoma are also active areas of research. The characterization of defects in TIGR and potential interacting genes could thus play crucial roles in our diagnostic and potentially therapeutic armamentarium in the coming years.

In summary, discoveries relating to the TIGR gene offer potentially useful leads to understanding basic mechanisms involved in the development of a variety of open-angle glaucomas. Defects in the TIGR coding region, and sequence variants in the gene's promoter, along with factors that could contribute increased environmental stress are currently being assessed for their roles in disease pathogenesis. This information, combined with other genes associated with secondary glaucoma (such as pigment dispersion, exfoliation material, etc.) offer exciting prospects for the coming years, with implications for diagnosis, monitoring, selection of specific therapies, and improving education and awareness of the disease. As we approach the frontier of genetic testing in glaucoma, including the availability of a variety of tests to screen for glaucoma in adults as well as children, it is essential to realize that many different factors could modulate/influence gene expression. This means that a given genetic test should often be understood as indicating that an increased risk of glaucoma may be present, or some protective factor may also apply. The timing of symptoms and penetration of the genetic base into clinical consequences can be modified by other genes and environmental influences. This implies that the role of clinical observation and acumen will be what really helps bring the value of the tests forward to individuals, and ophthalmology as a discipline. Further considerations of TIGR, as well as other prevalent genes/factors that are likely to be discovered with current efforts into glaucoma genetics and physiology, are likely to produce additional insights.

Acknowledgements. The many discoveries of colleagues and collaborators is greatly appreciated. The recent findings reported here were primarily supported by the Glaucoma Research Foundation, That Man May See, Inc. From UCSF, and NIH grant EY02477. The first author also received support from InSite Vision and has a financial interest in the TIGR gene research.

References

Nguyen TD, Chen P, Huang WD, Chen H, Johnson D, Polansky JR (1998) Gene structure and properties of TIGR, an olfactomedin-related glycoprotein cloned from glucocorticoid-induced trabecular meshwork cells. J Biol Chem 273:6341–6350

Polansky J, Nguyen TD (1998) The TIGR gene, pathogenic mechanisms, and other recent advances in glaucoma genetics. Curr Opin Ophthalmol 11:15–23

Polansky JR, Fauss DJ, Chen P, Chen H, Lutjen-Drecoll E, Johnson D, Kurtz RM, Ma ZD, Bloom E, Nguyen TD (1997) Cellular pharmacology and molecular biology of the trabecular meshwork inducible glucocorticoid response gene product. Ophthalmologica 211:126–139

Rozsa FW, Shimizu S, Lichter PR, Johnson AT, Othman MI, Scott K, Downs CA, Nguyen TD, Polansky J, Richards JE (1998) GLC1A mutations point to regions of potential functional importance on the TIGR/MYOC protein. Mol Vision 4:20

Stone EM, Fingert JH, Alward WLM, Nguyen TD, Polansky JR, Sunden SLF, Nishimura D, Clark AF, Nystuen A, Nichols BE, Mackey DA, Ritch R, Kalenak JW, Craven ER, Sheffield VC (1997) Identification of a gene that causes primary open angle glaucoma. Science 275:668–670

Gene Therapy for Glaucoma: Anterior and Posterior Segments Targets, Delivery Systems, Constraints

X. Liu, C.R. Brandt, B.T. Gabelt, and P.L. Kaufman

Introduction

Therapeutic pharmacology in glaucoma has been directed at intraocular pressure (IOP) reduction, based on the consensus that reduced IOP decreases the risk of glaucomatous visual loss. It has been generally accepted that trabecular meshwork (TM) cells, the extracellular matrix (ECM), and their interactions are essential for maintenance of normal outflow resistance [1]. In the TM from patients with primary open angle glaucoma (POAG), histological and immunological studies have noted excess accumulation of ECM materials [2,3]. However, TM function might be modified by pharmacologically changing the distribution and organization of cytoskeleton in TM cells and ECM molecules [4,5]. Agents such as H-7 and LAT-A are believed to exert their facility-increasing effects, at least in part, by interfering with actin cytoskeleton and associated intracellular and cell-ECM interactions in TM. The rapid expansion in knowledge about the molecular mechanisms of such compounds, and the advancement of molecular genetic technology, may allow genetic "resetting" of the outflow or inflow tissues to a desired "performance" level as an alternative to classical, exogenous, small molecule pharmacotherapy.

The molecular genetics of glaucoma is being unraveled at an astonishing rate. The abnormal presence of ECM materials in the TM of some eyes with POAG, juvenile open angle glaucoma (JOAG) and glucocorticoid (GC) induced glaucoma is probably related to corresponding genetic defects. For example, a gene lying within chromosome 1q23-1q24 and encoding a TM-inducible glucocorticoid response protein (TIGR/myocilin) has been identified [6]. From the genetic analysis of chromosome 1q-linked glaucoma families and other glaucoma patients, mutations in this gene responsible for some juvenile and adult forms of glaucoma have been found [7]. As an extracellular molecule (secreted glycoprotein) sensitive to matrix metalloproteinase 2 (MMP2) [8], TIGR is overexpressed in the GC-treated TM [6], perhaps indicating a role in outflow obstruction. The physiological role of the TIGR protein and pathophysiologic effects of its overexpressed or mutated pattern are not yet clear. To study the mechanism by which the genetic abnormalities lead to POAG or JOAG, overexpression or inhibition of specific gene products or introduction of antisense genes in the TM in vivo could be very helpful. Delivering a recombinant TIGR into the TM, or upregulating expression of MMPs, to remodel the ECM may be glaucoma management alternatives to conventional pharmacotherapy, which requires frequent repetitive administration, as well as to surgery.

Other possibilities for ocular gene transfer targeted at glaucoma management are delivering genes into the ciliary muscle (CM) to enhance uveoscleral outflow, the ciliary processes to reduce aqueous humor secretion, and the retina to protect the ganglion cells (RGCs). $PGF_{2\alpha}$ analogs enhance uveoscleral outflow by signaling for an enzymatically mediated remodeling of the connective tissue between the CM bundles [9–11]. Since $PGF_{2\alpha}$ and the downstream enzymes, and the various kinases which regulate the assembly and disassembly of the actin cytoskeleton and associated adherens junctions [12–16], are endogenously synthesized, altering the related transgene protein expression and controlling their production or degradation become at least theoretically possible. The ciliary epithelial bilayer is known as the main site responsible for active secretion of aqueous humor [17,18]. Therefore, the bilayer and its functionally related factors including cell-cell tight junctional complexes [19], ion channels and transporters (e.g. Cl^-) [20], cotransporters (e.g. $Na^+/K^+/2Cl^-$) and enzymes (e.g. carbonic anhydrase, Na,K-ATPase) [17,21,22] may be targets for genetic modulation of secretion.

Dysfunction and death of optic nerve axons/RGCs are directly responsible for glaucomatous visual loss. The molecular processes leading to the death of RGCs are varied and not completely defined [23], but may be intervened by molecular approaches for neuroprotection and neurorescue. Gene transfer/transgene expression in the RGCs or nearby cells may facilitate the investigation of these processes at the molecular level and lead to upregulation or supplement of survival promoting factors that could protect and/or regenerate RGCs. For example, Bennett et al. using adenovirus (AV) vectors expressing rod cGMP phosphodiesterase gene, were successful in delaying photoreceptor cell death in homozygous *rd* mutant mice for 6 weeks [24].

The Prospect of Gene Transfer to the Eye

The eye is an attractive target for gene therapy because of its well-defined anatomy, immunoprivilege and accessibility. In highly myelinated tissue with a compact cellular structure (e.g. the brain cortex) the spread of the viral vector is limited to the area close to the injection site [25]. In the eye, with its laminar structure, the gene may be transduced into a sufficient number of cells to have a therapeutic effect. The transparent media allow excellent visualization of the transfer process. Intraocular injection is a relatively safe and easy approach. Other possible strategies for ocular gene delivery include corneal inoculation, scleral or choroidal gene implants or episcleral injection [26]. The immune privileged environment [27] may contribute to the mildness of the inflammatory response following gene transfer [28], and may delay or prevent immune mediated shutdown of transgene expression.

Potential obstacles to ocular gene transfer include difficulties in localizing and delivering the gene to the appropriate target cells. Most cell types in the mature human eye have very limited division activity or are postmitotic, such as neuroretinal cells [29]. This obviates certain forms of gene transfer strategies (such as retrovirus-mediated) that require replication of target cells for efficient incorporation of the foreign gene into the host chromosome [30]. However, AV and herpes simplex virus type1 (HSV-1) have the ability to infect a wide variety of dividing and postmitotic or terminally differentiated cells, and to express foreign genes to a detectable or abundant level [31], making them potential vectors for ocular gene transfer.

Animal models are essential to evaluate the efficacy, safety, and potential for gene transfer for glaucoma and other ocular disorders. Gene delivery mediated by different systems into the living eye has been accomplished in lower species such as rodents [32–35], but only a few studies have attempted to introduce a foreign gene into living primate eyes, using methods such as fusogenic liposomes but not viral systems. Very recently, Borrás and colleagues reported AV-mediated *LacZ* gene transfer into the anterior segment of perfused organ-cultured post-mortem human eyes [36]. The human eye differs in many aspects from that of lower mammals [37,38], but in most ways closely resembles that of other higher primates [37–39]. Since the ultimate goal of gene transfer studies is to apply gene therapy in humans, the monkey can be considered the most desirable experimental animal model for facilitating the evaluation process.

Gene Delivery Strategies

The central impediment to successful gene therapy is the development of gene transfer systems for specific tissues. Table 1 is a summary of both non-viral and viral methods commonly used for in vitro and in vivo gene delivery. Therapeutic efficacy will require transgene expression to an appropriate level and for considerable duration. This feature requires the promoter systems used to respond to appropriate regulatory signals. The advantages of using virus-derived vectors include efficient entry, nuclear uptake, relatively stable transgene expression and large capability for incorporation of foreign DNA [30,31].

Table 1. Summary of methods for gene delivery

Nonviral methods
- Ligand-DNA conjugate: DNA conjugated with ligands that can be recognized by receptors on the cell surface.
- Liposome-mediated transfer: Positively charged liposomes have high efficiency for entrapping and transferring DNA into cells. Liposomes undergo cellular uptake through endocytosis. Low toxicity, low cost, convenience.
- Calcium-phosphate precipitation: DNA uptake by cultured cells is greatly enhanced by co-precipitation with calcium phosphate.
- Ultrasound-mediated tranfer: Transfection stimulated by exposure to ultrasound, which permeabilizes the cell membrane, allowing passive diffusion of plasmid into cells.
- Electroporation of cells in the presence of DNA. Enhanced by DEAE-dextran.
- Direct injection of pasmid containing expression cassette into tissue. Cells take up plasmid and express gene.

Virus-Mediated
- Herpes simplex virus (HSV)
  - Amplicon vectors: plasmids bearing an HSV origin replication and packaging signal, plus E. coli origin of replication. Helper virus needed
  - Replication defective HSV (deletion of one or more essential genes)
  - Replication competent HSV, attenuated mutant virus
- Retrovirus: ideal for ex vivo application of gene therapy.
- Adenovirus: efficiently infects non-dividing cells, e.g., retinal ganglion cells.
- Adeno-associated virus (AAV): defective parvovirus requiring cotransfection with either adenovirus or HSV.
- Vaccina virus.
- Epstein-Barr virus: eukaryotic cell episomes allowing vector replication.

Non-viral Methods

A number of non-viral methods have been used for delivering genes into the eye, including receptor-mediated endocytosis. Most of them rely on normal mechanisms used by mammalian cells for the uptake and intracellular transport of macromolecules. The commonly used methods are calcium-phosphate precipitation, DEAE-dextran, ligand-DNA conjugates, cationic lipids, electroporation and direct injection of DNA [30]. One promising method of non-viral transfer uses a mixture of a liposome and an expression plasmid complexed with the nonhistone chromosome nuclear high mobility group 1 (HMG1) protein, which was then coated with the envelope of inactivated Sendai virus to increase the fusion with the cell membrane. Transgene expression was observed in the TM and iris-ciliary body of rats and in the TM of monkeys after intracameral injection of the Sendai liposome solution. *LacZ* expression was also demonstrated in the photoreceptors of rat as long as 30 days after intravitreal and subretinal injections. No inflammation or toxic effects secondary to the Sendai liposomes were detected on histologic examination [40,41].

Virus-Mediated Methods

In recent years, extensive progress has been made in the development of virus-based gene transfer vectors. Genetically engineered viral vectors used to successfully effect foreign gene expression in ocular tissues of live animals include retrovirus, AV, adeno-associated virus (AAV) and HSV. As discussed, retrovirus-derived vectors can be used to transduce dividing cells such as ocular tumors or other proliferating cells but are not at present useful for differentiated cells such as TM, CM cells and neuroretinal cells. The advantage and disadvantages of the available viral vectors have been discussed elsewhere [30,42,43].

We have tested the feasibility of delivering a gene into rat, cat and monkey eyes using a replication-competent HSV type 1 ribonucleotide reductase mutant (hrR3) expressing the E. coli *LacZ* [32,44,45]. Briefly, cynomolgus monkey eyes received viral injections into the anterior chamber (2×10^7 plaque forming units, pfu) and/or the vitreous (5×10^7), and the distribution of cells expressing *LacZ* was evaluated. Our results showed that intracameral and/or intravitreal virus injection resulted in transgene expression in TM, ciliary non-pigmented epithelial (NPE) and retinal pigmented epithelial (RPE) cells, and sporadically in RGC cells (Fig. 1). No *LacZ* activity was found in the CM (although *LacZ* expression was detected in the CM of the cat in similar experiments (Fig. 2)). We observed significant inflammation, primarily lymphocytic, in the anterior chamber, TM, and CM in the virus-injected eyes, along with mild vitritis and retinitis. No *LacZ*-positive staining and no obvious inflammatory infiltration was found in the control eye. Similar results have been obtained in the rat or mouse with hrR3 [45]. Little long-term damage to ocular structures has been noted in rodent studies [45,46]. To determine the efficiency of in vitro HSV-mediated gene transfer, cultured human TM and CM cells were infected with hrR3; both displayed multiplicity-dependent *LacZ* activity. Figure 2 shows hrR3 virus-mediated transgene expression in the TM of the cat eye, the RPE of the rat eye, and in cultured TM cells. When considered together, these studies raise the possibility of using a replication-

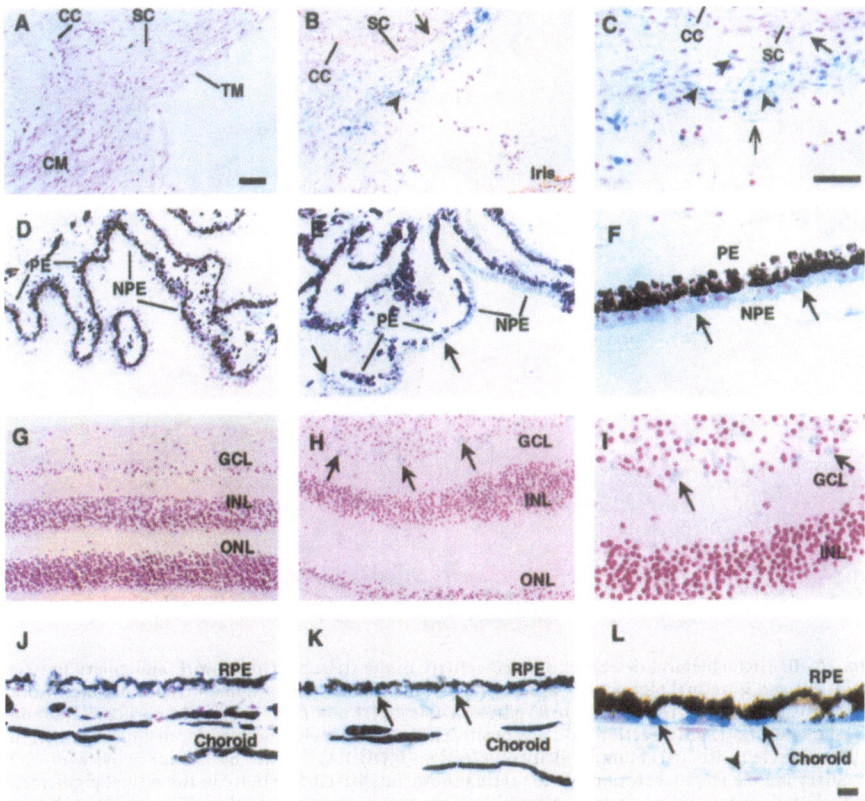

Fig. 1A–L. Histochemical detection of *LacZ* activity in various ocular cell types from monkeys killed 3 days after intraocular injection of hrR3 virus. A, D, G, J Different areas in the vehicle-injected eye. Virus treated eyes show transgene expression in: (B, C) endothelial cells in the corneoscleral (*arrowsheads*), uveal (*open arrow*) and juxtacanalicular (*arrow*) regions of the trabecular meshwork; (E, F) ciliary non-pigmented epithelial cells (*arrow*) in the pars plicata (E) and in the pars plana (F); (H, I) retinal ganglion cells (*arrows*); K, L retinal pigmented epithelial cells (*arrows*). All specimens were stained with nuclear fast red. *CC*, collector channel; *SC*, Schlemm's canal; *CM*, ciliary muscle; *NPE*, ciliary non-pigmented epithelium; *PE*, ciliary pigmented epithelium; *GCL*, ganglion cell layer; *INL*, inner nuclear layer; *ONL*, outer nuclear layer; *RPE*, retinal pigmented epithlium. *Bar* = 50µm (A,B,D,E,G,H), 20µm (C,F,I,J,K) or 10µm (L)

competent HSV-1 virus for delivery and expression of a functioning gene in ocular tissues for glaucoma gene therapy. However, before the potential of gene therapy can be realized, efficacy of gene delivery, stability of transgene expression, specificity of target tissue (cell) expression, and, most importantly, safety should be carefully addressed.

Acknowledgements. This work was supported in part by the National Institutes of Health (EY02698, PLK); the Glaucoma Research Foundation, San Francisco, CA (PLK, XL); the Retina Research Foundation, Houston, TX (CRB), and Research to Prevent Blindness, New York, NY (PLK, CRB).

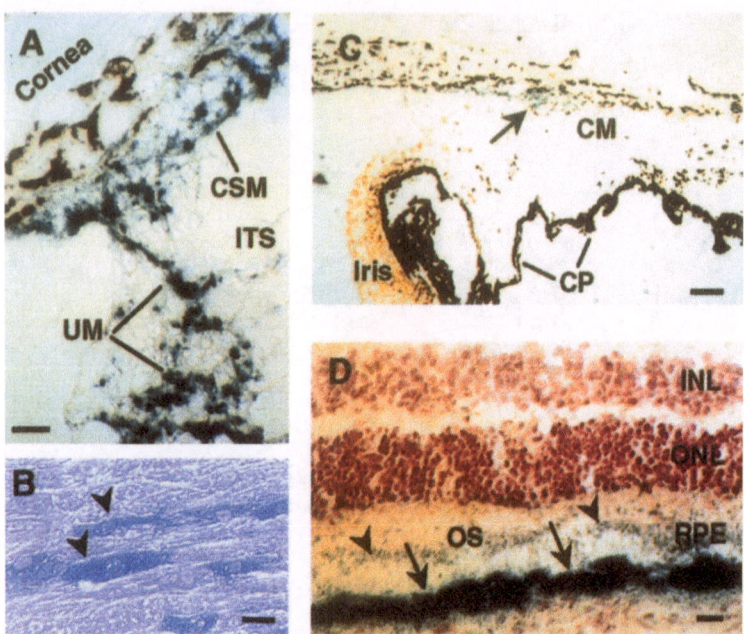

Fig. 2A–D. Histochemical detection of *LacZ* activity in the trabecular meshwork and ciliary muscle of cat eye and in retinal pigmented epithelium of albino rat eye, and in human trabecular meshwork cells in culture when treated with hrR3 virus. **A** Cat eye shows *LacZ* activity in corneoscleral and uveal meshwork (sagittal section). **B** *LacZ* positive human trabecular meshwork cells (*arrowheads*) in culture infected with hrR3 at multiplicity of infection (MOI) 1. **C** Cat eye shows *LacZ* activity (*arrow*) in ciliary muscle (sagittal section). **D** Rat retina shows intense *LacZ* activity in the retinal pigmented epithelium (*arrows*; RPE of normal and vehicle control eyes is unpigmented in this species), and photoreceptor outer segments (*arrowheads*). (**A**, **C** and **D** reprinted with permission from [47]. *CSM*, corneoscleral meshwork; *UM*, uveal meshwork; *ITS*, intertrabecular space; *CM*, ciliary muscle; *CP*, ciliary process; *GCL*, ganglion cell layer; *INL*, inner nuclear layer; *ONL*, outer nuclear layer; *OS*, photoreceptor outer segment; *RPE*, retinal pigmented epithelium. *Bar* = 20µm (**A**), 100 µm (**B–D**)

References

1. Acott TS (1992) Trabecular extracellular matrix regulation. In: Drance SM, van Buskirk EM, Neufeld AH eds: Pharmacology of glaucoma. Baltimore; Williams and Wilkins, pp 125–157
2. Lütjen-Drecoll E, Shimizu T, Rohrbach M, Rohen JW (1986) Quantitative analysis of "plaque material" in the inner and outer wall of Schlemm's canal in normal and glaucomatous eyes. Exp Eye Res 42:443–455
3. Acott TS (1994) Biochemistry of aqueous humor outflow. In: Kaufman PL, Mittag TW (eds) Glaucoma. In: Podos SM, Yanoff M (eds) Textbook of ophthalmology. London, Mosby, pp 1.47–1.78
4. Hernandez MR, Gong H (1996) Extracellular matrix of the trabecular meshwork and optic nerve head. In: Ritch R, Shields MB, Krupin T (eds) The Glaucomas, 2nd edition: Basic Sciences, London, Mosby, pp 199–243
5. Hernandez MR, Weinstein BI, Schwartz J, Ritch R, Gordon GG, Southern AL (1987) Human trabecular meshwork cells in culture: Morphology and extracellular matrix components. Invest Ophthalmol Vsi Sci 28:1655–1660
6. Polansky JR, Fauss DJ, Chen P, Chen H, Lütjen-Drecoll E, Johnson D, Kurtz RM, Ma ZD, Bloom E, Nguyen TD (1997) Cellular pharmacology and molecular biology of the trabecular meshwork inducible glucocorticoid response gene product. Ophthalmologica 211:126–139

7. Stone EM, Fingert JH, Alward WLM, Nguyen TD, Polansky JR, Sunden SLF, Nishimura D, Clark AF, Nystuen A, Nichols BE, Mackey DA, Ritch R, Kalenak JW, Craven ER, Sheffield VC (1997) Identification of a gene that causes primary open angle glaucoma. Science 275:668–670

8. Nguyen TD, Chen P, Chen H, Huang WD, Polansky JR (1997) Molecular biology and genetic studies of the major extracellular glucocorticoid (GC)-induced glycoprotein cloned from the human trabecular meshwork (HTM) cells (ARVO Abstract). Invest Ophthalmol Vsi Sci 38:S 473

9. Lindsey JD, Kashiwagi K, Kashiwagi F, Weinreb RN (1997) Prostaglandin action on ciliary smooth muscle extracellular matrix metabolism – implications for uveoscleral outflow. Surv Ophthalmol 41(Suppl 2): S 53–S 59

10. Lütjen-Drecoll E, Tamm E (1988) Morphological study of the anterior segments of cynomolgus monkey eyes following treatment with prostaglandin $F_{2\alpha}$. Exp Eye Res 47:761–769

11. Camras CB, Friedman AH, Rodrigues MM, Tripathi BT, Tripathi RC, Podos SM (1988) Multiple dosing of prostaglandin F_{2a} or epinephrine on cynomolgus monkey eyes. III. Histopathology. Invest Ophthalmol Vis Sci 29:1428–1436

12. Smith WL (1989) The eicosanoids and their biochemical mechanisms of action. Biochem J 259:315–324

13. Geiger B, Yehuda-Levenberg S, Bershadsky AD (1995) Molecular interactions in the submembrane plaque of cell-cell and cell-matrix adhesions. Acta Anat 154:46–62

14. Ryder MI, Weinreb RN, Alvarado J, Polansky J (1988) The cytoskeleton of the cultured human trabecular cell. Invest Ophthalmol Vis Sci 29:251–260

15. Theriot JA (1994) Regulation of the actin cytoskeleton in living cells. Cell Biol 5:193–199

16. Gips SJ (1994) Growth factor receptors, phospholipases, phospholipid kinases and actin reorganization. Cell Biol 5:201–208

17. Nilson SFE, Bill A (1994) Physiology and neurophysiology of aqueous humor inflow and outflow. In: Kaufman PL, Mittag TW (eds) Glaucoma. In: Podos SM, Yanoff M (eds) Textbook of ophthalmology. London, Mosby, pp 1.17–1.34

18. Morrison JC, Freddo TF (1996) Anatomy, microcirculation, and ultrastructure of the ciliary body. In: Ritch R, Shields MB, Krupin T (eds) The glaucomas, 2nd edition: Basic Sciences, London, Mosby, pp 125–138

19. Lütjen-Drecoll E (1982) Functional morphology of ciliary epithelium. In: Lütjen-Drecoll E (ed) Basic aspects in glaucoma research. Stuttgart, New York; Schattauer-Verlag p 96

20. Jacob TJ, Civan MM (1996) Role of ion channels in aqueous humor formation. Am J Physiol 271:C703–720

21. Lindskog S (1997) Structure and mechanism of carbonic anhydrase. Pharmacol Therapeutics 74:1–20

22. Coca-Prados M, Fernandez-Cabezudo MJ, Sanchez-Torres J, Crabb JW, Ghosh S (1995) Cell-specific expression of the human Na+,K(+)-ATPase beta 2 subunit isoform in the nonpigmented ciliary epithelium. Invest Ophthalmol Vis Sci 36:2717–2728

23. Yoles E, Schwartz M (1998) Potential neuroprotective therapy for glaucomatous optic neuropathy. Surv Ophthalmol 42:367–372

24. Bennett J, Tanabe T, Sun D, Zeng Y, Kjeldbye H, Gouras P, Maguire AM (1996) Photoreceptor cell rescue in retinal degeneration (rd) mice by in vivo gene therapy. Nature Medicine 2: 649–654

25. Hermens WJTMC, Giger RJ, Holtmaat AJGD, Dijkhuizen PA, Houweling DA, Verhaagen J (1997) Transient gene transfer to neurons and glia: Analysis of adenoviral vector performance in the CNS and PNS. J Neurosci Meth 71:85–98

26. Yang NS (1992) Gene transfer into mammalian somatic cells in vivo. Critical Reviews in Biotechnology 12:335–356

27. Jiang LQ, Jorquera M, Streilein W (1993) Subretinal space and vitreous cavity as immunologically privileged sites for retinal allografts. Invest Ophthalmol Vis Sci 34:3347–3354

28. Cousins SW, McCabe MM, Danielpour D, Streilein JW (1991) Identification of transforming growth factor-beta as an immunosuppressive factor in aqueous humor. Invest Ophthalmol Vis Sci 32:2201–2211

29. Li T, Adamian M, Roof DJ, Berson EL, Dryja TP, Roessler BJ, Davidson BL (1994) In vivo transfer of a reporter gene to the retina mediated by an adenoviral vector. Invest Ophthalmol Vis Sci 35:2543–2549

30. Mulligan RC (1993) The basic science of gene therapy. Science 260:920–932

31. Pepose JS, Leib D (1994) Herpes simplex viral vectors for therapeutic gene transfer delivery to ocular tissues. Recent breakthroughs in the molecular genetics of ocular diseases. Invest Ophthalmol Vis Sci 35:2662–2666

32. Kaufman PL, Jia WWG, Tan J, Gabelt B, Booth V, Tufaro F, Cynader M (1996) LacZ expression in ciliary muscle and trabecular meshwork of the living cat eye following anterior chamber injection of replication-deficient HSV-1 (ARVO Abstract). Invest Ophthalmol Vis Sci 37:S 444

33. Abraham NG, da-Silva JL, Lavrovsky Y, Stoltz RA, Kappas A, Dunn MW, Schwartzman ML (1995) Adenovirus-mediated heme oxygenase-1 gene transfer into rabbit ocular tissue. Invest Ophthalmol Vis Sci 36:2202–2210

34. Borrás T, Tamm ER, Zigler J Jr (1996) Adenovirus gene transfer varies in efficiency and inflammatory response. Invest Ophthalmol Vis Sci 37:1282–1293

35. Budenz DL, Bennett J, Alonso L, Maguire A (1995) In vivo gene transfer into murine corneal endothelial and trabecular meshwork cells. Invest Ophthamol Vis Sci 36:2211–2215

36. Borrás T, Matsumoto Y, Epstein DL, Johnson DH (1998) Gene transfer into human trabecular meshwork by anterior segment perfusion. Invest Ophthalmol Vis Sci 39:1503–1507

37. Rohen JW (1982) The evaluation of the primate eye in relation to the problems in glaucoma. In: Lutjen-Drecoll (eds) Basic aspects of glaucoma research. Schattauer, Stuttgart pp 3–33

38. Bito LZ (1984) Species differences in the response of the eye to irritation and trauma; a hypothesis of divergence in ocular defense mechanisms, and the choice of the experimental animals for eye research. Exp Eye Res 39:807–829

39. Rohen JW (1961) The histologic structure of the chamber angle in primates. Am J Ophthalmol 52:529

40. Hangai M, Kaneda Y, Tanihara H, Honda Y (1996) In vivo gene transfer into the retina mediated by a novel liposome system. Invest Ophthalmol Vis Sci 37:2678–2685

41. Hangai M, Tanihara H, Honda Y, Kaneda Y (1998) Introduction of DNA into the rat and primate trabecular meshwork by fusogenic liposomes. Invest Ophthalmol Vis Sci 39:509–516

42. Anderson WF (1998) Human gene therapy. Nature 392:25–30

43. Martin Duque MP, Sanchez-Prieto R, Lleonart M, Ramon Y, Cajal S (1998) Perspectives in gene therapy. Histol Histopathol 13:231–242

44. Liu X, Brandt CR, Gabelt BT, Kaufman PL (1999) Herpes simplex virus mediated gene transfer to primate ocular tissues Exp Eye Res (in press)

45. Spencer B, Agarwalla S, Miskullin M, Brandt CR. Herpes simplex virus mediated gene delivery to the rodent visual system (submitted)

46. Brandt CR, Imesch P, Spencer BI, Eliassi-Rad B, Syed NA, Untawale S, Robinson NL, Albert DM (1997) The herpes simplex virus type 1 ribonucleotide reductase is required for acute retinal disease. Arch Virol 142:883–896

47. Kaufman PL, Tia WWG, Tan J, Chen Z, Gabert BT, Booth C, Tufaro F, Cynader M (1999) A perspective of neuroprotection and gene therapy in the glaucomas. Surv Ophthalmol (in press)

CHAPTER 12

Morphology of the Trabecular Meshwork

E. Lütjen-Drecoll

It is well estabilished that in primate eyes most of the resistance to aqueous humor outflow needed for maintenance of a pressure gradient between intraocular pressure of ~ 15 mm Hg and the episcleral venous pressure of ~ 10 mm Hg is located within the trabecular meshwork. A correlation of morphological measurements with physiological data has shown that the extracellular material of the cribriform or subendothelial layer underneath the inner wall of Schlemm's canal (SC) forms most of the outflow resistance (for review see [1,2,3,4]) (Fig. 1).

Increase in aqueous outflow resistance found in primary open-angle glaucoma (POAG), steroid-induced glaucoma and pseudoexfoliation (PEX) glaucoma seems to

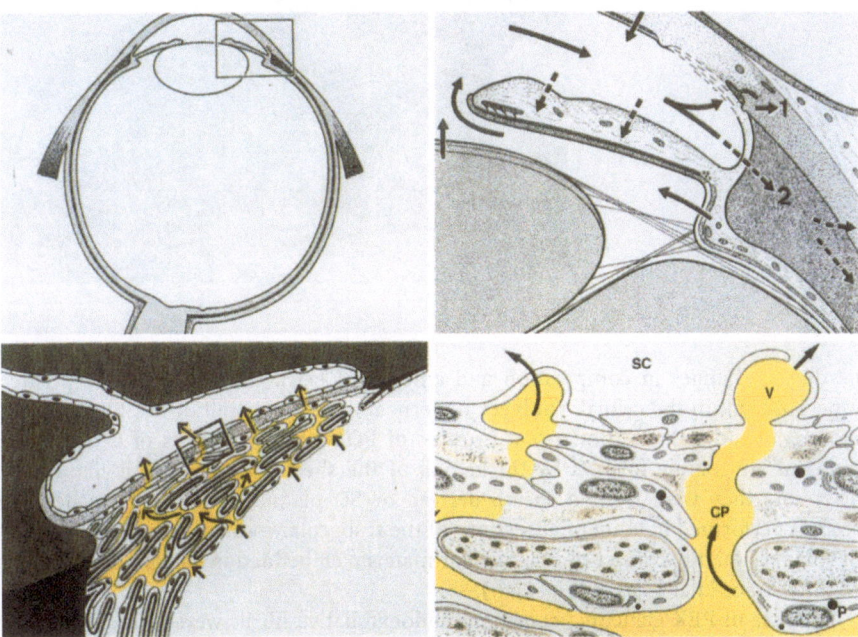

Fig. 1. Schematic drawings of the human outflow tissues in increasing magnifications. The aqueous humor pathways (CP) through the lamellated portion of the trabecular meshwork, the subendothelial or cribriform region and finally through the vacuoles (V) of the inner wall endothelium into Schlemm's canal (SC) are marked by *arrows* and *yellow* color. *1,* conventional outflow route; *2,* uveoscleral outflow route

Fig. 2 a, b. Electron micrographs of sagittal sections through the inner wall of Schlemm's canal in primary open angle glaucoma. **a** An 82 year old female. The lamellated portion of the trabecular meshwork is continuous with a subendothelial elastic network (*arrow*) which is connected to the inner wall endothelium by connecting fibrils (*arrow heads*) (x 1900).
b An 80 year old male. Higher magnification of the subendothelial elastic network (*arrows*) and the thickened connecting fibrils (*arrow heads*) forming the "plaques" underneath the inner wall of Schlemm's canal (SC) (x 7500)

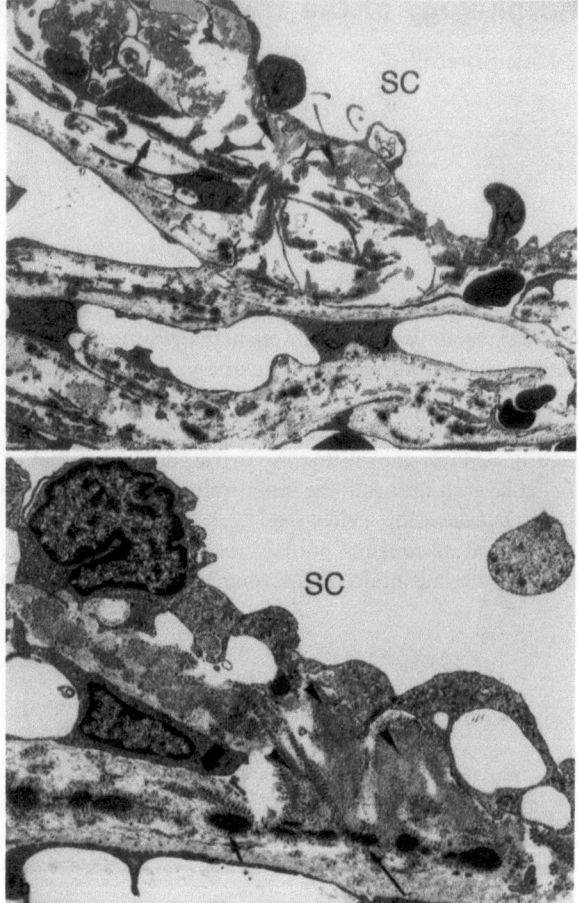

be due to changes in composition and amount of extracellular material deposited especially within the cribriform layer underneath the inner wall of SC. Electron microscopic studies have shown that in cases of POAG these deposits of extracellular material are mainly formed by thickening of the sheaths of the elastic-like fibers. Therefore they were termed sheath-derived or SD plaques. Enzyme-histochemical studies performed in tangential sections of the trabecular meshwork indicate that the SD plaques mainly consist of fine fibrillar material embedded in various components of the extracellular matrix (Fig. 2a,b).

In cases of PEX glaucoma specific pseudoexfoliative fibrils were found which are (if deposited to a greater extent within the aqueous pathways) responsible for an increase in outflow resistance. Interestingly the amount of SD plaques characteristic for POAG is not significantly increased in cases of PEX glaucoma (Fig. 3a,b).

Recently we had the opportunity to investigate trabeculectomy specimens and eyes from patients suffering from steroid-induced glaucoma. In these cases the morphol-

Fig. 3 a, b. Electron micrographs of a sagittal section through the inner wall of Schlemm's canal (SC) in pseudoexfoliation glaucoma in an 83 year old female.
a Accumulation of the typical pseudoexfoliation fibrils (*arrows*) underneath the inner wall of SC (x 7500);
b higher magnification of pseudoexfoliation fibrils (x 34 000)

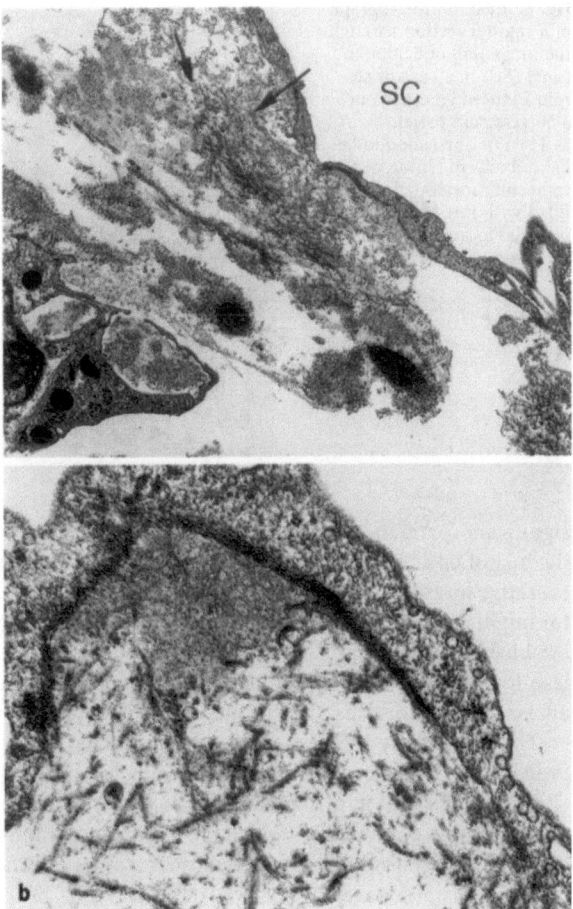

ogy of the cribriform region differed significantly from both POAG and PEX glaucoma. We found, e.g., immediately underneath the inner wall of SC, an accumulation of densely packed fine fibrils, and, in addition, in the inner portion of the cribriform layer fingerprint-like arranged material resembling basement membranes (Figs. 4,5). In most eyes with steroid-induced glaucoma an augmentation of SD plaque material was not found. PEX fibrils were also not present in these cases.

In trabeculectomy specimens derived from eyes of Japanese patients suffering from juvenile glaucoma both the SD plaque material characteristic for POAG and the fine fibrillar and basement membrane-like material characteristic for steroid-induced glaucoma were significantly increased (Fig. 5). These findings led to the conclusion that the development of glaucoma could well be due to several pathogenetic factors which induce increased extracellular material and intraocular pressure (for review see [1,2,3,4]).

We investigated the morphology of the trabecular meshwork and optic nerve in a number of glaucomatous eyes fixed at different stages of POAG and PEX. We found a

Fig. 4. Electron micrograph of a sagittal section through the inner wall of Schlemm's canal (SC) in a case of steroid induced glaucoma in a 50 years old patient (x 11 900). The subendothelial cribriform region of the trabecular meshwork is filled with fine fibrillar material located between activated trabecular cells

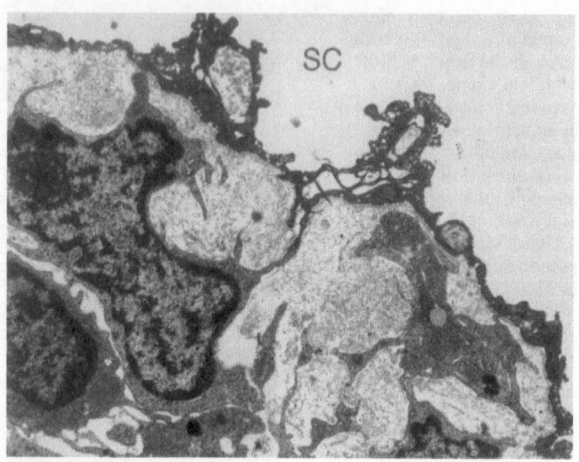

significant correlation between the amount of SD plaque material or PEX material and the loss of optic nerve fibers [5,6]. Since the extracellular material itself is not directly causative for the loss of nerve axons, these findings could indicate, that a common factor might cause both kinds of changes. This factor is not yet known. It is, however, well established that in monkeys a sustained increase of intraocular pressure (IOP) can lead to optic nerve damage comparable to that seen in human POAG. Therefore IOP is an essential factor causative for glaucomatous optic nerve deterioration.

The reason why IOP is increased in glaucomatous eyes is still not known. It is not even known how aqueous outflow is regulated normally.

It is known that in primate eyes with a well-developed accommodation apparatus, ciliary muscle contraction can lead to expansion of the trabecular meshwork thereby enhancing the filtration area of the inner wall of SC and outflow facility. The expan-

Fig. 5. Electron micrograph of a sagittal section through the inner wall of Schlemm's canal (SC) in a case of juvenile glaucoma in a 31 year old female (x 11 900). In addition to "plaques" and fibrillar material (not shown) abundant extracellular material resembling whirls of basement membranes within the trabecular meshwork is seen

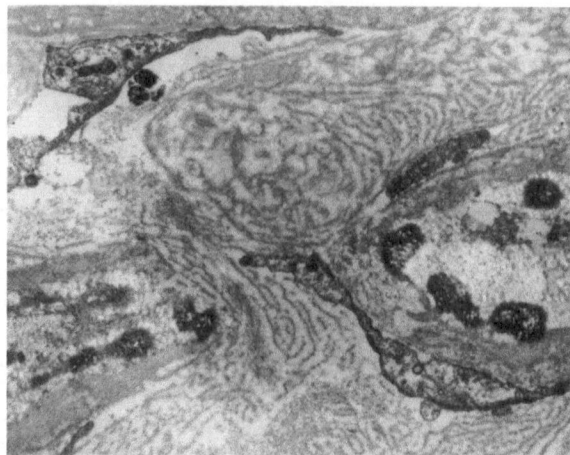

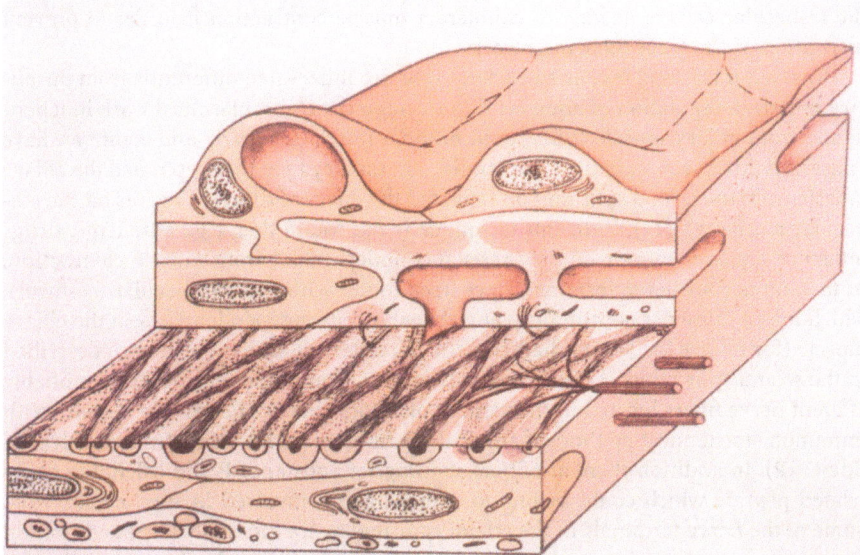

Fig. 6. Schematic drawing of the cribriform elastic network and its connection to the inner wall endothelium

sion of the trabecular meshwork depends on the point of insertion of ciliary muscle tendons which insert not only at the scleral spur and the connective tissue cores of the trabecular beams but also by bent "connecting fibrils" at the inner wall endothelium of SC. These connecting fibrils are presumably straightened during muscle contraction thereby widening the lumen of SC and the outflow pathways in the subendothelial region (for review see [1,2,3,4]) (Fig. 6).

The trabecular lamellae are, however, not only connected to each other by connective tissue strands but also by the trabecular cells which brigde the intertrabecular spaces and thus contribute to the formation of the sponge-like three-dimensional meshwork. The cells covering the beams of the corneoscleral portion of the trabecular meshwork are connected to the cribriform and subendothelial cells which finally are also in contact with the endothelial lining of SC. Immunohistochemical studies reveal that in human eyes trabecular cells stain with antibodies against smooth muscle (sm) α-actin and myosin. Ultrastructurally they resemble myofibroblasts ([7], for review see [4]). The number of these stained cells decreases with age but even in old eyes, sm α-actin-positive cells are still present in the posterior portion of the meshwork and in the scleral spur [8,9]. As has been shown by Wiederholt and his group, in organ cultures of anterior eye segments, agents that cause relaxation of trabecular cells increase outflow facility [10]. These data indicate that there might be a certain antagonism between ciliary muscle and trabecular meshwork contractility in the sense that ciliary muscle contraction enlarges the intertrabecular spaces, thereby increasing outflow facility, whereas trabecular meshwork contraction might decrease the size of the intertrabecular spaces, thereby decreasing outflow facility (Fig. 1). As the ciliary muscle inserts into a relatively soft tissue, it is possible that contraction of the trabecular cells is needed to counteract muscle contraction in order to prevent disruption of the trabecular meshwork.

However, if trabecular cells and scleral spur are innervated differently from the ciliary muscle, a regulation of aqueous flow through the trabecular meshwork independently from ciliary muscle tone would become possible. Barany and Kaufman have addressed this question in previous studies. In monkey eyes they separated the ciliary muscle from the scleral spur and investigated the effect of different agents on the trabecular meshwork [11]. With this technique it was found that, e.g., adrenergic drugs influence aqueous humor outflow resistance independent from muscle contraction. In fact, numerous nerve terminals have been found within the trabecular meshwork which might influence contractility of trabecular cells independently from the ciliary muscle (for review see [12]). Characteristic nerve terminals have also been described in the scleral spur region [13]. E. Tamm from our group found terminals of probably efferent nerve fibers located in the vicinity of myofibroblasts in the scleral spur. With immunohistochemical methods many of these fibers stain for vasointestinal polypeptide (VIP). In addition there are fibers staining for substance P and calcitonin generelated peptide which could belong to afferent axons involved in, e.g., nociception. Some of the nerve terminals in the scleral spur region are especially large and contain numerous vesicles and mitochondria [13]. They are incompletely surrounded by Schwann cells. Immunohistochemically there is a positive staining for neurofilaments and synptophysin but not for the other neurotransmitters. Both the ultrastructure and the staining pattern of these terminals resemble mechanoreceptors found in other parts of the body (Fig. 7). Further physiological studies have to clarify whether there is in fact a relationship between the afferent nerves which could measure mechanical stretching of the sclera or scleral spur and the efferent terminals might regulate contractility of the trabecular meshwork.

Nerve terminals have also been found in the episclera of various mammals including humans [14,15]. Some of these nerve fibers terminate at the numerous arterio-venous anastomoses present in the episcleral vasculature. Therefore, resistance to aqueous outflow might also be influences by changes in episcleral venous pressure.

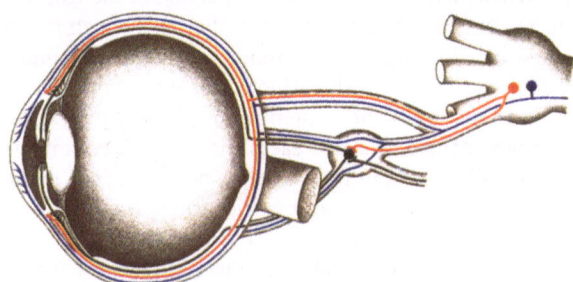

Fig. 7. Schematic drawing of the nerve terminals in the scleral spur region (*red*) presumably mechanoreceptors. The related nerve cells are located within the trigeminal ganglion. It is possible that axons from these ganglion cells form synapses with the ganglion cells of the ciliary ganglion (*black*) innervating the ciliary muscle and presumably contribute to the innervation of the contractile cells in the outflow pathways

In summary, it should be pointed out that still a great deal of work has to be done before the exact mechanisms of aqueous outflow regulation and their changes in glaucomatous eyes are clarified and before a more effective therapy of the various kinds of glaucoma can be developed.

References

1. Lütjen-Drecoll E, Rohen JW (1992) Functional morphology of the trabecular meshwork. In: W. Tasman and E.A. Jaegert (eds) Duane's foundation of clinical ophthalmology. J.B. Lippincott, Philadelphia, pp 1-33
2. Lütjen-Drecoll E, Rohen JW (1994) The normal anterior segment. Section I: anatomy of aqueous humor formation and drainage. In: PL Kaufman and TW Mittag (eds) Textbook of ophthalmology, Vol. 7, Mosby Year Book Europe, London
3. Lütjen-Drecoll E, Rohen JW (1996) Morphology of aqueous outflow pathways in normal and glaucomatous eyes. In: R Ritch, MB Shields, Th Krupin (eds) The glaucomas, 2nd edn, Vol. 1, Mosby, St. Louis, pp 80-123
4. Lütjen-Drecoll E (1998) Functional morphology of the trabecular meshwork in primate eyes. Progress in Retinal and Eye Research 18:91-119
5. Gottanka J, Flügel-Koch C, Martus P, Johnson DH, Lütjen-Drecoll E (1997a) Correlation of pseudoexfoliative material and optic nerve damage in pseudoexfoliation syndrome. Invest Ophthalmol Vis Sci 38:2435-2446
6. Gottanka J, Johnson D, Martus P, Lütjen-Drecoll E (1998) Severity of optic nerve damage in eyes with POAG is correlated with changes in the trabecular meshwork. J Glaucoma 6:123-132
7. Flügel C, Tamm E, Lütjen-Drecoll E, Stefani FH (1992) Age-related loss of α-smooth muscle actin in normal and glaucomatous human trabecular meshwork of different age groups. J Glaucoma 1:165-173
8. Tamm E, Flügel C, Stefani FH, Rohen JW (1992) Contractile cells in the human scleral spur. Exp Eye Res 54:531-542
9. Lütjen-Drecoll E (1995) Innervation of myofibroblast-like scleral spur cells in human monkey eyes. Invest Ophthalmol Vis Sci 36:1633-1644
10. See for Wiederholt in this volume.
11. Kaufman PL, Barany EH (1976) Residual pilocarpine effects on outflow facility after ciliary muscle disinsertion in the cynomolgus monkey. Invest Ophthalmol 15:558
12. Stone, RA, Laties AM (1987) Neuroanatomy and neurorendocrinology of the chamber angle. In: GK Krieglstein (ed) Glaucoma update III. Springer-Verlag, Berlin Heidelberg
13. Tamm ER, Flügel C, Stefani FH, Lütjen-Drecoll E (1994) Nerve endings with structural characteristics of mechanoreceptors in the human scleral spur. Invest Ophthalmol Vis Sci 35:1157
14. Funk RH, Gehr J, Rohen JW (1996) Short-term hemodynamic changes in episcleral arteriovenous anastomoses correlate with venous pressure and IOP changes in the albino rabbit. Curr Eye Res 15:87-93
15. Funk RH, Rohen JW (1996) Scanning electron microscopic study of episcleral arteriovenous anastomoses in the owl and cynomolgus monkey. Curr Eye Res 15:321-327

CHAPTER 13

Contractility of the Trabecular Meshwork: A Target for Treatment of Glaucoma?*

M. Wiederholt, H. Thieme, J. U. Nass, and F. Stumpff

Classical Concept of Outflow Regulation

It is generally assumed that contraction of ciliary muscle (CM) fibers extending into the trabecular meshwork (TM) influences outflow, and hence intraocular pressure (IOP). Application of muscarinic agonists such as carbachol or pilocarpine contract the CM. This has been directly shown for human and bovine CM strips (Fig. 1). Contraction of CM may expand and spread the TM, thus increasing the filtration area which leads to an increase of outflow (Fig. 1). In this well established model, the TM was thought to have no direct effect on aqueous humor outflow. Here, we review our arguments for the fact that TM acts in addition to CM in regulating outflow (for a detailed review see [1,2]).

Fig. 1. Classical concept of the effect of pilocarpine on reduction of intraocular pressure (IOP). The insert demonstrates that pilocarpine dose-dependently contracts isolated ciliary muscle strips. (From [8])

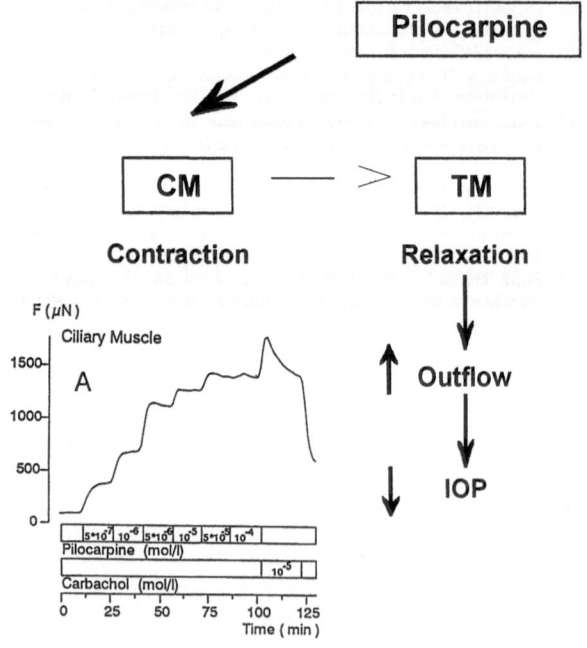

* Supported by the Deutsche Forschungsgemeinschaft (DFG Wi 328/19)

Arguments for an Active Contribution of the Trabecular Meshwork on Outflow Regulation

1. It has been demonstrated that TM tissue and cultured TM cells from human eyes and eyes of various animals contain contractile filaments suggestive of a smooth-muscle-like function of the TM. It has only recently been postulated that TM contractility may directly affect outflow resistance [3].

2. Human and bovine TM cells have electrical properties similar to those of smooth muscle cells. As in smooth muscle cells, depolarization of TM cells by various maneuvers induces voltage spikes. These voltage spikes are dependent on extracellular calcium and can be blocked by calcium channel blockers such as nifedipine [3,4]. The membrane voltage measurements suggest that human and bovine TM cells possess functional muscarinic, α- and β-adrenergic, and endothelin receptors [1,3,4]. Using patch-clamp techniques, various channels have been described directly [1,5]. Among several K^+ channels present in TM cells, the maxi-K^+ channel (K_{Ca}) is most important, because it plays a key role in regulating the balance between relaxation and contraction in smooth muscle cells. In TM cells, this channel is regulated by intracellular Ca^{2+}, ATP, cyclic GMP, and protein tyrosine kinase. The maxi-K^+ channel may be an important target for vasoactive substances such as nitrovasodilators and naturally occuring tyrosine kinase inhibitors that modify TM contractility [6,7] and thus probably aqueous humor outflow.

3. The contractile properties of isolated trabecular meshwork strips could be measured directly [8]. Measurements of bovine TM were compared with recording of CM strips and revealed similarities and significant differences between TM and CM strips. For the first time, a direct effect of pilocarpine on TM contractility was demonstrated (Fig. 2). Of the cholinergic agonists carbachol was more potent than aceclidine, pilocarpine and acetylcholine. Compared to pilocarpine (100%), carba-

Fig. 2. Original registration demonstrating a direct effect of pilocarpine (and carbachol) on isolated trabecular meshwork strips (from [8]). In isolated anterior segments with intract trabecular meshwork and no ciliary muscle, pilocarpine reduces aqueous humor outflow and thus should increase intraocular pressure (from [11])

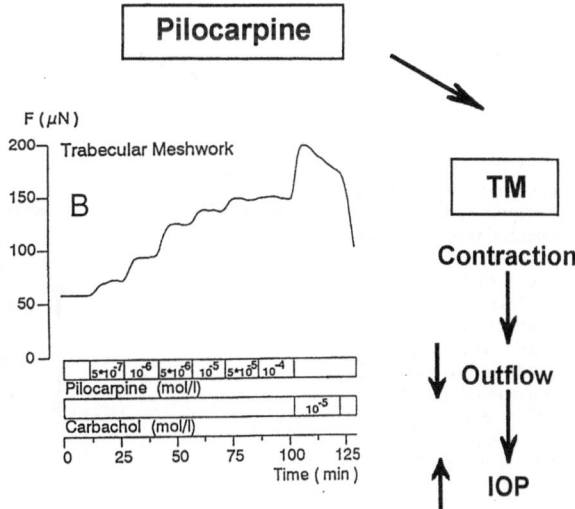

chol evoked a maximal contraction of 165 % in TM and CM strips. The functional muscarinic receptors were mainly of the M_3 subtype [8,9].

4. Aqueous humor outflow was measured in perfused anterior segments of the bovine eye with a morphological intact TM but no CM [10]. The relative outflow was significantly reduced by carbachol and pilocarpine. Epinephrine reduced outflow at high concentrations while slightly increasing it at lower concentrations. The increase in outflow was fully blocked by the β-antagonist metipranolol. Endothelin-1 dose-dependently inhibited relative outflow [10]. Thus, substances that contract isolated TM strips (carbachol, pilocarpine, endothelin, and high-dose epinephrine) reduce the outflow rate in the perfused segment with an intact TM but no CM. By contrast, substances that relax isolated TM strips (low-dose epinephrine, ethacrynic acid, cytochalasin D) increase the outflow rate [10,11]. Most of the data obtained in perfused bovine anterior segments are compatible with data obtained in perfused human anterior segments; however, some data are conflicting [12–14]. Whether these differences are due to species differences or to a varying contribution of CM fibers extending into the outflow pathway of the perfused human anterior segment is an open question.

Functional Antagonism Between Trabecular Meshwork and Ciliary Muscle on Aqueous Humor Outflow Regulation

From the data obtained with isolated TM strips and perfused anterior segments, the concept of functional antagonism in contractility between the trabecular meshwork and ciliary muscle was postulated (Fig. 3). This concept may be extended to the human eye, as both human and bovine eyes contain TM cells that are morphologically, electrically, and functionally comparable. Thus, in the intact eye, the contractil-

Fig. 3. A functional antagonism in contractility between trabecular meshwork (TM) and ciliary muscle (CM) on regulation of aqueous humor outflow and intraocular pressure is postulated. In addition to the effect of pilocarpine on CM, pilocarpine acts directly on the contraction of TM cells. This contraction is independent of the pilocarpine effect on CM. The overall pilocarpine effect on aqueous humor dynamics and IOP depends on the contractility balance between CM and TM *thick arrow*, strong effect; *thin arrow*, weak effect. (From [1,2])

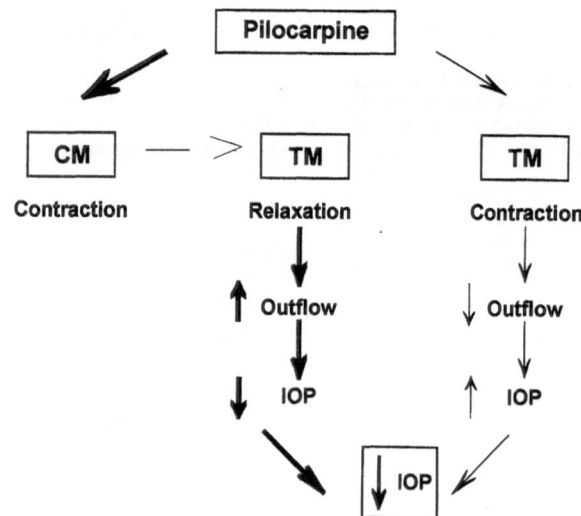

ity balance between TM and CM may determine the total aqueous humor outflow, as exemplified by the effect of pilocarpine (Fig. 3). There is substantial morphological and functional evidence that pilocarpine increases aqueous humor outflow by contracting the CM. This well-established model has to be modified. The overall outflow increase and resultant IOP decrease induced by pilocarpine are probably due to a more pronounced direct effect of pilocarpine on the CM. Although this functional antagonism between TM and CM may seem surprising at first, most regulatory processes are negative feedback mechanisms. The overall effect of various drugs on outflow is thus determined by the balance between their relative influence on CM and TM contractility. Furthermore, the recent findings of Tamm et al. [15] should be considered in connection with our concept of a functional antagonism between CM and TM. In the human scleral spur there are contractile cells that are probably functionally independent of the contractile elements of the TM and the CM. Thus, at least in the human eye, three different contractile elements may modify aqueous humor outflow through the trabecular meshwork.

Pharmacology of Regulation of TM Contractility

Concerning electro- and pharmacomechanic coupling, there are important similarities and differences in the influence of various substances on TM and CM contractility. Qualitative and quantitative differences have been discussed in detail [1,11]. Table 1 summarizes various substances tested on contractility of isolated TM strips. Contraction resulted from high extracellular K^+, muscarinic agonists, α-adrenergic (mainly α_2) agonists, endothelin, prostaglandin agonists of the thromboxane type (TP), and indomethacin. Relaxation resulted from β-adrenergic agonists, cyclic GMP/NO, prostaglandin agonists of the EP_2 type, the diuretic ethacrynic acid, substances such as cytochalasin D that interfere with the cytoskeleton, low extracellular Ca^{2+}, calcium channel blockers, blockers of nonselective cation channels, and activation of the maxi-K^+ channel by cGMP or by inhibitors of protein tyrosine kinase (genistein, tyrphostin). Furthermore, relaxation could be induced by interaction with protein

Table 1. Summary of various drugs and substances on contracility of isolated trabecular meshwork strips

Contraction	Relaxation
• Muscarinic agonists: Carbachol, pilocarpine, acetylcholine	• Adrenergic agonists (β): isoproterenol
• Adrenergic agonists (α): epinephrine, brimonidine	• cGMP / NO activation
• Endothelin: ET_A agonists	• Prostanoids: EP_2 agonists
• Prostanoids: TP agonists	• Diuretics: ethacrynic acid
	• Cytoskeleton: cytochalasin, ethacrynic acid
No effects	• Ca^{2+} channel blockers: nifedipine, verapamil
• Diuretics: furosemide, hydrochlorothiazide	• Nonselective cation channel blocker: flufenamic acid
• Carbonic anhydrase inhibitors: methazolamide, diclofenamide, dorzolamide	• Maxi K^+ channel activation: genistein, tyrphostin, cGMP, flufenamic acid
• Prostanoids: $PGF_{2\alpha}$, 17-phenyl-$PGF_{2\alpha}$	• PKC inhibitor: chelerythrine, H 7
	• PKG / PKA inhibitor: H 8
	• Tyrosine kinase inhibitor: genistein, tyrphostin

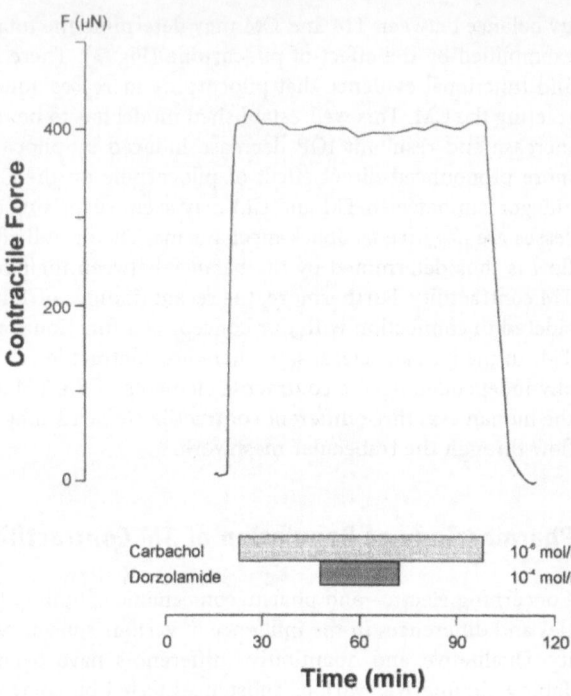

Fig. 4. Original trace registering the contraction of an isolated trabecular meshwork strip. In the tissue precontracted by carbachol, the carbonic anhydrase inhibitor dorzolamide had no effect

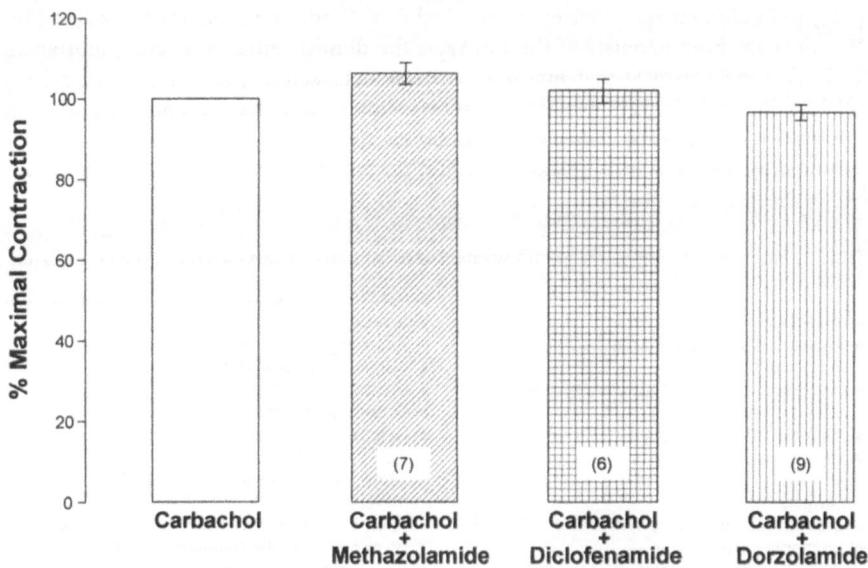

Fig. 5. Summary of the effects of carbonic anhydrase inhibitors (10^{-4} mol/l) on trabecular meshwork contractility relative to contraction induced by 10^{-6} mol/l carbachol (= 100 %)

kinase C, protein kinase G/A, and by interaction with various protein tyrosine kinases [1,2,5-11].

Table 1 also summarizes some substances which had no effect on contractility of TM and CM. It was recently demonstrated that modulation of the $Na^+ 2Cl^- K^+$ cotransporter alters TM cell volume and permeability of TM monolayers [16]. However, inhibition of the cotransporter could not be shown to have a direct effect on aqueous humor secretion and outflow in perfused monkey and human eyes or on contractility of isolated TM and CM preparations [17]. Diuretics belonging to the group of carbonic anhydrase inhibitors have been used systemically to lower IOP. Recently, locally applicable carboanhydrase inhibitors such as dorzolamide have been introduced successfully [18]. In trabecular and CM cells of the human eye and eyes of various species, a significant carbonic anhydrase activity could not ne detected [19]. Furthermore, a significant activity could also be excluded in vessels of the CM [19], while in retinal capillaries the membrane-bound carbonic anhydrase activity was demonstrated [20]. Because of the possible relaxing effect of carbonic anhydrase inhibitors on contractile elements, we tested several carbonic anhydrase inhibitors on contractility. Figure 4 demonstrates that dorzolamide (obtained from MSD Sharp & Dohme, München) has no effect on TM contractility. In addition to dorzolamide, we tested the optimal membrane penetrating carbonic anhydrase inhibitor metazolamide and the clinically widely used inhibitor diclofenamide (obtained from Dr. Mann Pharma, Berlin). Figure 5 and Figure 6 summarize our data. It can be concluded that inhibitors of carbonic anhydrase have no effect on contractility of TM and CM, thus, their effect on the reduction of IOP is mainly due to an inhibition of the secretion of aqueous humor.

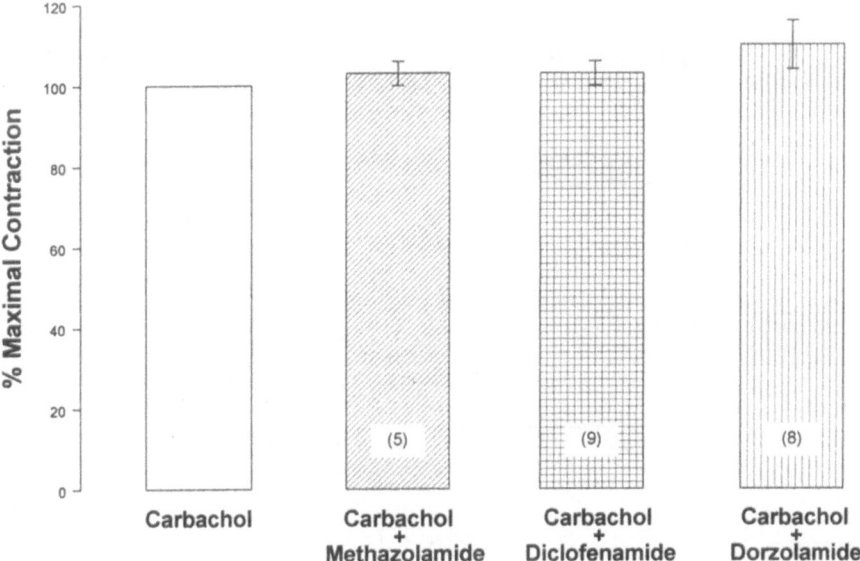

Fig. 6. Summary of the effects of carbonic anhydrase inhibitors on ciliary muscle strips contracted by carbachol

Search for New Drugs to Improve Outflow

Our new concept of aqueous humor outflow regulation derived from direct measurements of TM contractility assumes a modulation of contractile proteins in the trabecular meshwork by electro- and/or pharmacomechanical coupling. In addition, there is an increasing interest in agents that modify the cytoskeleton of TM cells, the structural complexes between cells, and the interaction between trabecular meshwork cells and the extracellular matrix [21]. Agents that affect these parameters may increase aqueous humor outflow through the TM. The increase in outflow facility induced by ethacrynic acid has been associated with changes in the cytoskeleton of TM cells [22], and in addition to these observed changes, ethacrynic acid probably interferes with contractile proteins and induces relaxation of TM [1,10]). Currently, we are searching for new substances that directly interfere with the contractility of TM cells. The contractility of cells can be modulated by interference with transporters, channels, receptors, and membrane voltage or by interference with the various single transduction pathways. Figure 7 is a schematic representation of channels, transporters, and receptors involved in the regulation of transport properties of TM cells and thus intracellular Ca^{2+} and contractility (for review see [1]). Very little is known about the intracellular second messengers and the various single transduction pathways in TM cells. Table 2 summarizes our current approach to describe new substances for modulation of TM contractility. Some of the effects of substances on ion channels have been reported [1,5,10]. Most recently, we have focused on the effect of various protein

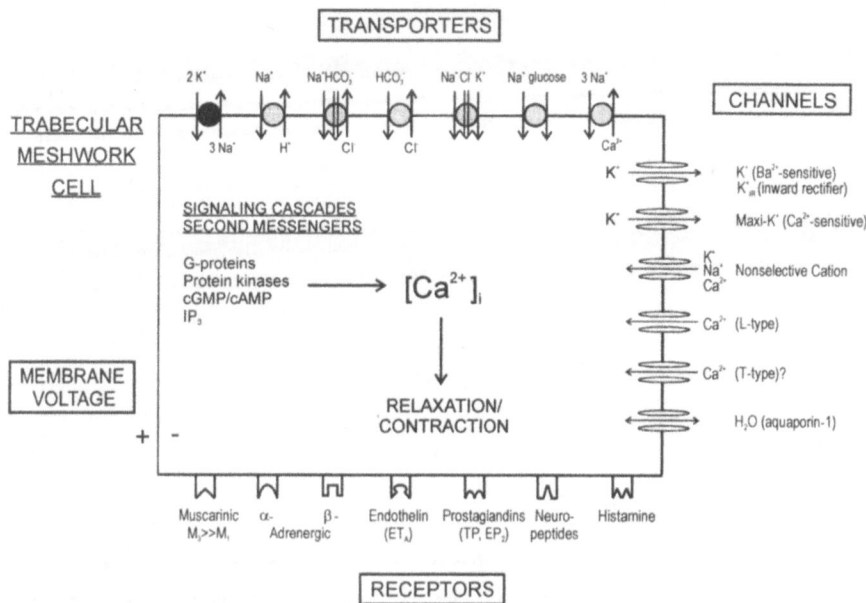

Fig. 7. Summary of functional characterization of transports, channels, and receptors in trabecular meshwork cells. (From [1])

Fig. 8. The signal transduction pathway in trabecular meshwork (and ciliary muscle) cells. Receptors are activated by carbachol or epidermal growth factor (EGF), serine/threonine and tyrosine protein kinases are involved in the signal transduction. The final cellular response, contractility, is modulated by intracellular calcium and ion channels. Inhibitors of serine/threonine (chelerythrine, NPC, H8) and tyrosine protein kinases (genistein, tyrphostin) were used. (From [7])

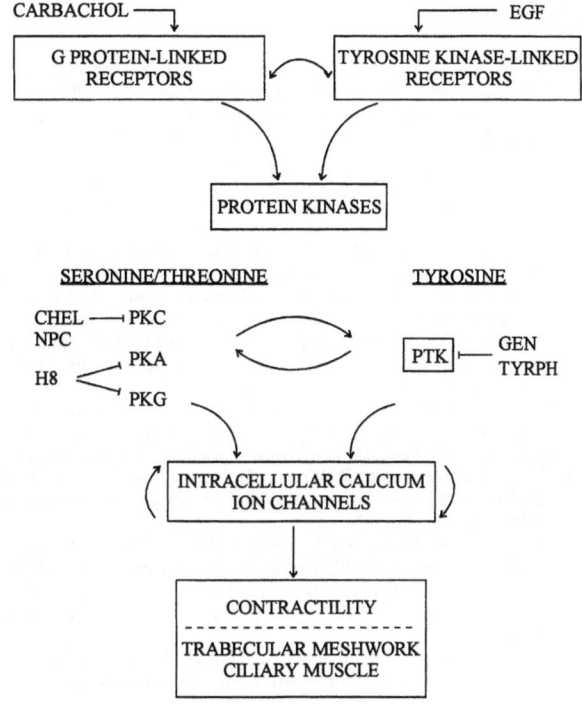

Table 2. New concepts for regulation of aqueous humor outflow by modulation of TM contractility

---

- Modulation of ion channels
  Ca^{2+}: verapamil ($\perp$)*, nifedipine ($\perp$)
  Nonselective cation: flufenamic acid ($\perp$)
  Maxi-K^+: iberiotoxin ($\perp$), genistein ($\uparrow$)*, tyrphostin 51 ($\uparrow$), cGMP ($\uparrow$), flufenamic acid ($\uparrow$)

- Modulation of signal transduction
  PKC: chelerythrine ($\perp$), staurosporine ($\perp$), H 7 ($\perp$), DAG ($\uparrow$), phorbol ester ($\uparrow$)
  PKG / PKA: H 8 ($\perp$)
  Tyrosine kinase: genistein ($\perp$), tyrphostin ($\perp$), EGF ($\uparrow$)

---

*$\perp$, inhibitors; $\uparrow$ activators.

kinases and their inhibitors on contractility [7]. It could be shown that inhibition of protein tyrosine kinase induces more prominent relaxation in TM than in CM. The relaxing effect of inhibiting protein tyrosine kinases is independent of protein kinase C and protein kinase A/G. The signaling cascade after activation of a tyrosine kinase receptor by epidermal growth factor (EGF) is differently modulated in TM and CM. The results are schematically summarized in Fig. 8 [7]. Protein tyrosine kinase inhibitors such as genistein are promising agents for the development of novel antiglaucoma drugs.

References

1. Wiederholt M, Stumpff F (1998) The trabecular meshwork and aqueous humor reabsorption. In: Civan MM (ed) Current topics in membranes, vol. 45 The eye's aqueous humor: From secretion to glaucoma. Academic Press, San Diego 163–202
2. Wiederholt M (1998) Direct involvement of trabecular meshwork in the regulation of acqueous humor outflow. Curr Opinion Ophthalmol 9; II: 46–49
3. Coroneo MT, Korbmacher C, Stiemer B, Flügel C, Lütjen-Drecoll E, Wiederholt M (1991) Electrical and morphological evidence for heterogenous populations of cultured bovine trabecular meshwork cells. Exp Eye Res 52:375–388
4. Lepple-Wienhues A, Rauch R, Clark AF, Grässmann A, Berweck S, Wiederholt M (1994) Electrophysiological properties of cultured human trabecular meshwork cells. Exp Eye Res 59:305–311
5. Stumpff F, Strauß O, Boxberger M, Wiederholt M (1997) Characterization of maxi-K-channels in trabecular meshwork and their regulation by cGMP. Invest Ophthalmol Vis Sci 38:1883–1892
6. Wiederholt M, Sturm A, Lepple-Wienhues A (1994) Relaxation of trabecular meshwork and ciliary muscle by release of nitric oxide. Invest Ophthalmol Vis Sci 35:2515–2520
7. Wiederholt M, Groth J, Strauß O (1998) Protein tyrosine kinase pathways and the regulation of trabecular meshwork and ciliary muscle contractility. Invest Ophthalmol Vis Sci 39:1012–1020
8. Lepple-Wienhues A, Stahl F, Wiederholt M (1991) Differential smooth muscle-like contractile properties of trabecular meshwork and ciliary muscle. Exp Eye Res 53:33–38
9. Wiederholt M, Schäfer R, Wagner U, Lepple-Wienhues A (1996) Contractile response of the isolated trabecular meshwork and ciliary muscle to cholinergic and adrenergic agents. German J Ophthalmol 5:146–153
10. Wiederholt M, Dörschner N, Groth J (1997) Effect of diuretics, channel modulators, and signal interceptors on contractility of the trabecular meshwork. Ophthalmologica 211:153–161
11. Wiederholt M, Bielka S, Schweig F, Lütjen-Drecoll E, Lepple-Wienhues A (1995) Regulation of outflow rate and resistance in the perfused anterior segment of the bovine eye. Exp Eye Res 61:223–234
12. Erickson-Lamy K, Korbmacher C, Schuman JS, Nathanson JA (1991) Effect of endothelin on outflow facility and accommodation in the monkey eye in vivo. Invest Ophthalmol Vis Sci 32:492–495
13. Erickson-Lamy K, Nathanson JA (1992) Epinephrine increases facility of outflow and cyclic AMP content in the human eye in vitro. Invest Ophthalmol Vis Sci 33:2672–2678
14. Gilabert R, Gasull X, Pales J, Belmonte C, Bergamini MV, Gual A (1997) Facility changes mediated by cAMP in the bovine anterior segment in vitro. Vision Rev 37:9–15
15. Tamm ER, Koch TA, Mayer B, Stefani FH, Lütjen-Drecoll E (1995) Innervation of myofibroblast-like scleral spur cells in human and monkey eyes. Invest Ophthalmol Vis Sci 36:1633–1644
16. O'Donnell ME, Brandt JD, Curry F-RE (1995) NaCl cotransport regulates intracellular volume and monolayer permeability of trabecular meshwork cells. Am J Physiol 268:C1067–C1074
17. Gabelt BT, Wiederholt M, Clark AF, Kaufman PL (1997) Anterior segment physiology after bumetanide inhibition of Na-K-Cl cotransport. Invest Ophthalmol Vis Sci 38:1700–1707
18. Sugrue MF (1995) The preclinical pharmacology of dorzolamide hydrochloride, a topical carbonic anhydrase inhibitor. J Ocular Pharmacol 12:363–376
19. Lütjen-Drecoll E, Lönnerholm G, Eichhorn M (1983) Carbonic anhydrase distribution in the human and monkey eye by light and electron microscopy. Graefe's Arch Clin Exp Ophthalmol 220:285–291
20. Terashima H, Suzuki K, Kato K, Sugai N (1996) Membrane-bound carbonic anhydrase activity in the rat corneal endothelium and retina. Jpn J Ophthalmol 40:142–153
21. Kaufman PL (1992) Pharmacologic trabeculocanalotomy. Arch Ophthalmol 110:34–36
22. Liang LL, Epstein DL, de Kater AW, Shasafaei A, Erickson-Lamy KA (1992) Ethacrynic acid increases facility of outflow in the human eye in vivo. Arch Ophthalmol 110:106–109

CHAPTER 14

The Actin Cytoskeleton and Aqueous Outflow*

B. Tian, J. A. Peterson, B. T. Gabelt, B. Geiger, and P. L. Kaufman

Introduction

The actin-based cytoskeleton, consisting of actin filaments and associated proteins, plays an essential role in the regulation of cellular events, including the stability of cell shape and cell-cell (C-C) and cell-extracellular matrix (C-ECM) adherens junctions. These C-C and C-ECM adherens junctions contain complex transmembrane interactions between the external cell surface and the actin-based cytoskeleton, mediated by specific adhesion receptors (integrins and cadherins) and a variety of submembrane anchor proteins, such as vinculin [1] and catenins [2], which link the microfilaments to the membrane in these sites. In addition to structural proteins these cell adhesion also contain a variety of signal transduction molecules such as protein kinase C and different tyrosine kinases, which can affect cell function [3]. The cellular adhesions are dynamic structures which change in number, location on the cell membrane, configuration, protein composition and "tightness" in response to a variety of factors, including hormones, drugs and physical stresses [3–5].

Actin filaments are a major component of the cytoskeleton and the submembrane plaque of adherens junctions in many cell types, and are abundantly present in the cells of the corneoscleral and juxtacanalicular portions of trabecular meshwork (TM) and the inner wall of Schlemm's canal in cynomolgus and rhesus monkeys and in humans [6]. In the TM, adhesions between cells and between cells and extracellular matrix contribute to TM geometry and flow resistance [7,8]. Logically, compounds that affect the actin cytoskeleton can alter the shape of cells in the TM and thereby change the overall geometry and decrease the flow resistance. In the late1970s, Kaufman and coworkers demonstrated that cytochalasins, a group of fungal metabolites that disrupt actin filaments by a complex mechanism [9–12], dramatically increase outflow facility in cynomolgus monkeys [13–15]. Morphologic studies demonstrated that separation of cells in the juxtacanalicular region of the meshwork and the inner

* This study was supported by the National Institutes of Health, Bethesda, MD (grant EY02698, PLK); the Glaucoma Research Foundation, San Francisco, CA (Catalyst Program Award, PLK and BG); Research to Prevent Blindness, New York, NY (Senior Scientific Investigator Award and Unrestricted Department grant, PLK); the Ocular Physiology Research & Education Foundation, Madison, WI (BT); Yeda Research & Development, Ltd.; the Ruth Belilos Foundation, and the E. Neter Chair in Cell and Tumor Biology (BG). The University of Wisconsin, the Weizmann Institute of Science and the Research Foundation of State University of New York have filed patent applications related to this presentation. Accordingly, Drs. Kaufman and Geiger may have a proprietary interest.

wall of Schlemm's canal, with subsequent ruptures in the inner wall, and washout of extracellular material [16,17], accompanied the decreased flow resistance across the TM.

More recently, it was shown that other compounds, such as serine-threonine protein kinase inhibitors and latrunculins, could disrupt actin cytoskeleton by different mechanisms [18–20]. We therefore studied the effects of the protein kinase inhibitor H-7 and latrunculin A on outflow facility in cynomolgus monkeys.

Protein Kinase Inhibitor H-7

H-7 (1-(5-isoquinolinyl-sulfonyl)-2-methylpiperazine), a broad spectrum serine-threonine kinase inhibitor, blocks the phosphorylation activity of diverse protein kinases including protein kinase C, myosin light chain kinase (MLCK) and rho kinase [21,22]. Exposure of H-7 to cultured cells disrupts the actin-based cytoskeleton and inhibits acto-myosin contractility, leading to deterioration of the actin microfilament system and perturbation of its membrane anchorage, which in turn weakens C-ECM and to a lesser degree C-C contacts in various cell types [18,23,24].

In living monkeys, total outflow facility was measured by two-level constant pressure perfusion of the anterior chamber (AC). A bolus infusion of 10 µl of 5 mM H-7 (initial 500 µM in the ~ 100 µl cynomolgus AC [25]) significantly increased the facility by 26 % during a 60-min post-drug perfusion (Fig. 1). After an AC exchange followed by an intracameral infusion with 10–500 µM H-7 (Fig. 2) or after topical application of 20 µl of 90–650 mM H-7 (Fig. 3), a dose- and time-dependent increase in outflow facility occurred. In AC exchange perfusion, 10, 100 or 300 µM H-7 concentration are

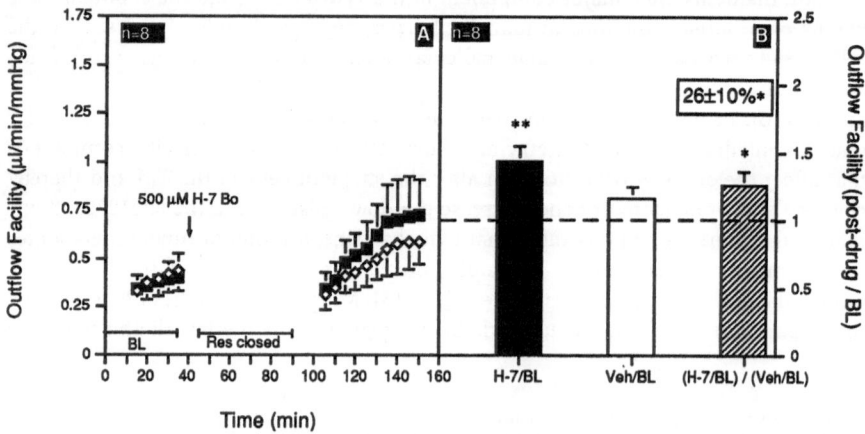

Fig. 1 A,B. A Effect of intracameral bolus (*Bo*) injection with 10 µl of 5 mM H-7 (500 µM in the 100 µl cynomolgus AC) on outflow facility in monkeys (*BL*, baseline; *Res*, reservoir) Data are mean±SEM (facility units on *left ordinate*; ratios on *right ordinate*) for *n* animals, each contributing one H-7- and one vehicle (*Veh*)-treated eye. Percentage in B shows the increase of overall facility in H-7-treated eyes within 60 min post-drug perfusion, compared to contralateral vehicle-treated eyes and corrected for corresponding baselines. *Dashed line* represents ratio = 1.0. * $P < 0.05$, ** $P < 0.005$ for ratios different from 1.0 by the 2-tailed paired t-test

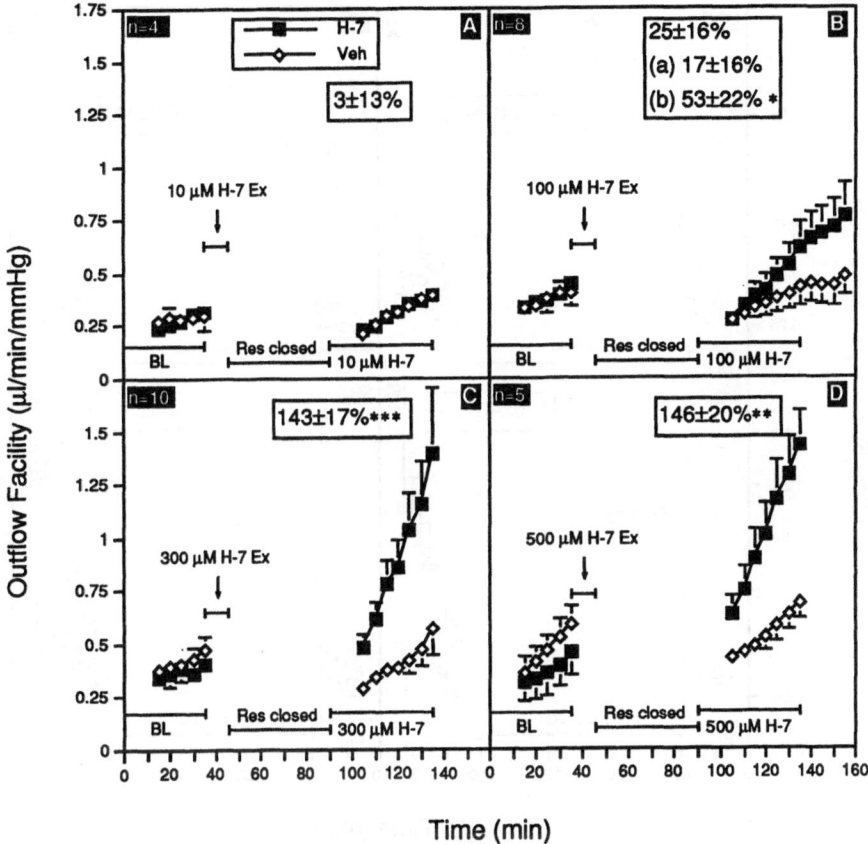

Fig. 2A–D. Effect of intracameral exchange (*Ex*) infusion with 10–500 μM H-7 on outflow facility in monkeys (*BL*, baseline; *Res*, reservoir). Data are mean±SEM μl/minHg for *n* animals, each contributing one H-7- and one vehicle-treated eye. Percentages show the increases of overall facility in H-7-treated eyes within 45 min post-drug perfusion, compared to contralateral vehicle-treated eyes and corrected for corresponding baselines (in **B**, item (*a*) represents the increase for the first 30 min, item (*b*) represents the increase for the second 30 min). * $P < 0.05$, ** $P < 0.001$ for ratios different from 1.0 by the 2-tailed paired t-test

subthreshold, just threshold and maximal facility-effective doses respectively, with 300 μM and 500 μM concentrations producing the same facility increase. Topical doses of 90, 150, 400 and 650 mM (0.3, 1.1, 2.9 and 5.7 mg) H-7 increased facility by 21%, 59%, 126% or 86% within 45 min, respectively. The 20 μl 150 mM topical dose produces an ~ 300 μM concentration in the ~ 100 μl cynomolgus AC [24,25]. The facility-effective dose range (~ 100-300 μM in the AC) was identical to those for actin filament and adherens junctions alterations in cultured cells [18], suggesting that H-7 increased facility by a cytoskeletal-cell junctional mechanism. As expected from findings in cultured cells [19,26], the increased outflow facility by H-7 is reversible within ~ 2 h (data not shown), consistent with transient alterations in cytoskeletal organization and cell adhesions rather than irreversible toxicity. A recent study has confirmed

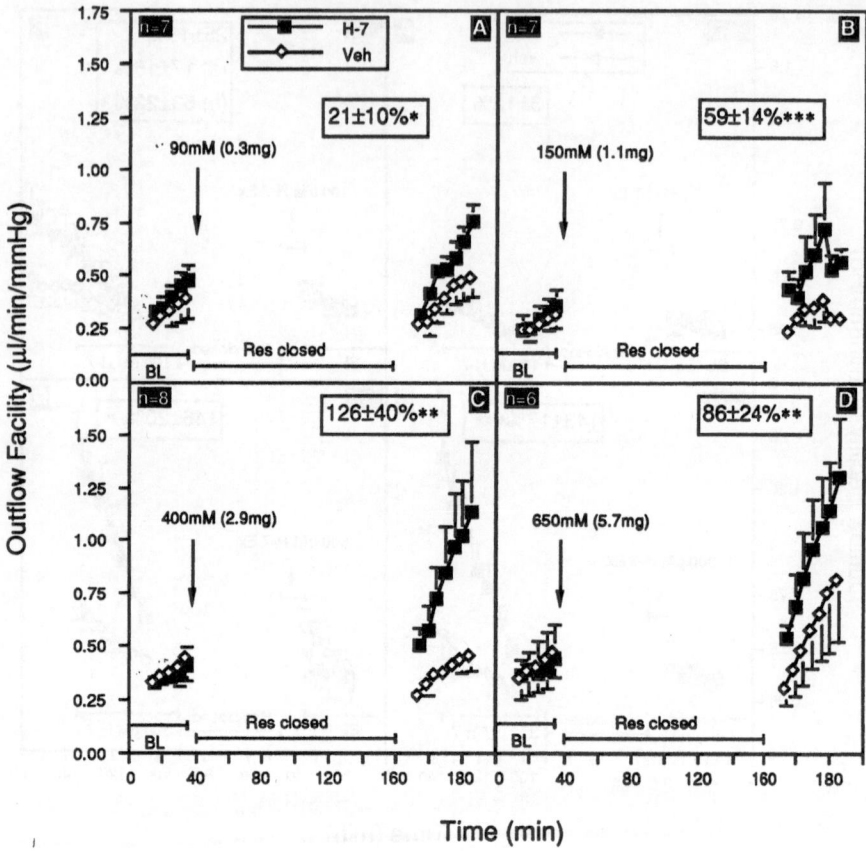

Fig. 3A–D. Effect to topical H-7 on outflow facility in monkeys (*BL*, baseline; *Res* reservoir). Data are mean±SEM µl/min/mmHg for *n* animals, each contributing one H-7- and one vehicle-treated eye. Percentages show the increases of overall facility in H-7-treated eyes within 45 min post-drug perfusion, compared to contralateral vehicle-treated eyes and corrected for corresponding baselines. * $P<0.1$, ** $P<0.05$, *** $P<0.01$ for ratios different from 1.0 by the 2-tailed paired t-test

that the facility-increasing effect is consequent to direct drug action on the TM rather than on other structures in the living eye [27].

Latrunculin A

Latrunculin A (LAT-A), a marine macrolide derived from Red Sea sponges, destroys microfilaments by binding to G-actin and blocking filament nucleation and elongation [20]. Exposure of cultured cells to LAT-A induces cell shape and junction disruption (mainly C-C junctions, but to a lesser extent C-ECM junctions). In living monkeys, AC exchange perfusion with 0.5–5 µM LAT-A or perfusion after topical administration of 21–42 µg LAT-A causes a dose- and time-dependent facility increase similar to H-7 (data not shown) [28,29].

Discussion

Cytochalasins increase outflow facility, distend the TM, separate the cells and enhance the washout of extracellular material in the TM [16,17] by disrupting the actin microfilaments in the TM cells. H-7 and LAT-A affect the actin cytoskeleton in several types of cultured cells by different mechanisms, but, similar to cytochalasins, increase outflow facility in cynomolgus monkey eyes, indicating that the actin-based cytoskeleton plays an important role in the regulation of outflow resistance in the TM.

H-7- and LAT-A-induced perturbation of cell contractility and consequent cytoskeleton alterations and weakening of cell adhesions in the TM might lead to elevated outflow facility, if fluid flow across a TM structure "loosened" by such agents further loosened and separated TM layers and cells, enhancing intercellular flow. Thus, following a bolus intracameral infusion, AC exchange infusion or topical application of H-7 or LAT-A, initial facility values were only slightly (Fig. 1–3), but dose-dependently elevated (Figs. 2, 3). Substantial facility elevation required continued perfusion, suggesting that the deterioration of the actin filament network destabilizes cell junctions within the TM and produces slight resistance reduction at low transtrabecular pressure gradients and flow rates. However, at higher pressure gradients or flow rates (e.g. during perfusion), the destabilized TM architecture is further disrupted to substantially reduce flow resistance. Under this scenario, such actin filament-disrupting agents may be effective in glaucoma patients with elevated IOP, especially if they are not receiving secretory suppressants, and digital ocular pressure may enhance the effect.

References

1. Geiger B, Tokuyasu KT, Dutton AH, Simger SJ (1980) Vinculin, an intracellular protein localized at specialized sites where microfilament bundles terminate at cell membranes. Proc Natl Acad Sci USA 77:4127–4131
2. Ozawa M, Baribault H, Kemler R (1989) The cytoplasmic domain of the cell adhesion molecular uvomorulin associates with three independent proteins structurally related in different species. EMBO J 8:1711–1717
3. Geiger B, Yehuda-Levenberg S, Bershadsky AD (1995) Molecular interactions in the submembrane plaque of cell-cell and cell-matrix adhesions. Acta Anat 154:46–62
4. Polansky JR, Bloom E, Konami D, Weinreb RN, Alvaraco JA (1984) Cultured human trabecular cells: evaluation of hormonal and pharmacological responses in vitro. In: Ticho U, David R (eds) Recent advances in glaucoma. Elsevier Science, Amsterdam, The Netherlands: pp 201–206
5. Perkins TW, Alvarado JA, Polansky JR, Stilwell L, Maglio M, Luster R (1988) Trabecular meshwork cells grown on filters: conductivity and cytochalasin effects. Invest Ophthalmol Vis Sci 29:1836–1846
6. Gipson IK, Anderson RA (1979) Actin filaments in cells of human trabecular meshwork and Schlemm's canal. Invest Ophthalmol Vis Sci 18:547–561
7. Lütjen-Drecoll E, Rohen JW (1996) Morphology of aqueous outflow pathways in normal and glaucomatous eyes. In: Ritch R, Shields MB and Krupin T (eds) The glaucomas, Basic Sciences (2nd edition). Mosby, St. Louis, pp 89–123
8. Hernandez MR, Gong H (1996) Extracellular matrix of the trabecular meshwork and optic nerve head. In: Ritch R, Shields MB and Krupin T (eds) The glaucomas, Basic Sciences (2nd edition). Mosby, St. Louis, pp 213–249
9. Brenner SL, Korn ED (1979) Substoichiometric concentrations of cytochalasin D inhibit actin polymerization: Additional evidence for an F-actin treadmill. J Biol Chem 254:9982–9985
10. Brown SS, Spudich JA (1981) Mechanism of action of cytochalasin: evidence that it binds to actin filament ends. J Cell Biol 88:487–491

11. Davies P, Allison AC (1978) Effects of cytochalasin B on endocytosis and exocytosis. In: Tannenbaum SW (ed) Cytochalasins: biochemical and cell biological aspects. Elsevier/North-Holland, Amsterdam pp 143–160

12. Godman GC, Miranda AF (1978) Cellular contractility and the visible effects of cytochalasin. In: Tannenbaum SW (ed) Cytochalasins: biochemical and cell biological aspects. Elsevier/North-Holland, Amsterdam pp. 277–429

13. Kaufman PL, Bárány EH (1977) Cytochalasin B reversibly increases outflow facility in the eye of the cynomolgus monkey. Invest Ophthalmol Vis Sci 16:47–53

14. Kaufman PL, Bill A, Bárány EH (1977) Effect of cytochalasin B on conventional drainage of aqueous humor in the cynomolgus monkey. Exp Eye Res 25 suppl: 411–414

15. Kaufman PL, Erickson KA (1982) Cytochalasin B and D dose-outflow facility response relationship in the cynomolgus monkey. Invest Ophthalmol Vis Sci 23:646–650

16. Johnstone M, Tanner D, Chau B, Kopecky K (1980) Concentration dependent morphologic effects of cytochalasin B in the aqueous outflow system. Invest Ophthalmol Vis Sci 19:835–841

17. Svedbergh B, Lütjen-Drecoll E, Ober M, Kaufman PL (1978) Cytochalasin B-induced structural changes in the anterior ocular segment of the cynomolgus monkey. Invest Ophthalmol Vis Sci 17:718–734

18. Volberg T, Geiger B. Citi S, Bershadsky AD (1994) Effect of protein kinase inhibitor H-7 on the contractility, integrity, and membrane anchorage of the microfilament system. Cell Motil Cytoskel 29:321–338

19. Yu JC, Gotlieb AI (1992) Disruption of endothelial actin microfilaments by protein kinase C inhibitors. Microvasc Res 43:100–111

20. Coué M, Brenner SL, Spector I, Korn ED (1987) Inhibition of actin polymerization by latrunculin A. FEBS Lett. 213:316–318

21. Hidaka H, Inagaki M, Kawamoto S, Sasaki Y (1984) Isoquinolinesulfonamides, novel and potent inhibitors of cyclic nucleotide dependent protein kinase and protein kinase C. Biochemistry. 23:5036–5041

22. Chrzanowska-Wodnicka M, Burridge K (1996) Rho-stimulated contractility drives the formation of stress fibers and focal adhesions. J Cell Biol 133:1403–1415

23. Mobley PL, Hedberg K, Bonin L, Chen B, Griffith OH (1994) Decreased phosphorylation of four 20-kDa proteins precedes staurosporine-induced disruption of the actin/myosin cytoskeleton in rat astrocytes. Exp Cell Res 214:55–66

24. Tian B, Kaufman PL, Volberg T, Gabelt BT, Geiger B (1998) H-7 disrupts the actin cytoskeleton and increases outflow facility. Arch Ophthalmol 116:633–643

25. Erickson-Lamy KA, Kaufman PL, McDermott ML, France NK (1984) Comparative anesthetic effects on aqueous humor dynamics in cynomolgus monkey. Arch Ophthalmol 102:1815–1820

26. Birrell GB, Hedberg KK, Habliston DL, Griffith OH (1989) Protein kinase C inhibitor H-7 alters the actin cytoskeleton of cultured cells. J Cell Physiol 141:74–84

27. Tian B, Gabelt BT, Peterson JA, Kiland JA, Kaufman PL (1999) H-7 increases trabecular facility and facility after ciliary muscle disinsertion in monkeys. Invest Ophthalmol Vis Sci 40:239–242

28. Peterson JA, Tian B, Kiland JA, Gabelt BT, Bersharsky A, Geiger B, Kaufman PL (1996) Latrunculin (LAT)-A & staurosporin, but not swinholide (SWIN)-A, increase outflow facility in the monkey. Invest Ophthalmol Vis Sci 37 (ARVO abstracts) S. 825

29. Peterson JA, Tian B, Kiland JA, Geiger B, Spector I, Kaufman PL (1997) In cynomolgus monkeys latrunculin (LAT)-A, LAT-B increase outflow facility, LAT-A decreases intraocular pressure and initially increases aqueous humor formation. Invest Ophthalmol Vis Sci 38 (ARVO abstract) S 243

CHAPTER 15

Glaucoma Screening:
A Vehicle for Continuing Medical Education

R. P. Mills

Introduction

Glaucoma 2001 is a national public service project of the American Academy of Ophthalmology. Its aspirational goal is to eliminate blindness from undetected glaucoma by the year 2001. The practical goal is to reduce glaucoma blindness by earlier detection of the disease. Fully 50 % of persons who have glaucoma are unaware that they have it. The project's three components are education of primary care physicians about the risk factors for development of glaucoma, no-charge ophthalmological examinations of patients identified at high risk for glaucoma by participating ophthalmologists, and public information about this common blinding disease.

One of the most popular programs in the project has been the Glaucoma Awareness Program, in which screening eye exams by volunteer ophthalmologists are provided to attendees at major medical meetings. The goal of the program is to disseminate knowledge of glaucoma risk factors among primary care and other physicians so they will make referrals of high risk patients to ophthalmologists, allowing earlier detection of glaucoma. To date, these have been run at two American Medical Association, two National Medical Association, one Allergy and Immunology, and one American Academy of Family Practice national meetings (200–400 screenees per meeting), and tens of state and local medical meetings. In each case, undetected glaucoma has been diagnosed and referral accomplished, in addition to detection of other important eye disease. More important from the standpoint of the goals of Glaucoma 2001, one-to-one discussions of the risk factors for glaucoma have taken place between ophthalmologists and attendees (largely physicians). However, no attempt to collect data on the effectiveness of this education in raising awareness of risk factors has been made at any previous screening.

This program evaluation seeks to answer the question, "Is the Glaucoma Awareness Program effective in creating enduring knowledge of glaucoma among attendees at a glaucoma screening at a national medical meeting?" The question is chosen because of concerns over the cost-effectiveness of the Glaucoma Awareness Program. Each screening has direct costs of about $ 15,000 for exhibit booth rental and setup costs and staff time and travel. Additional costs to be considered are time donated by volunteer ophthalmologists, and opportunity costs for Glaucoma 2001 and the American Academy of Ophthalmology.

While literature exists on strategies for physician education about risk factors from the diabetes translation programs [1] to efforts of pharmaceutical companies and professional societies about lipid risk factors in cardiovascular disease [2], and measuring the effect of traditional continuing medical education programs [3], there is no study of the effectiveness of a public screening as a vehicle to attract physicians who are then educated about risk factors.

Subjects and Methods

Screening Logistics

The Glaucoma Awareness program (glaucoma screening) was carried out under the auspices of the American Academy of Ophthalmology Glaucoma 2001 project at the National Medical Association (NMA) meeting, Sheraton-Waikiki Hotel in Honolulu, Hawaii on August 3–5, 1997. The populations to be studied were the attendees at this meeting who volunteered for screening and a random sample of the NMA membership who did not volunteer for screening. Formerly the Negro Medical Association, the NMA membership is comprised predominantly of African-American physicians, who themselves are at especially high risk for glaucoma. Meeting attendees included physician members of the NMA, spouses, nurses, and vendors. The sampling method was nonrandom; all persons volunteering for a free glaucoma screening were offered enrollment in the study. From prior experience with glaucoma screenings, we know that people who know they have glaucoma tend to volunteer to see if they still have it, or to get a free second opinion; people who are aware of it because of an afflicted family member or friend are attracted; and people who know that glaucoma is a blinding eye disease may also be more likely to volunteer. Thus, the sample tends to be enriched with people already aware of glaucoma, though they may not necessarily be highly aware of risk factors for the disease.

The exhibit hall where the screening booth was located was open from 9:30 am to 2 pm daily. Ophthalmologists from the Honolulu area with valid Hawaii medical licenses were recruited to donate 90 min shifts; there were two slit-lamps and two ophthalmoscopes, plus an automated fundus imaging device and a screening visual field test device.

The budget for this Glaucoma Awareness Project was approximately $ 20,000 (higher than average because of Hawaii venue), and financed by the American Academy of Ophthalmology. Two staff members from the American Academy of Ophthalmology, one technician from an ophthalmic imaging company, 18 volunteer ophthalmologists, and the author were the personnel involved. Equipment was loaned by national ophthalmic instrument companies, or hand-carried for personal use by the volunteer ophthalmologists. The booth space was approximately 225 ft^2.

Evaluation Design

The evaluation reported here is a single group pretest/post-test impact evaluation design, enhanced by a static comparison group of randomly selected members of the NMA who did not volunteer for screening who were administered the post-test only. The logistics of the screening did not allow for a true experimental design with a control group of screenees who did not receive education. However, it is not important whether the education, the screening, the questionnaire, or another factor caused any change in awareness of glaucoma risk factors; it is the program in its entirety that is being evaluated.

The comparison group of organization members was included to provide information on the differences in knowledge between those meeting attendees who volunteered for screening and the broader population of physician members who did not, addressing issues of selection bias.

The comparison of the static comparison group to the screened group was intended to address threats to external validity; was the population volunteering for screening too different from the rest of the meeting attendees to allow generalizability? Were the characteristics of the nonvolunteers different in any consistent way from the volunteers? In addition, the static comparison group post-test was compared to the screening group pretest. With similar results, the implication is that the knowledge level did not change over the duration of the study among the noneducated, and that there was no selection bias on glaucoma knowledge between the volunteers and the nonvolunteers.

Questionnaire Design

The questionnaire consisted of three questions, one each about glaucoma risk factors, intraocular pressure, and signs of glaucoma damage. Brevity was the principal objective, since potential screenees would not be willing to complete a long instrument in a busy exhibit hall. Moreover, when the same questions were sent in a follow-up, the expectation was that no more than 60 s would be available for completion. The questions were pretested among several primary care physicians and nurses, and their comments were helpful in the final instrument design. Although the three questions were the same in both formats, the pretest format (Appendix 1) was appropriate for administration at the screening site, and the post-test format (Appendix 2) was designed for maximum response in a FAX or mail survey, according to recommendations of Salant and Dillman [4].

Screenees

Approximately 240 physicians and accompanying persons were screened, of whom approximately 50 % were physicians and members of the NMA, and nearly all were African-American. Each screenee filled out a brief demographic form, provided informed consent and permission to contact later by FAX, phone, or mail, and completed the glaucoma risk factor questionnaire. No potential screenee declined to participate or refused later contact by the investigator. Screenees then waited in queue for an examining ophthalmologist, and during that time their answers on the questionnaire were discussed with them by the author. This education about glaucoma risk factors lasted approximately 2 min on a noisy exhibit floor with many distractions. All of the information needed to answer the three questions correctly was transmitted during the education, though the information was not necessarily received by the screenee. It is important to point out that the environment in which the instrument was administered was adverse to concentration; even educably normal individuals develop an acquired attention deficit disorder in the exhibit hall of a major convention. An examining ophthalmologist then performed the screening, and as time allowed, reinforced the education as it related to the screenee's personal circumstances.

The information below will be kept confidential and used only for purposes of this study.

Name _____	☐ Male ☐ Female
Phone_____	Ethnicity (check closest choice):
FAX_____	
City, State_____	☐ African-American ☐ Caucasian
What is your present occupation (specialty)?	☐ Other black American ☐ Native American
_____	☐ Hispanic ☐ Asian
	☐ Other
☐ Clinic-based or ☐ Hospital-based	NMA Member? (yes/no)

Glaucoma 2001 Questionnaire

1. Place a check mark next to the items below that you consider to be major risk factors for primary open angle glaucoma (check as many as apply):

    ☐ systemic hypertension
    ☐ advanced age
    ☐ chronically red eyes
    ☐ family history of glaucoma
    ☐ African-American ancestry
    ☐ elevated serum cholesterol
    ☐ stress at home or work
    ☐ no recent eye exam

2. In your opinion, is screening for elevated intraocular pressure is a reliable way to decide whether glaucoma is present in an individual patient? (check one):

    ☐ Yes
    ☐ No

3. In your opinion, detection of glaucoma damage can be found through (check all that apply):

    ☐ visual field testing
    ☐ ophthalmoscopy (looking at the optic nerve in the eye)
    ☐ visual acuity measurement
    ☐ measuring intraocular pressure
    ☐ refraction
    ☐ history of visual difficulties
    ☐ history of pain

Appendix 1. Pretest questionnaire

1. Place a check mark next to the major risk factors for primary open angle glaucoma (check as many as apply):

- ☐ systemic hypertension
- ☐ advanced age
- ☐ chronically red eyes
- ☐ family history of glaucoma
- ☐ African-American ancestry
- ☐ elevated serum cholesterol
- ☐ stress at home or work
- ☐ no recent eye exam

NMA Member? (yes/no)

Ethnicity (check closest choice)

- ☐ African-American
- ☐ Other black American
- ☐ Hispanic
- ☐ Caucasian
- ☐ Native American
- ☐ Asian
- ☐ Other

2. Screening for elevated intraocular pressure is a reliable way to decide whether glaucoma is present in an individual patient   (check one):
- ☐ True
- ☐ False

The information below will be kept confidential and used only for purposes of this study.

Name _____

Phone _____

3. Detection of glaucoma damage can be found through (check all that apply):
- ☐ visual field testing
- ☐ ophthalmoscopy (looking at the optic nerve in the eye)
- ☐ visual acuity measurement
- ☐ measuring intraocular pressure
- ☐ refraction
- ☐ history of visual difficulties
- ☐ history of pain

FAX   _____

City, State _____

_____

What is your present occupation (specialty)?

Appendix 2. Post-test questionnaire

Follow-Up Questionnaire

Four months after the meeting, on December 6, 1997, screenees were contacted by FAX or mail on American Academy of Ophthalmology letterhead and thanked for their participation. Included was the three item questionnaire with the same questions as on the pretest and a request to take 2 min to complete it and FAX it back to the Academy offices.

Since the contact was not anonymous, no attempt was made to preserve anonymity in the questionnaire responses. Respondents were deleted from the list of persons to recontact, and a repeat FAX or mail was used as a second request to nonrespondents on January 10, 1998, and a third request to continued nonrespondents was sent on March 5, 1998.

The NMA generously agreed to provide the author with a randomly selected list, including FAX numbers, if available, of 300 NMA members. Participants in the screening were deleted from the list, and the remainder served as a comparison population, all of whom were physicians. On January 10, 1998, a cover letter and the questionnaire were sent to the comparison group by mail or FAX. Although a list of meeting attendees who did not participate in the screening might have been preferable, the NMA was unable to generate a list limited to attendees. A second and final letter with questionnaire was sent to the comparison group on March 5, 1998.

Analysis Strategy

The questionnaires were scored to provide one point for each correct answer on each component of the three questions. Thus, for question 1, a score of 8 was possible, 4 from correctly checking the four true risk factors, and 4 from correctly not checking the four distractor risk factors. For question 2, a score of 1 was possible by correctly answering the true-false question. For question 3, a possible score of 7 could be achieved by checking the two correct findings, and not checking the five distractors. Item-by-item responses were entered into a spreadsheet and scores automatically calcuated for each of the three questions and for a total score.

The screenees were divided into two groups for analysis: physicians and nonphysicians. For each group of screenees, a pretest, post-test and demographic and historical information was available. The third analysis category was the physician comparison group on whom post-test scores and demographic information alone were available. Since there was no intervention in the comparison group and no known intervening glaucoma education to which they were exposed, the comparison group post-test was assumed to be the equivalent of a control group pretest.

Distributions of all variables were examined to ensure appropriateness of parametric statistical analysis. Pretest scores were compared between the physician and nonphysician screenees, and between the pretest scores of physician screenees and the post-test scores of the physician comparison group using the independent sample t test. Linear regression was performed with total or individual question scores as the dependent variables and demographic and historical information as predictor variables. Appropriate dummy variables were constructed for variables with two or more categories of response.

Pretest and post-test scores of the physician and nonphysician screenees were compared using paired sample t tests, with change in score as the primary outcome (dependent) variable. Secondary outcome analyses were performed using scores by question or item as the dependent variable. Linear regression was conducted on the differences between the pretest and post-test scores as the dependent variable and the historical and demographic data as predictor variables. Finally, the post-test scores of the physician screenees were compared to the post-test scores of the physician control group to determine if a difference in glaucoma knowledge existed using an independent sample t test.

Results

Post-test responses were received from 31 physician screenees (26 % response rate), 17 nonphysician screenees (14 % response rate), and 26 physicians from the comparison group (10 % response rate). Pretest responses revealed a wide range of difficulty of the items on the three questions, with mean correct answers ranging from 4 % to 100 % (Table 1). Most of the respondents correctly identified family history of glaucoma and rejected red eyes as a risk factor for glaucoma. However, less than 50 % of physicians and nonphysicians correctly rejected systemic hypertension as a risk factor for glaucoma. Less than 10 % of all respondents knew that intraocular pressure was not a reliable way to decide whether glaucoma was present in an individual patient. Interestingly, there was little difference on individual items among the three groups of respondents, except that in contrast to the two physicians groups, fewer of the nonphysicians thought that pain was a feature of glaucoma damage, and more of the nonphysicians thought that visual difficulty was a feature of glaucoma damage.

Table 1. Pretest correct responses

Question 1: Place a check mark next to the major risk factors for primary open angle glaucoma (check as many as apply):

Risk factor	Correct answer	Physician screenees (n = 31)	Nonphysician screenees (n = 17)	Physician "controls" (n = 26)
Systemic hypertension	False	42 %	41 %	35 %
Advanced age	True	74 %	76 %	73 %
Red eyes	False	84 %	88 %	77 %
Family history of glaucoma	True	97 %	100 %	88 %
African-American	True	90 %	65 %	69 %
Elevated cholesterol	False	84 %	82 %	77 %
Stress at home/work	False	68 %	71 %	85 %
No recent eye exam	True	55 %	71 %	50 %

Question 2: Screening for elevated intraocular pressure is a reliable way to decide whether glaucoma is present in an individual patient (check one):

Correct answer	Physician screenees (n = 31)	Nonphysician screenees (n = 17)	Physician "controls" (n = 26)
False	6 %	6 %	8 %

Question 3: Detection of glaucoma damage can be found through (check all that apply):

Finding	Correct answer	Physician screenees (n = 31)	Nonphysician screenees (n = 17)	Physician "controls" (n = 26)
Visual fields	True	61 %	76 %	54 %
Ophthalmoscopy	True	84 %	65 %	62 %
Visual acuity	False	52 %	59 %	69 %
Intraocular pressure	False	6 %	18 %	4 %
Refraction	False	77 %	82 %	73 %
History of visual difficulty	False	48 %	24 %	35 %
History of pain	False	58 %	82 %	62 %

Table 2. Pretest scores

	Mean correct*	Standard deviation	t value	p value
Nonscreened physicians (n = 26)	9.2	1.9	-1.23	0.22
Screened physicians (n = 31)	9.8	2.2		
Screened physicians (n = 31)	9.8	2.2	-0.29	0.77
Screened nonphysicians (n = 17)	10.1	2.1		

Mean score on 3 individual questions

	Question 1 (8 possible)	Question 2 (1 possible)	Question 3 (7 possible)
Nonscreened physicians (n = 26)	5.5	0.08	3.6
Screened physicians (n = 31)	5.9	0.06	3.9
Screened nonphysicians (n = 17)	5.9	0.06	4.1

*Total correct (16 possible); independent sample t tests.

Table 3. Linear regression on total pretest score

Variable	B statistic	t statistic	p value
Gender	0.63	0.84	0.40
Age category	−0.16	−0.32	0.75
Race	0.79	0.33	0.74
History vascular disease	−1.32	−1.50	0.14
History of eye problem	0.49	0.38	0.70
History of myopia	0.25	0.18	0.86
Family history glaucoma	0.17	0.22	0.83
Reason for exam: prevention	−0.64	−0.66	0.51
Reason for exam: personal risk	−0.07	−0.07	0.94
Region of residence (East vs other)	0.40	0.58	0.57
(Constant)	9.92	4.80	0.0000

Total R-squared = 0.13, $p = 0.86$.

There was no significant differences in the total scores or the scores on any of the three questions between the physician and nonphysician screenees and between the physician screenees and the physician comparison group (Table 2). Linear regression of total pretest score of all 48 physician and nonphysician screenees against demographic and historical variables revealed no significant relationship, and the resulting model explained only 13 % of the observed variation (Table 3). Examination of the differences between physician screenees and physicians from the comparison group revealed no significant differences by demographic characteristics of age, gender, and race. However, there was a significant differences between screened physicians and screened nonphysicians (Table 4), with significantly more nonphysicians being female ($p = 0.003$).

Among the screened physicians there was a significant improvement in glaucoma knowledge as judged by the overall score change between the pretest and post-test, and this improvement was evident for all three questions. However, the nonphysicians did not show significant improvement; in fact, on all three questions there was a nonsignificant deterioration in performance (Table 5). A comparison of the scores of the screened physicians on the post-test to the scores of the control, nonscreened physicians demonstrated a better performance on all three questions, with a significantly higher total score (Table 6).

Table 4. Intergroup demographic differences: screened physicians compated to nonscreened physicians and to screened nonphysicians (independent sample t-tests)

Demographic	Nonscreened physicians ($n = 26$)	p value	Screened physicians ($n = 31$)	p value	Screened nonphysicians ($n = 17$)
Gender (% male)	68 %	0.44	77 %	0.003	35 %
Age*	1.46	0.32	1.65	0.79	1.59
Race (% African-American)	100 %	0.32	97 %	0.46	100 %
History of vascular disease	NA	NA	26 %	0.86	24 %
History of eye problem	NA	NA	35 %	0.25	53 %
Family history of glaucoma	NA	NA	45 %	0.80	41 %

*$1 \le 50$; $2 = 50$–64; $3 = 65$–74; $4 \ge 74$

Table 5. Change in knowledge from pretest to post-test

	Mean pretest score	Mean post-test score	p value
Screened physicians ($n = 31$)			
Total score	9.9	10.9	0.016
Q1	5.9	6.2	
Q2	0.06	0.23	
Q3	3.9	4.5	
Screened nonphysicians ($n = 17$)			
Total score	10.1	9.6	0.41
Q1	5.9	5.7	
Q2	0.06	0.00	
Q3	4.1	3.9	

Table 6. Comparison of post-test of screened physicians to pretest of nonscreened physicians

	Post-test screened physicians ($n = 31$)	Pretest nonscreened physicians ($n = 26$)	p value
Total score	10.9	9.2	0.002
Q1	6.2	5.5	
Q2	0.23	0.08	
Q3	4.5	3.6	

Table 7. Linear regression on change of score from pretest to post-test

Variable	B statistic	t statistic	p value
Gender	−0.47	−0.58	0.57
Age category	−0.78	−1.48	0.15
Race	0.47	0.19	0.85
History vascular disease	0.61	0.65	0.52
History of eye problem	0.47	0.33	0.74
History of myopia	0.63	0.42	0.67
Family history glaucoma	−0.47	−0.59	0.56
Reason for exam: prevention	0.85	0.82	0.41
Reason for exam: person at risk	1.93	1.80	0.08
Region of residence (East vs other)	−0.12	−0.16	0.88
Referral for further testing	−1.73	−1.53	0.14
(Constant)	2.33	0.89	0.37

Total R-squared $= 0.19$; $p = 0.68$.

Linear regression of the change in total score was performed against demographic and historical variables among both groups of screenees (Table 7). No significant relationship was demonstrated for gender, age, race, personal histories of vascular disease or eye problems, family history of glaucoma, U.S. region of residence, or whether a referral for further testing of that individual resulted from the screening. Overall, the regression model explained only 19 % of the variance and was not statistically significant from zero.

Discussion

The answer to the primary question posed by this impact evaluation is that the Glaucoma Awareness Program is effective in improving the level of knowledge of glaucoma among physicians attending glaucoma screenings at a national medical meeting, when measured 4–6 months after completion of the program. This beneficial effect of the program could not be demonstrated among medically sophisticated nonphysicians who volunteered for screening, despite the fact that they started with similar knowledge levels and received the same education as the physicians. However, since the target population of the Glaucoma Awareness Program is primary care physicians, the demonstrated positive impact on nonophthalmic physicians would appear to provide justification for its continuance.

Considering the patched, single group, pretest/post-test design enhanced with a static comparison group used in this impact evaluation, there were several threats to internal validity, but other potential threats were not operative. No history-selection interaction effects were anticipated. Maturation effects limited to the screened population were unlikely, except among participants identified as abnormal on screening (who could be identified and stratified) who might have been motivated to learn more independently. Testing effects were probably operative, even though the interval of 4–6 months between tests was long.

Instrumentation effects were absent because the pretest and post-test were identical. Participants were not selected because of their performance on the test, so no regression artifacts were anticipated. Differential response rate of the screened group and the comparison group were expected and observed, and efforts to increase yield were more productive in the screened group.

Threats to external validity related principally to whether the group of screenees differed in any material way from those who did not volunteer for screening, and hence the results observed would not be generalizable to the larger universe of physician members of the NMA. The comparison group of physicians drawn as a random sample of NMA members was not significantly different from those volunteering for screening on a number of demographic and historical criteria, and there was no difference in the total score on the questionnaire. The similar questionnaire scores were obtained at different time points: previous to education in August, 1997 for the screenees, and in early 1998 for the comparison group. The similar scores observed would imply, first, that the screenees, whether they were motivated to attend the screening because they were aware of personal risk for glaucoma or not, did not have a greater knowledge of the disease than those who did not volunteer. Second, it implies that there was no event between August 1997 and early 1998 that produced improved knowledge in all physicians members of the NMA that was attributed statistically to our educational intervention.

It might have been preferable to have designed this study with a true control group, in which attendees appearing for screening were randomized into those receiving glaucoma education and those not receiving education. Because of the logistics of the screening, such a design was not possible. Besides, there was less interest in whether the education per se resulted in improved knowledge than whether the program in its entirely did so. Thus control by randomization of other variables such as increased attention to glaucoma-related information appearing between the screening and the post-test was not necessary.

There was no comparison group of nonscreened nonphysicians available to survey. It was clear that the screened nonphysicians did not represent a cross-section of the lay public, since their knowledge on the pretest was at least as good as the physicians. Examination of their occupations revealed that most worked in the medical field, as office assistants, nurses, public health officials, and pharmaceutical representatives. Assembling a comparison group with comparable backgrounds would have been difficult, even with a list of meeting registrants, which the NMA was not willing to provide.

The results reported here are preliminary, representing an overall response rate of 20 % among the screenees and 10 % among the comparison group. The reasons for the low response rate in early returns may relate to the fact that the respondents are physicians and other medical professionals that characteristically have low response rates to mail (or FAX) surveys. This low response rate leaves open the possibility that screenees who responded were more likely to do so because they experienced an improved awareness of glaucoma and were therefore motivated to complete the questionnaire. The fact that post-test responses were individually paired with the same person's pretest responses eliminates the possibility that screenees who knew more about glaucoma completed the post-test and were compared to a larger population of pretest scores from screenees less knowledgeable about glaucoma.

While only very limited demographic and historical data were collected in the interests of brevity, there was no relationship between any of these variables and level of knowledge of glaucoma on the pretest. This result runs counter to the intuitive deduction that people who have personal risk factors for glaucoma would be more knowledgeable about the disease, having been motivated to learn more about it out of self-interest.

Examination of the pretest by item revealed a wide range of correct responses. As expected, few of the respondents knew that intraocular pressure was an unreliable indicator of glaucoma in an individual patient. (Most pressures in the population in the abnormally high range are found in normals without glaucoma [ocular hypertensives], and 50 % of glaucoma patients have normal intraocular pressure when tested with a single reading.) Although post-test results indicated some improvement in knowledge on this question, the effect of years of emphasis of intraocular pressure in glaucoma teaching proved difficult to erase in a single encounter. In a similar vein, more than half of the respondents thought incorrectly that systemic hypertension was a risk factor for glaucoma, perhaps relying on historical wisdom that the two diseases are related. Interestingly, physicians and nonphysicians scored similarly on most items, except that nonphysicians incorrectly overemphasized the role of symptomatic visual difficulty in detecting glaucoma damage, while correctly underemphasizing the role of pain. The fact that the nonphysicians were medically sophisticated probably explains this similar overall performance. Interestingly, participants were uniformly intrigued by whether their answers to the questions were correct, giving a focal point for the ophthalmologist's instruction before screening, so the pretest will probably be retained as a feature of the education program even after the evaluation phase is concluded.

Change in glaucoma awareness between pretest and post-test was significant only for physicians. There is no apparent explanation for the failure of the program to improve the knowledge level of nonphysicians; in fact, the trend of knowledge was downward, so small sample size alone cannot be invoked. Limited demographic and historical variables did not appear to correlate with change in score in a regression model, except that persons attending the screening for a preventive exam (in a dummy variable with personal risk, information, and curiosity as the alternative) seemed to show better score improvement. The glib explanation that people with a preventive, public health focus are better learners is probably not justified. Again, an intuitive deduction was not supported by the evidence: people who received a referral for further glaucoma testing as a result of an abnormal screening might be motivated to learn more about glaucoma than those not referred.

While there was a significant difference in knowledge attributable to the Glaucoma Awareness Program, the mean change in score was just over one on a scale of 16. It might be argued that a change of such minor degree was not worth the resources expended on the project. However, it is difficult to demonstrate an enduring effect from a single brief intervention, and the fact that significance was reached with a modest sample size is encouraging, indeed. Perhaps a larger effect, broader effect among the membership, and/or longer lasting knowledge change would result from repetition of the project at sequential meetings over several years.

The implications of this impact evaluation are that the Glaucoma Awareness Program has a demonstrable positive effect on knowledge level of the primary target population of nonophthalmic physicians. Coupled with the subjective improvement of attitude towards ophthalmology for being at the meeting and donating time and energy, and the detection of cases of glaucoma and other eye disease among busy professionals, there is ample evidence supporting continuation of the project. Not only will the American Academy of Ophthalmology be more likely to continue its sponsorship, but pharmaceutical companies or foundations with an interest in glaucoma may be interested in funding the project into the future. Dissemination of the results of this evaluation, when completed with results from additional respondents, will be of interest not only to the Academy of Ophthalmology, but to the wider scientific community and local organizations of ophthalmologists considering staging similar programs.

References

1. Etzwiler DD (1994) Diabetes Translation – a blueprint for the future. Diabetes Care 17:1–4
2. Shepherd J, Pratt M (1996) Prevention of coronary heart disease in clinical practice: commentary on current treatment patters in six European countries in relation to published recommendations. Cardiology 87:1–5
3. Anderson FA Jr, Wheeler HB, Goldbery RJ, Hosmer DW, Forcier A, Patwardhan NA (1994) Changing clinical practice. Prospective study of the continuing medical education and quality assurance programs on the use of prophylaxis for venous thromboembolism. Arch Intern Med 154:669–677
4. Salant P, Dillman DA (1994) How to conduct your own survey. John Wiley and Sons, NY pp 102–121

Disc Damage as a Prognostic and Therapeutic Consideration in the Management of Patients with Glaucoma

G. L. Spaeth, S. Hwang and M. Gomes

Introduction

Some patients with glaucoma do not get worse, some get worse slowly, and some get worse rapidly. It would be desirable to know what characteristics allow accurate prediction of who will not get worse, who will get worse slowly, and who will get worse rapidly. Analyses have been done using various criteria (Table 1). Many of these have been done in an effort to determine what will provide the most sensitive indicator for future worsening of glaucoma.

Regardless of the conclusions of these studies, current practice still focuses on the level of intraocular pressure and only secondarily on other factors, such as the amount of optic nerve damage or visual field loss.

Because lowering intraocular pressure is the only proven method of preventing patients with glaucoma from getting worse, attention has clearly been directed overwhelmingly to how and how much to lower intraocular pressure. Over the years this has changed (Table 2). Current recommendations are to lower intraocular pressure to a "target pressure", which is largely determined as an absolute or percentage decrease

Table 1. Factors implicated in patients with glaucoma whose condition deteriorates

1. Level of intraocular pressure
2. Other factors such as
   a. Family history, genes, race
   b. Diagnostic entity – pigment dispersion syndrome, exfoliation syndrome
   c. Obesity, cardiovascular system
   d. Myopia
3. Amount of disc damage present

Table 2. Strategies of caring for patients with glaucoma

1. Lower the intraocular pressure below 21 mm Hg.
2. Lower intraocular pressure until there is no continuing deterioration of visual field.
3. Lower intraocular pressure until there is no continuing deterioration of the optic nerve.
4. Lower intraocular pressure to a specifically calculated "target pressure".
5. Lower intraocular pressure until the optic disc or visual field improves.
6. Use the amount and type of disc damage as the basis for determining the intensity of therapy.
7. Use the amount and type of disc damage as the basis for determining the intensity of therapy modified by various risk factors.

in intraocular pressure from baseline intraocular pressure, sometimes modified by lowering the target pressure still further if optic nerve damage is severe [1-3].

There have been studies to determine whether reducing the level of intraocular pressure is an effective way of managing glaucoma, though these studies are difficult to perform and are surprisingly few in number [4-11].

Lowering intraocular pressure does benefit some patients. The higher the intraocular pressure the greater the likelihood that the glaucoma will progress. When people have intraocular pressure consistently below 15 mm Hg, the likelihood of continuing deteriorations is small [11]. Nevertheless, there is still no way to predict accurately what specific intraocular pressure will be appropriate for a specific patient. The population studies provide guidelines, but only guidelines.

It is not appropriate to lower the intraocular pressure to 15 mm Hg or less in all patients. In the first place many patients do not need to have their intraocular pressure lowered to 15 mm Hg in order to avoid getting worse, and second, both medical and surgical treatments cause side effects and complications. Third, low pressure itself can be associated with significant problems: hypotony maculopathy, poor sight due to unstable refraction, increased incidence of retinal vein occlusion, and more rapid loss of visual field.

Just how much the intraocular pressure needs to be lowered in a specific patient, then, is still a matter which has not been resolved. One suggestion has been to lower intraocular pressure until there is an improvement in disc or visual field [12, 13].

However, valid improvement in visual field is difficult to document because of the variability of the test. Definite improvement in the appearance of the optic nerve also is difficult to document, not only because of limitations in our ability to see such improvement, but also because once the disc has become badly damaged, improvement is less likely to occur. A prospective way to determine how much the intraocular pressure needs to be lowered in a specific patient prior to the initiation of therapy would be a major help.

It has long been believed that patients with marked optic nerve damage are at greater risk for getting worse than patients with lesser amounts of optic nerve damage [11, 14, 15]. That is, patients with "healthy-appearing" optic discs appear to be less likely to end up with serious visual problems than are patients who start with "unhealthy"-appearing optic discs.

Here, we present a pilot study designed to evaluate use of optic disc damage as a predictive indicator of deterioration of vision in patients with glaucoma and a proposal for a method of management based on the presumed health of the optic disc and factors that affect the health of the optic disc.

Materials and Methods

We reviewed 500 charts selected at random from the files in the office of the author. In order to be included in this series of charts reviewed, the patient had to have been seen within the past year and to have been followed for a minimum of 10 years. All patients had to have a diagnosis of glaucoma, or to be considered suspect for having glaucoma on the basis of an elevated intraocular pressure. The patients' optic discs were classified according to the system indicated in Table 1. In this staging system

Table 3. Stages of glaucoma: 500 cases

Stage	Optic disc characteristics	Number (%)
0	Healthy-appearing, without apparent cupping or pallor	141 (28)
I	Suspect (cup asymmetry 0.1 to 0.2 c/d, rim width at inferior pole 0.2–0.3 c/d, cup 0.5 c/d or geater, vertical cup 0.1 c/d larger than horizontal cup)	147 (29)
II	Questionable damage (asymmetry 0.2–0.3 c/d; rim width 0.1 to 0.2 c/d; questionable notch, questionable saucer	64 (13)
III	Definite damage (asymmetry 0.4 or greater; rim loss in one quadrant; definite notch, definite acquired pit, disc hemorrhage crossing rim)	41 (8)
IV	Marked damage (rim lost in two or more quadrants, superior and inferior notches)	106 (20)
Total		500 (100)

healthy-appearing discs were considered as stage 0, and patients with far-advanced cupping at stage IV, with intermediate stages between (Table 3). Additional information collated included age, race, sex, intraocular pressure, positive family history of glaucoma, presence or absence of systemic hypertension, presence or absence of cardiovascular disease.

Results

Shown in Table 4 is the number of cases in which patients showed a deterioration of the optic disc by at least one stage. Nineteen of the 500 patients showed a deterioration of two stages or more. A review of these charts showed that:

1. In five patients the deterioration was associated with a complication of surgery (four, a complication of cataract extraction, and one, a complication of a tube-shunt procedure).
2. In four patients the progressive damage occurred despite pressure that were thought to be in a "satisfactory range", all four of these patients had "low-pressure glaucoma" (maximum intraocular pressure was 15 mm Hg).
3. In four patients management of glaucoma with medicines was nerve considered to have brought the intraocular pressure into a range that was definitely satisfactory, pressures remaining in the 20s despite significant damage; the patients were advised to have surgery, but chose not to have surgery (one had chronic angle-closure glaucoma, another a combination of angle-recession glaucoma and pigmentary glaucoma, and the remaining two, primary open-angle glaucoma).

Table 4. The number of cases in which patients showed a deterioration of the optic disc by at least one stage

Stage	Number (percentage)
0	11 (8)
I	8 (6)
II	26 (40)
III	20 (50)
IV	? (?)

4. Two patients stopped coming for their appointments for an interval during which they did not use medication; during that interval their glaucoma became worse.
5. One patient with a primary open-angle glaucoma in which the disc had focal damage did not use her medications routinely, as a result of which the intraocular pressure was unstable.
6. One patient (whose right eye had been enucleated for complications associated with essential iris atrophy) had an apparently stable primary open-angle glaucoma in the left eye for 12 years; however, the optic disc and visual field of the left eye quite rapidly deteriorated within a period of 1 year, during which time the intraocular pressure did not appear to be higher than it had been for the 12 years that the patient had shown no deterioration. The maximum intraocular pressure during the period of apparent stability was 18 mm Hg. Following surgery, which lowered the intraocular pressure in the left eye to around 12 mm Hg, further deterioration did not occur.
7. One patient, a physician with myopia, chose not to use medications while the pressure was in the 20s or low 30s, until the deterioration became unmistakable, at which time therapy was started.
8. In one patient, who had a combined-mechanism type of glaucoma, an angle-closure attack occurred, causing significant deterioration.

Discussion

The results of this retrospective study, in which the difference between the stages is quite arbitrary, and in which no attempt was made to make the groups comparable, are only suggestive. However, deterioration was clearly far more likely to occur in patients with more marked damage than in those with less marked damage.

The present report is not a critical study of the factors that predispose to patients getting worse. In considering the 19 patients in whom a deterioration of more than two stages occurred, there was no conspicuous pattern of causality. There did not appear to be a relationship between intraocular pressure, family history, or any of the other information available on the charts. While "elevated" intraocular pressure appeared to play a role in the deterioration of eight of the 500 patients who got worse, five got worse despite intraocular pressures in a range around 15 mm Hg or below.

One might argue that the present system of management based on lowering intraocular pressure until one achieves stability of disc and field is an adequate method, and therefore a different management algorithm is not necessary. But in fact, this system guarantees overtreatment or undertreatment of some patients. One estimates a target pressure, tries to get the intraocular pressure into that range, and then monitors the disc and visual field. If these get worse, then the target pressure is lowered and more vigorous treatment given. If the discs and visual fields do not get worse, it is assumed that the target pressure is in a satisfactory range, and the therapy is continued in a way designed to keep the patient's intraocular pressure at that same level. What is the consequence of this method? In some patients the target pressure will certainly be higher than required and in others it will actually be actually lower than required to maintain stability. The former group of patients are undertreated and lose visual field, while the latter group of patients are overtreated and, while stable, have unnecessary side effects or complications.

Table 5. Disc staging system

Stage	Extent of disc damage	Findings						
		R/L asym-metry	Thinnest width of rim[a]	Notch present	Disc hemor-rhage present	Vertical/horizontal dimen-sions	Shape[b] (APON)	Rim thinner than before
0	No damage	0	More than 0.2	No	No	Isn't[c]	Normal	No
1	Probably normal	0.1+	0.2	No	No	0.1[d]	Normal	No
2	Possibly normal	0.2+	0.15	No	No	0.2[d]	?	No
3	Probable damage	0.3+	0.1	Possibly	Yes	0.3[d]	?	No
4	Mild damage	–	0.01-0.1	Yes	Yes	–	Abnormal	Less than 0.1
5	Moderate damage	–	0 for less than 60° AND	Yes or	Yes	– or	Abnormal	Less than 0.2
6	Marked damage	–	0 for 61°-120° AND	–	Yes	– or	Abnormal	–
7	Far advanced damage	–	0 for greater than 121° AND	–	Yes	–	Abnormal	–

+ In terms of c/d ratio.
[a] Graded in terms of rim radius (greatest measurement possible = 0.5; thus, 0.5 = no loss and 0.0 = complete loss, no remaining rim
[b] Shape refers to pattern of cupping and whether this appears "glaucomatous" – HRT grade may be used.
[c] Relative width of rim should be thickest inferiorly, next superiorly, next nasally, and thinnest temporally.
[d] Refers to size of vertical c/d – horizontal c/d ratio.

What is proposed here is a system of management based on the belief that patients with healthier discs are less likely to deteriorate than those with less healthy discs. Additionally, various risk factors are incorporated as modifiers.

In order to increase the sensitivity of the disc grading scale, and to allow smaller amounts of damage to be recorded as a change, the number of stages has been increased from that utilized in the pilot study reported earlier here. Specifically, seven stages of damage are specified in Table 5. The risk factors that serve as modifiers are shown in Table 6. These risk factors are weighed according to an arbitrary scale indicated in Table 5. Management, then, is based on adding the grade of disc damage of the severity of the risk factors. The higher the total score the more likely the patient is to develop sufficient damage that the patient's health will be harmed by the presence of the glaucoma. The risk factors, then, include the duration that the patient will be at risk for getting damage, since this is an essential aspect in estimating the likelihood that the patient's function will be affected by the glaucoma.

Table 6. Modifying risk factors used with the disc staging system

- the duration in years during which the patient is expected to be at risk for getting worse
- the family history
- the race
- the level of intraocular pressure
- the presence of the pigment dispersion syndrome
- the presence of the exfoliation syndrome
- the presence and degree of myopia
- whether or not the patient is obese

There are obvious shortcomings to the method of management by "disk and risk" proposed here. The significance of one risk factor may be far greater in one patient than in another. The weighting of the risk factors is highly arbitrary. Furthermore, the desires and needs of the patient and of the physician must both be considered in arriving at a rational therapeutic plan. An additional significant shortcoming relates to the fact that healthy optic discs vary markedly, and visual field loss can occur even in the absence of an apparent deterioration of the optic disc.

An additional shortcoming of this plan of management is that it is directed toward the *control of glaucoma in one eye* rather than to *preservation of health in the patient*. It assumes that the goal is to prevent significant loss in *either* eye. This is, in fact, the way therapy is directed at present. However, this method also needs to be examined critically. In my opinion it is more appropriate to manage patients on the basis of preservation of the patient's entire health, of which visual function is one important part, but only one part. It may be appropriate to "allow" the optic nerve to deteriorate in some patients. The costs to the patient's health of trying to prevent any unilateral deterioration may be far greater than the costs associated with worsening of the nerve. However, that subject, though appropriate, is deferred for another discussion. The results of the CIGTS study should provide important help in this regard [3].

Neuronal damage needs to be fairly extensive before visual field loss becomes detectable using the most sensitive methods available [18]. Additional neuronal damage is required before the visual field loss becomes noticeable to the patient, and still additional damage before the visual field loss becomes sufficiently extensive that it interferes with the patient's ability to function (Fig. 1). It is obvious that the healthier the disc the greater is the complement of neurons that needs to be lost prior to the patient developing detectable visual field loss, symptomatic visual field loss, or loss of visual function. Since patients have no visual symptoms from glaucoma when their discs are entirely healthy, the only justification for initiating treatment in a patient with a healthy disc is the intent to prevent the development of functional loss in the future.

It is believed that discs that are already damaged are more susceptible to continuing damage than are discs that are not already damaged [11, 14–16]. This can be supported on theoretical grounds, but there is no meaningful clinical evidence to support this. The fact that patients with damage discs tend to get worse more rapidly than patients who do not have damaged discs may not be a factor of the disc being damaged already, but rather a factor of the sensitivity of the disc to becoming damaged. Discs that are more damaged may have become more damaged merely because they are more susceptible to damage. However, there is evidence that the disc can sustain damage to the point of developing visual field loss and yet recover, with apparently no lasting damage [5, 19, 20]. If the existence of existing damage, even in the early stages, made the optic nerve more susceptible to continuing damage, then more patients with stage II optic nerve damage should have deteriorated than those with stage I damage. Yet that was not found in the current study. That is was not found may be a consequence of relatively small numbers or of lack of validity of the staging system. In any case the present study did *not* support the hypothesis that early damage to the optic nerve makes the optic nerve more susceptible to continuing damage.

Putting all this together, it is hard to justify treating patients with undamaged appearing optic discs merely because of the theoretical belief that perhaps one might be more successful in preventing functional damage in the future. However, when

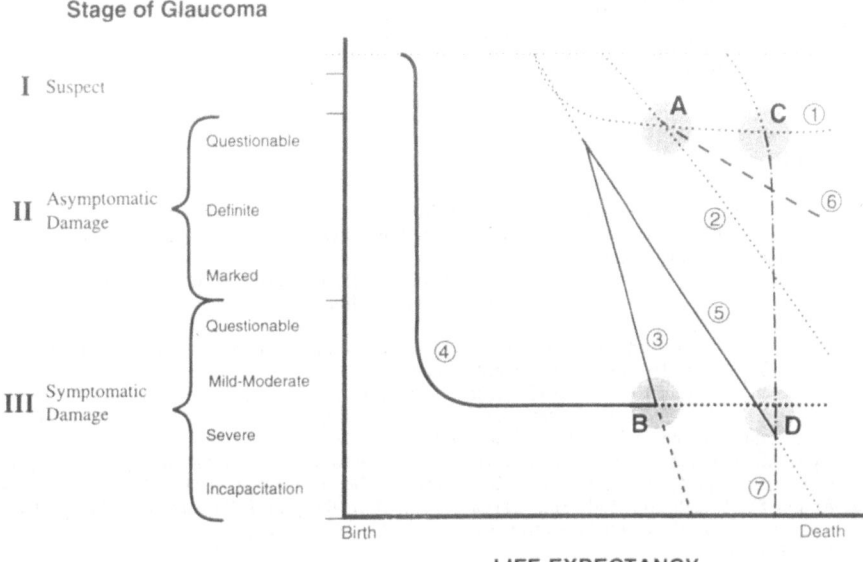

Fig. 1. Glaucoma graph. The glaucoma graph is a way of determining and understanding the clinical course of glaucoma in an individual patient. On the *y axis* of the graph is the stage of the glaucoma, and on the *x axis* is the life expectancy. The slope and the curve of each of the individual lines are determined and graphed in different ways: *Dotted lines* indicate that the slope and the curve have been determined by plotting the results of serial studies, such as repeated disc photographs taken yearly or repeated visual field examinations. *Solid lines* depict the clinical course as described in the patient's history. *Dashed lines* are extrapolations that are presumed to represent what will happen in the future. These hypothetical, extrapolated future courses are based on the nature of the previous courses and on knowledge of what has happened since a known point in time. This illustration shows the courses of seven different patients with different manifestations of glaucoma: A patient at point "A" has minimal glaucoma, and about one third of his or her life still to live. A patient at point "B" has advanced glaucoma and has about one third of his or her life still to live. A patient at point "C" has very early glaucoma and only a few years to live. A patient at point "D" has advanced glaucoma and only a few years to live. For further details, see Appendixes 1 and 2

patients have developed moderate or marked damage, they do indeed appear to be at far greater risk for developing continuing damage. Whether this is due to an increased sensitivity of the optic nerve, or whether it is a sign of an optic nerve that is predisposed to damage, the conclusion is that such patients need more vigorous therapy than patients with earlier stages of disc damage.

This study and a few considerations from the literature suggest that there is little justification for vigorous treatment of patients with healthy-appearing optic discs, and there may be no need for therapy at all. In contrast, patients with advanced cupping not only have a greater disposition to get worse, but also they are more likely to be affected by any worse thing that occurs. Consequently, as a general guideline it appears justified to treat such patients vigorously [11, 15, 16].

It is the thesis of this report that a major change needs to be introduced into the basic guidelines for therapy. These guidelines should not be primarily related to the level of intraocular pressure *but rather to the amount of disc damage that is present,* the rate at which the disc damage is progressing, and the duration for which the disc damage is expected to occur. This method already has been proposed, and the current report provides further support.

References

1. American Academy of Ophthalmology. (1) Primary Open-Angle Glaucoma (1996). (2) Primary Open-Angle Glaucoma Suspect (1995). Preferred Practice Patterns. San Francisco: American Academy of Ophthalmology
2. The Advanced Glaucoma Intervention Study Group (1998) The Advanced Glaucoma Intervention Study (AGIS): 4. Comparison of treatment outcomes within race. Seven-year results. Ophthalmology 105:1146–1164
3. Wilson MR, Gaasterland D (1996) Translating research into practice: controlled clinical trials and their influence on glaucoma management. J Glaucoma 5:139–146
4. Kronfeld PC, McGarry HI (1948) Five year follow up of glaucomas. JAMA 136:957–965
5. Shiose Y, Kanda T (1974) Quantitative analysis of "optic cup" and its clinical application. Part II. Consideration on clinical cases. Jpn J Clin Ophthalmol. 28:367–374
6. Jay L, Allan D (1989) The benefit of early trabeculectomy vs conventional management in primary open-angle glaucoma relative to the severity of the disease. Eye 3:528–535
7. Araujo SV, Spaeth GL, Roth SM, Starita RJ (1995) A Ten-year Follow-up on a Prospective, Randomized Trial of Postoperative Corticosteroids after Trabeculectomy. Ophthalmology 102:1753–1759
8. Migdal C, Gregory W, Hitchings R (1994) Long-term functional outcome after early surgery compared with laser and medicine in open-angle glaucoma. Ophthalmology 101:1651–1656
9. Glaucoma Laser Trial Research Group (1990) The Glaucoma Laser Trial (GLT). 2. Results of argon laser trabeculoplasty vs topical medications. Ophthalmology 97:1403–1413
10. Normal-Tension Glaucoma Study Group (1999) Results of the Normal-Tension Glaucoma Study. Am J Ophthalmol (in press)
11. Grant WM, Burke JF Jr. (1982) Why do some people go blind from glaucoma? Ophthalmology 89:991–998
12. Spaeth GL (1994) Reversible changes in the optic disc and visual field in glaucoma. Curr Opinion in Ophthalmol 5:36–56
13. Spaeth GL, Fellman RL, Starita RL et al. (1985) A new management system for glaucoma based on improvement of the appearance of the optic disc or visual field. Trans Am Acad Ophthalmol Otolaryngol 83:269–284
14. Burgoyne CF, Quigley HA, Thompson HW, Vitale S, Varma R (1995a) Early changes in optic disc compliance and surface position in experimental glaucoma. Ophthalmology 102:1800–1809
15. Chandler P, Grant WM (1965) Lectures on glaucoma. Lea and Febiger, Philadelphia, p. 14
16. Chandler PA (1960) Long-term results in glaucoma therapy. Am J Ophthalmol 49:221–246
17. Gliklich RE, Steinmann WC, Katz LJ et al. (1987) Primary open-angle glaucoma and visual field changes. Invest Ophthalmol Vis Sci 12:63
18. Quigley HA, Adicks EM, Green WR, Maumenee AE (1981) Optic nerve damage in human glaucoma II. The site of injury and susceptibility of damage. Arch Ophthalmol 99:635–649
19. Greenidge KC, Spaeth GL, Traverso CE (1985) Change in appearance of the optic disc associated with lowering of intraocular pressure. Ophthalmology 92(7):897–903
20. Katz LJ, Spaeth GL, Cantor LB et al. (1989) Reversible optic disc cupping and visual field improvement in adults with glaucoma. Am J Ophthalmol 107:485–492

Appendix 1. The Glaucoma Graph

See Fig. 1.

- Patient no. 1, considered at point "A" has one third of his or her life to live and is an early stage of glaucoma. About one third of his or her life earlier, this patient was noted to have elevated pressure and followed without treatment. The patient continued to be followed without treatment and no damage to the optic nerve or visual field was ever noted. It is reasonable to assume that, if the patient continues to have intraocular pressures around the same level as those noted initially, he or she will probably follow the course described by line 1, and will die without any evidence of glaucoma damage.

- Patient no. 2, also considered at point "A", ie, having minimal damage with one third of his or her life left to live. In this case, however, the patient's intraocular pressure rose continuously, and the patient was noted to develop early disc field damage, which then continued at the rate depicted by the dashed line 2. This patient, if untreated, would develop definite asmyptomatic damage. However, the patient would have no functional loss at the time of his or her death.

- Patients nos. 3 and 4, at point "B": both have advanced glaucoma and one third of their lives left to live. However, patient no. 3 is deteriorating rapidly and will be blind long before he or she dies, whereas patient no. 4, who had a blow to eye as a child and lost vision to a steroid-induced glaucoma at that time, has had stable vision for most of his or her life, and it is reasonable to expect that it will continue to be stable.

- Patients at points "C" and "D" both have only a few years to live, but those at point "C" (like patients nos. 1 and 2 at point "A") have minimal damage, and those at point "D" (like patient no. 4 at point "B") have marked damage.

- Patient no. 5 started with a clinical course similar to that of patient no. 3 (advanced glaucoma and deteriorating rapidly), but around the midpoint of his or her life, the glaucoma became less severe. Nevertheless, this patient will be blind at the time of his or her death unless there is effective intervention. Compare patient no. 4, who at point "D" has the same life expectancy and the same amount of damage as patient no. 5 (only a few years to live and advanced glaucoma). Patient no. 4, however, has a stable clinical course and does not appear too need a change in therapy. In contrast, patient no. 5 needs lowering intraocular pressure urgently.

- Patient no. 6, at around point "C" also has only a few years of life remaining, bus has a glaucoma that is getting worse a little bit more slowly than that affecting patients no. 2 and 5. However, since patient no. 6 has so little damage to start with, no treatment is necessary, even though he or she is getting worse. Even without treatment, he or she will not have enough damage or visual loss due to glaucoma at the time of death that he or she will have any awareness of being sick, and will have no limitation in function.

- Patient no. 7 at point "C" has only a few years left to live, but has a type of glaucoma which is deteriorating so rapidly that even though he or she has only a short period of time of live, he or she will be blind well before the time of death.

Using the glaucoma graph to define and characterize the nature of the clinical course helps the physician and patient to understand that:

- Patients nos. 1, 4, and 6 do not need any treatment at all; patient no. 1 will never develop damage, patient no. 4 has marked damage but it is not getting worse, and patient no. 6 is getting worse so slowly that it will not interfere with his or her life.

- Patients nos. 3, 5, and 7 can be seen to need treatment urgently in order to prevent them from becoming totally blind prior to the time of their deaths.

- Patient no. 2: The need for treatment is controversial. Since this patient would never develop glaucoma, perhaps he or she should not be treated at all. But since he or she would develop some damage, those who want to prevent any damage at all would advise therapy.

Appendix 2. Specifics of grading scale for Glaucoma Graph

Stage 0: No risk factors or finding.

I. SUSPECT

    A. Less likely
       Disc findings:
       a. Asymmetry 0.1 c/d
       b. Width of inferior or superior rim 0.3 c/d
       c. c/d 0.4–0.6
       d. Vertical c/d 0.1 greater than horizontal

    B. More likely
       Disc findings:
       a. Asymmetry 0.2 c/d
       b. Width of inferior or superior rim 0.2 c/d
       c. c/d greater than 0.6
       d. Vertical c/d 0.2 greater than horizontal c/d

II. DAMAGE (refers to one eye except as specified under II C, II D, and II E)

    A. Questionable
       Disc findings:
       a. Asymmetry 0.3 c/d
       b. Rim 0.1
       c. c/d greater than 0.6
       d. Vertical c/d 0.2 greater than horizontal
       e. Questionable notch
       f. Questionable saucer
       g. Questionable shape

    B. Early
       Disc findings:
       a. Documented rim thinning of superior or inferior rim of 0.1 c/d
       b. Asymmetry 0.4
       c. Rim present all areas but less than 0.1 in one quadrant
       d. Definite notch
       e. Definite acquired pit of optic nerve
       f. Disc hermorrhage crossing rim
       g. Shape glaucomatous

    C. Moderate (or grade II B in both eyes)
       Disc findings:
       a. Documented thinning of superior or inferior disc rim 0.2 c/d
       b. Rim lost in no more than one quadrant
       c. Shape abnormal

    D. Marked (or grade II C in both eyes)
       Disc findings:
       a. Rim lost in more than one but less than three quadrants
       b. Inferior and superior notches

    E. Far Advanced (or grade II D in both eyes)
       Disc findings:
       a. Rim lost in three or more quadrants

CHAPTER 17

Disc Hemorrhage as a Risk Factor for Progression of Normal-Tension Glaucoma

Y. Kitazawa, T. Yamamoto and K. Ishida

Introduction

The pathogenesis of normal-tension glaucoma (NTG) is believed to be multifactorial. A variety of clinical factors have been implicated in the progression of optic nerve change in NTG. Intraocular pressure (IOP) plays a substantial role even in NTG eyes, which is supported by clinical evidence [1–6]. Factors other than IOP also seem to be involved in the development of glaucomatous optic neuropathy in at least a considerable number of NTG eyes. Included as the positive evidence for such factors are: a higher incidence of disc hemorrhage (DH) [7–12], more pronounced peripapillary chorioretinal atrophy [13], a higher incidence of retinal occlusive vascular diseases [9, 14], the development of glaucoma-like cupping after anterior ischemic optic neuropathy caused by giant cell arteritis [15–17], the frequently observed coexistence of several immunocompromised conditions [18, 19], the increased resistance index in orbital vessels [20], and an alteration in the diurnal curve of systemic blood pressure [21, 22].

Recently we studied clinical factors associated with progression of visual field loss in NTG patients followed more than 2 years and found that DH was one of the most important risk factors for the visual field deterioration [23]. Here, we report on the relative importance of DH among risk factors and to what extent the visual field progression is affected by DH in NTG patients.

Patients and Methods

Normal-tension glaucoma was defined by: normal open-angle; peak IOP lower than or equal to 21 mm Hg at all times including a 24-h measurement; presence of typical glaucomatous visual field defects associated with glaucomatous optic nerve changes; and presence of optic neuropathy not attributable to other ocular or systemic pathology. The subjects were 110 NTG patients selected from our patient population, consisting of 211 consecutive NTG patients, who visited the Glaucoma Service, Gifu University Hospital, during a period between January 1985 and January 1995. The selection criteria were: a follow-up period at our clinic of at least 2 years at 1- to 3-month intervals; no previous intraocular surgeries performed; mean deviation (MD) better than –15.00 decibels (dB) without threat to fixation; visual acuity better than 20/40; and reliable perimetric results with a Humphrey Field Analyzer using the Central 30-2 program, i.e., fixation loss less than 20 %, and both false positive and false negative reactions less than 33 %. When both eyes of a patient met the criteria, the eye with a

Table 1. Patients' background

Age[a] (years)	56.9±10.8	(24–75)
Sex (M/F)	30/80	
Follow up[a] (months)	51.5±22.3	(24–112)
Past history (positive/negative) systemic hypertension	28/82	
Visual acuity[a]		(20/40–20/10)
Refraction[a] (D)	–1.53±3.47	(–15.13–+3.50)
IOP at 24-h measurement[a] (mm Hg)		
Maximum	16.3±2.2	(10–20)
Mean	13.8±2.1	(8.0–19.3)
Minimum	11.2±2.3	(4–16)
Magnitude of fluctuation	5.1±1.8	(1–14)
IOP during follow-up[a] (mm Hg)	14.4±1.7	(8.8–19.0)
MD[a] (dB)	–5.91±3.72	(–14.84–+2.08)
CPSD[a] (dB)	7.56±4.03	(0.00–16.81)
Disc typing (focal ischemic/total)	67/110	
Cold recovery[a] (T1: %)	52.4±14.8	(8.3–80.8)
Blood pressure[a] (mm Hg)		
Systolic	125.3±17.5	(92–184)
Diastolic	74.9±12.5	(45–102)
Mean	91.7±13.0	(64–123)
Pulse rate[a] (bpm)	74±10	(54–98)
DH (positive/negative)	52/58	
Ocular hypotensives (user/non-user)	22/88	

From [23], with the permission of Journal of Glaucoma, Lippincott, Williams and Wilkins.
CPSD, corrected pattern standard deviation.
[a] Mean ± SD (range).

better MD was subjected to analyses. If surgical treatment was performed, only the data from the period prior to the surgery were analyzed. The number of perimetric examinations analyzed ranged from 5 to 16 (mean: 8.7). The first two perimetric results were excluded from the analysis to obviate learning effects. A perimetric result with an obvious artifact was also excluded. The clinical backgrounds of the subjects are shown in Table 1.

Two different definitions of visual field loss progression were employed: one by the visual field MD change and another by pointwise comparison. Progression by the MD change was defined as a 3.00 dB or greater deterioration demonstrated twice during the follow-up. The pointwise progression was defined by deterioration of at least two contiguous points by 10.00 dB or greater and/or deterioration of at least three contiguous points by 5.00 dB or greater, at least one of them being 10.00 dB or greater, at two consecutive perimetric examinations. The uppermost four test points of the Central 30-2 program were excluded from the analysis of the pointwise progession. When the progression of visual field loss was rated positive according to the criteria, the follow-up was deemed to have reached its endpoint when the first perimetric abnormality was detected. The Kaplan-Meier life-table method was used for calculating the probability of a stable visual field defined by each progression criterion. In addition, the Cox proportional hazards model was applied to determine the factors associated with visual field loss progression. The PC-SAS system was used for the calculation. Explanatory variables for the Cox model included age, sex, past history of systemic hypertension and diabetes mellitus, visual acuity, refractive error, several IOP parameters of a 24-h measurement without any medications, i.e., maximum, mean and minimum IOPs and the magnitude of the IOP fluctuation, and those during the follow-up, type of optic nerve head changes [12], systemic blood pressure, pulse rate, presence/absence of DH during the follow-up, recovery rate from a cold exposure test of hand [24], and treatment modality (no treatment, calcium-channel blockers, such as nifedipine and brovincamine, and/or antiglaucoma medications). The percent recovery rate at 1 and 4 min of the cold exposure test was defined as $(Tt - Tmin) / (Tpre - Tmin) \times 100$ (%) where Tt, $Tmin$, and $Tpre$ represent finger temperature at time t, minimum finger temperature, and that before the testing, respectively. If calcium-channel blockers were employed for at least the later half of the entire follow-up period, the patient was rated positive for the treatment. The indication for an oral calcium channel-blocker was decided upon at the discretion of the responsible physicians (YK, TY), taking the individual condition of each patient into consideration, especially a recovery rate from the cold challenge and/or a low IOP during the 24-h measurement. Two patients who were prescribed a calcium-channel blocker for systemic hypertension were rated positive for the treatment. The calcium-channel blockers prescribed were nifedipine 10 mg *b.i.d.* in eight patients, brovincamine 20 mg *t.i.d.* in 26 patients, and nilvadipine 4 mg *b.i.d.* in two patients. Patients prescribed brovincamine in our previous study [24] were also enrolled in the current study. The antiglaucoma medications were used in a total of 22 patients: 16 patients with a topi-

Table 2. Patients' background divided by calcium-channel blocker use

	CCB users (36 cases)		CCB non-users (74 cases)	
Age[a] (years)	56.0±10.9	(37–72)	57.4±10.8	(24–75)
Sex (M/F)	7/29		23/51	
Follow-up[a] (months)	56.9±21.9	(26–112)	48.8±22.1	(24–107)
Past history (positive/negative) systemic hypertension	9/27		19/55	
Visual acuity[a]		(20/40–20/15)		(20/40–20/10)
Refraction[a] (D)	−1.55±3.37	(−10.00 – +3.50)	−1.52±3.54	(−15.00 – +3.13)
IOP at 24-h measurement[a] (mm Hg)				
Maximum	15.9±2.3	(10–19)	16.5±2.2	(12–20)
Mean	13.5±2.0	(9.7–17.3)	13.9±2.1	(8.0–19.3)
Minimum	11.2±2.0	(7–15)	11.2±2.5	(4–16)
Magnitude of fluctuation	4.8±1.5	(1–8)	5.2±2.1	(3–14)
IOP during follow up[a] (mm Hg)	14.3±1.5	(11.6–16.7)	14.4±1.9	(8.8–19.0)
MD[a] (dB)	−6.22±4.04	(−13.36 – +0.16)	−5.75±3.57	(−14.84 – +2.08)
CPSD[a] (dB)	7.90±4.65	(0.00–16.32)	7.39±3.72	(0.66–16.81)
Disc typing (Focal ischemic/total)	22/36		45/74	
Cold recovery[a] (T1: %)	47.5±14.2	(8.3–75.6)	54.9±14.5	(21.0–80.8)
Blood pressure[a] (mm Hg)				
Systolic	124.2±15.9	(92–159)	125.9±19.6	(93–184)
Diastolic	73.1±12.3	(52–100)	75.8±12.6	(45–100)
Mean	90.1±12.1	(64–113)	92.5±13.5	(66–123)
Pulse rate[a] (bpm)	72±8	(54–88)	75±10	(55–98)
DH (positive/negative)	19/17		33/41	
Ocular hypotensives (user/non-user)	9/27		13/61	

From [23], with the permission of Journal of Glaucoma, Lippincott Williams and Wilkins.
CPSD, corrected pattern standard deviation.
[a] Mean ± SD (range).

cal β-blocker only and six with a topical β-blocker and dipivefrin. The clinical backgrounds of the subjects divided by the use of calcium-channel blockers are shown in Table 2. No statistically significant difference was found between the two groups for each parameter. The follow-up period ranged from 24 to 112 months (mean: 51.5 months).

Results

Out of 110 eyes, 22 (20%) were judged as having visual field progression during the follow-up period using the MD definition; 47 eyes (43%) were rated progressive by the pointwise definition. The Kaplan-Meier life-table method estimated that the probability of visual field loss non-progession with a standard error was 76% ± 4% at a 112-month follow-up by the MD definition and 42% ± 7% at a 112-month follow-up by the pointwise definition (Fig. 1).

In a total of 110 cases, the Cox proportional hazards model indicated that progression by the MD definition was significantly correlated with calcium-channel blocker treatment, DH, recovery rate of a cold recovery test, systolic blood pressure, and corrected pattern standard deviation (CPSD) of visual field (Table 3a). By the pointwise definition calcium-channel blocker treatment, MD, and IOP fluctuation during 24-h measurement were identified as factors associated with the field loss progression (Table 3b).

The cases were subdivided into two groups by use or non-use of calcium-channel blockers, and the probability of field stability was calculated for each group using the Kaplan-Meier life-table method. The probability of visual field loss non-progression with a standard error was 91% ± 5% at a 112-month follow-up and 70% ± 6% at a

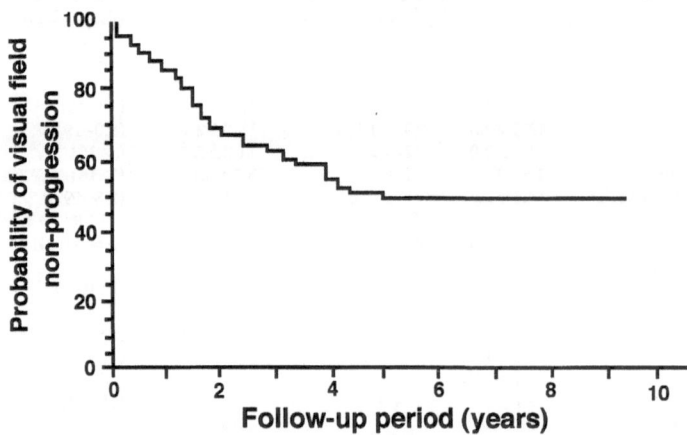

Fig. 1. Estimation of the probability of visual field loss non-progression by the Kaplan-Meier life-table method in the total 110 cases. The probability with a standard error was 76 ± 5% at a 112-month follow-up by the MD definition (*bold line*) and 48 ± 6% at a 112-month follow-up by the pointwise definition (*solid line*).
(From [23], with the permission of Journal of Glaucoma, Lippincott Williams and Wilkins)

Table 3. Factors identified to be associated with visual field loss progression by either definition of visual field progression

a. Based on the mean deviation definition; number of cases with progressive visual field loss was 22 of 110 eyes

Factor	Hazard ratio	95 % confidence	p value
CCB			
Untreated	1		
Treated	0.14	0.04–0.49	0.002
Percent recovery at 1 min in a cold recovery test by 1 % increase	0.96	0.83–0.99	0.005
Systolic blood pressure by 1 mm Hg rise	1.03	1.01–1.05	0.005
Disc hemorrhage			
Absent	1		
Present	3.62	1.40–9.32	0.008
CPSD by 1 dB increase	1.13	1.01–1.28	0.039

b. Based on the pointwise definition; number of cases with progressive field loss was 47 of 110 eyes

Factor	Hazard ratio	95 % confidence	p value
CCB			
Untreated	1		
Treated	0.47	0.20–0.83	0.014
Mean deviation by 1 dB better	0.91	0.85–0.99	0.031
IOP fluctuation during phasing[a] by 1 mm Hg increase	1.22	1.01–1.40	0.033

From [23], with the permission of Journal of Glaucoma, Lippincott Williams and Wilkins.
CCB, calcium-channel blocker; CPSD, corrected pattern standard deviation; IOP, intraocular pressure.
[a] Difference between peak IOP and trough IOP during diurnal intraocular pressure measurements.

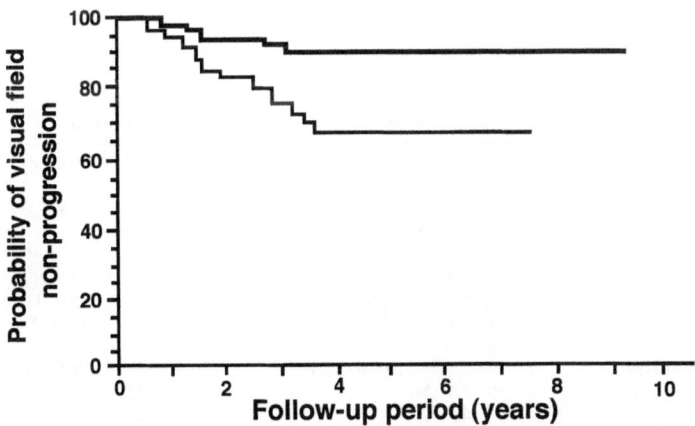

Fig. 2. Estimation of the probability of visual field loss non-progression by the Kaplan-Meier life-table method using the MD definition subdivided by the use of calcium-channel blockers. The probability with a standard error was 91 ± 5 % at a 112-month follow-up for 36 calcium-channel blocker users (*bold line*) and 68 ± 6 % at a 91-month follow-up for 74 non-users (*solid line*). The differences was statistically significant between the two groups (*p* = 0.019; Logrank test).
(From [23], with the permission of Journal of Glaucoma, Lippincott Williams and Wilkins)

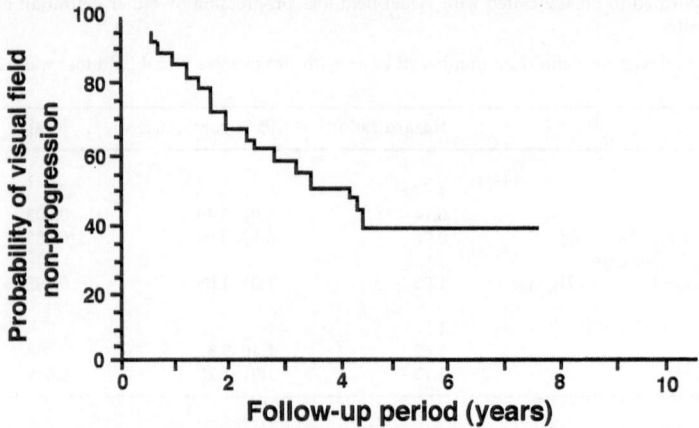

Fig. 3. Estimation of the probability of visual field loss non-progression by the Kaplan-Meier life-table method using the pointwise definition subdivided by the use of calcium-channel blockers. The probability with a standard error was 65 ± 10 % at a 112-month follow-up for 36 calcium-blocker users (*bold line*) and 39 ± 8 % at a 91-month follow-up for 74 non-users (*solid line*). The difference was statistically significant between the two groups (*p* = 0.009; Logrank test).
(From [23], with the permission of Journal of Glaucoma, Lippincott Williams and Wilkins)

91-month follow-up for calcium-channel blocker users and non-users, respectively, by the MD definition (Fig. 2). The difference was statistically significant (*p* = 0.024; Logrank test). It was 65 % ± 10 % at a 112-month follow-up and 35 % ± 7 % at a 91-month follow-up for calcium-channel blocker users and non-users, respectively, by the pointwise definition (Fig. 3). The difference was again highly significant between the two groups (*p* = 0.016; Logrank test).

Table 4. Patients' background

	DH – (38 cases)		DH + (36 cases)	
Age[a] (years)	57.1±11.0	(24–75)	57.6±10.7	(35–74)
Sex (M/F)[a]	16/22		7/29	
Follow-up[a] (months)	71.2±26.3	(30–133)	67.0±29.28	(24–138)
Refraction [b] (D)	−1.78±4.08		−1.25±2.88	
IOP at phasing[a] (mm Hg)				
Maximum	16.5±2.3	(10–20)	16.5±2.1	(12–20)
Mean	14.0±2.3	(9.7–17.3)	13.9±2.1	(8.2–17.7)
Minimum	11.4±2.4	(5–16)	11.0±2.6	(6–16)
Range	5.1±1.5	(3–9)	5.4±2.2	(3–14)
IOP during F/U[a] (mm Hg)	14.4±1.8	(8.8–19.0)	14.4±1.9	(8.9–17.2)
MD[b] (dB)	−6.53±3.96		−4.92±2.93	
CPSD[b] (dB)	8.31±3.87		6.41±3.33	
Cold recovery[a] (T1: %)	55.9±13.9	(24.2–80.8)	53.7±15.2	(21.0–75.2)
Mean BP[a] (mm Hg)	92.5±15.3	(67–123)	92.4±11.4	(70–106)
Pulse rate[a] (bpm)	73±11	(55–98)	74±10	(60–98)
Ocular hypotensives (user/non-user)	5/33		8/28	

[a] Mean ± SD (range).
[b] Mean ± SD.

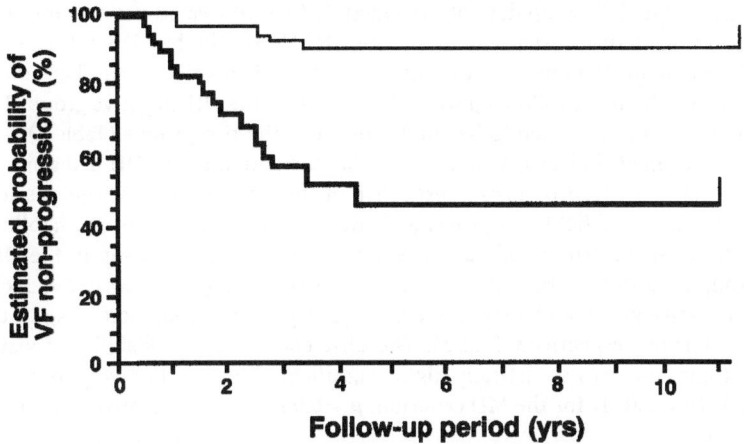

Fig. 4. Estimation of the probability of visual field (VF) loss non-progression by the Kaplan-Meier life-table method using the MD definition subdivided by the presence of disc hemorrhages. The probability patients without DH with a standard error was 89 ± 5 % at a 133-month follow-up for 38 (*solid line*) and 48 ± 9 % at a 138-month follow-up for 36 patients with DH (*bold line*). The difference was statistically significant between the two groups (*p* = 0.019; Logrank test)

Since the use of CCB was demonstrated to be a significant prognostic factor regardless of the criterion for the visual field progession, it became obvious that the significance of DH as a prognostic factor should be evaluated in patients who did not receive CCB treatment. Hence, we repeated the identical analyses in those patents who were not treated with CCB (CCB-untreated patients). The analysis was carried

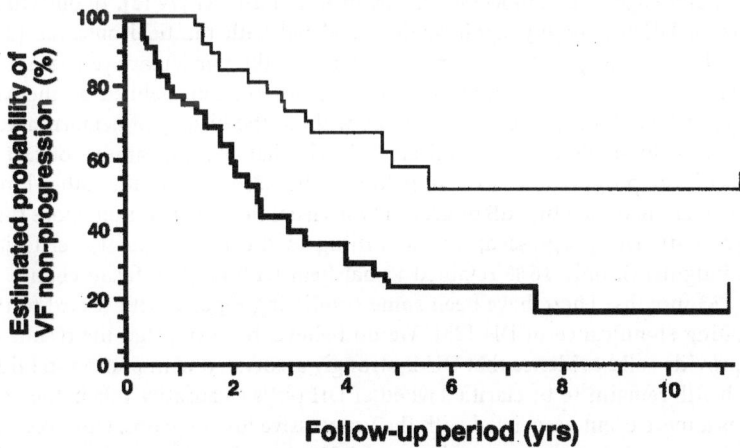

Fig. 5. Estimation of the probability of visual field (VF) loss non-progression by the Kaplan-Meier life-table method using the pointwise definition subdivided by the presence of disc hemorrhage. The probability with a standard error was 52 ± 6 % at a 133-month follow-up for 36 patients with DH (*solid line*) and 16 ± 9 % at a 138-month follow-up for 36 patients with DH (*bold line*). The difference was statistically significant between the two groups (*p* = 0.009; Logrank test)

out using the update follow-up data. We devided 74 CCB-untreated patients into two groups depending on the presence or absence of DH. Those who had DH at least once were rated positive for DH and were classified into the DH-positive group. Those who had no DH throughout the follow-up were classified into the DH-negative group. The patients' background was noted to be similar between the two groups (Table 4).

The life-table analysis clearly demonstrated that the patients with DH had a significantly worse visual field prognosis irrespective of the criterion for the progression. The probability of visual field non-progression was 89 % ± 5 % at a 138-month follow-up in the DH-negative group and 48 % ± 9 % at a 133-month follow-up in the DH-positive group according to the MD criterion, respectively (Fig. 4). It was 52 % ± 6 % in the DH-negative group and 16 % ± 9 % in the DH-positive group according to the pointwise criterion, respectively (Fig. 5). The difference in the probability of visual field non-progression was statistically highly significant between the two groups for each analysis ($p = 0.0001$ for the MD criterion; $p = 0.0018$ for the pointwise criterion; Logrank test).

Discussion

In the current study we were able to demonstrate that several factors other than IOP are significantly associated with the outcome of visual field loss progession in NTG. Of the associated factors identified by the Cox model, DH, calcium-channel blocker treatment, recovery rate of a cold recovery test, and systolic blood pressure, are considered to have little, if any, to do with IOP.

DH is well known to take place frequently in NTG patients. Although the exact mechanism of DH development is still unclear, many investigators report a significantly higher incidence of DH in NTG eyes than in other types of glaucoma and ocular hypertension and suggest a pathogenic linkage of DH and NTG [7–12]. In our study, the presence of DH was highly significantly correlated with the field outcome [23]: when an eye had a history of DH, it was estimated that the particular eye had a 3.62 times higher chance of developing visual field loss progression, defined by the MD deterioration of 3.00 dB or greater, than the one without the history of hemorrhage.

The results of life-table analysis indicated clearly that the appearance of DH is associated with the progression of visual field defects. According to the rather loose criterion (worsening of MD by 3 dB or greater) for visual field aggravation, more than 50 % of eyes with DH progressed; and according to the more sensitive criterion (pointwise judgment), only 16 % retained visual field without significant change at the end of 133 months. There have been some conflicting reports with regard to the prognosticating significance of DH [25]. We do believe, however, that the results of our study provide solid evidence that DH is strongly associated with poor visual field prognosis. It still remains to be clarified whether DH plays a causative role in the axonal loss or is a mere event associated with the progressive loss of axons. Our previous studies demonstrated that the vast majority of DH takes place in the vicinity of the border of retinal nerve fiber loss and adjacent, healthier-looking retina [26]. The finding suggests the possibility that the border of the area of nerve fiber loss reflects the most active site of pathological processes, most probably in the laminar region where there is ongoing distortion of laminar plate alignment which must be associated with the impaired return of venous blood resulting in the extravasation of blood or DH. However, the conjecture does not explain at all the distinctly higher incidence of DH in NTG as opposed to POAG or high-tension glaucoma. In these forms of glaucoma the disc changes and retinal nerve fiber loss are quite similar. Hence, the distinct difference in the prevalence of DH between POAG and NTG is hardly explainable based solely on the distortion of small vessels induced by the mechanical stress at the lamina cribrosa. Theoretically other factors including the integrity of blood vessels per se and/or blood contents probably might be different between NTG and POAG, such that hemorrhage may be more easily inducible in the former.

There has been increasing evidence that a substantial proportion of NTG patients demonstrate abnormal reactivity of small vessels to external stimuli, particularly to exposure to cold. The association of glaucoma and the abnormal response of blood flow in the finger following a cold challenge was first demonstrated by Drance and associates in 1988 [27]. They showed that both mean baseline flow and the mean flow after exposure to cold were lower in NTG patients and suggested that vasospasm has a role in the development of the disease. The association of vasospasm with NTG has also been suggested by other investigators [28], although it is still controversial [29]. Although the excessive vasospastic response cannot necessarily be associated with the loss of structural integrity of vessels, it may be taken for a sign of impaired functional integrity of vascular walls [30].

Vascular walls are affected in a variety of autoimmune diseases and in some of them blood coagulation is pathologically altered. The frequent association of autoimmune diseases with NTG also supports the notion that small vessels are more likely to be compromised in NTG patients [31].

Like NTG the majority of collagen diseases has a definite sexual preponderance, afflicting more females. In contrast, POAG evenly affects both sexes. The prevalence of DH markedly increases with aging in females, as shown in a recent study of a large number of individuals who underwent systemic and ocular examinations for the detection of geriatric diseases [32]. By contrast, the prevalence remains almost identical in adult males. The result seems to provide evidence, although circumstantial, for yet unidentified systemic factors which could be more prevalent in NTG than in POAG.

It should also be recognized that a blood clot, the result of hemorrhage, can release substances which bring about vasoconstriction, resulting in ischemia of adjacent neuronal tissue. For example, hemoglobin combines with nitric oxide and inactivates the vasodilating action of the latter [33].

The present study clearly revealed that DH indicates an ominous prognosis. It cannot be overemphasized that the pathogenesis of DH needs to be clarified in order to identify every possible means of halting the visual field progression.

References

1. Shiose Y, Kitazawa Y, Tsukahara S, Akamatsu T, Mizokami K, Futa R et al. (1991) Epidemiology of glaucoma in Japan. A nationwide glaucoma survey. Jpn J Ophthalmol 35:133–155
2. Cartwright MJ, Anderson DR (1988) Correlation of asymmetric damage with asymmetric intraocular pressure in normal-tension glaucoma (low-tension glaucoma). Arch Ophthalmol 106:898–900
3. Crichton A, Drance SM, Douglas DD, Schulzer M (1989) Unequal intraocular pressure and its relation to asymmetric visual field defects in low-tension glaucoma. Ophthalmology 96:1312–1314

4. Abedin S, Simmons RJ, Grant WM (1982) Progressive low-tension glaucoma. Treatment to stop glaucomatous cupping and field loss when these progress despite normal intraocular pressure. Ophthalmology 89:1–6
5. de Jong D, Greve EL, Hoyng PEJ, Geijssen HC (1989) Results of a filtering procedure in low tension glaucoma. Int Ophthalmol 13:131–138
6. Hitchings RA, Wu J, Poinoosawmy D, McNaught A (1995) Surgery for normal tension glaucoma. Br J Ophthalmol 79:402–406
7. Drance SM, Sweeney VP, Morgan RW, Feldman F (1973) Studies of factors involved in the production of low-tension glaucoma. Arch Ophthalmol 89:457–465
8. Chumbley LC, Brubaker RF (1976) Low-tension glaucoma. Am J Ophthalmol 81:761–767
9. Levene RZ (1980) Low tension glaucoma: A critical review and new material. Surv Ophthalmol 24:621–664
10. Gloster J (1981) Incidence of optic disc haemorrhages in chronic simple glaucoma and ocular hypertension. Br J Ophthalmol 65:452–456
11. Kitazawa Y, Shirato S, Yamamoto T (1986) Optic disc hemorrhage in low-tension glaucoma. Ophthalmology 93:853–857
12. Geijssen HC (1991) Studies on normal pressure glaucoma. Kugler, New York
13. Araie M, Sekine M, Suzuki Y, Koseki N (1994) Factors contributing to the progression of visual field damage in eyes with normal-tension glaucoma. Ophthalmology 101:1440–1444
14. Sonnsjö B, Krakau CET (1993) Arguments for a vascular glaucoma etiology. Acta Ophthalmol 71:433–444
15. Hayreh SS (1974) Pathogenesis of cupping of the optic disc. Br J Ophthalmol 58:863–876
16. Hayreh SS (1974) Anterior ischaemic optic neuropathy. II. Fundus on ophthalmoscopy and fluorescein angiography. Br J Ophthalmol 58:964–980
17. Sebag J, Thomas JV, Epstein DL, Grant WM (1986) Optic disc cupping in anterior ischemic neuropathy resembles glaucomatous cupping. Ophthalmology 93:357–361
18. Cartwright MJ, Grajewski AL, Friedberg ML, Anderson DR, Richards DW (1992) Immune related disease and normal-tension glaucoma. A case-control study. Arch Ophthalmol 110:500–502
19. Wax MB, Barrett DA, Pestronk A (1994) Increased incidence of paraproteinemia and autoantibodies in patients with normal-pressure glaucoma. Am J Ophthalmol 117:561–568
20. Harris A, Sergott RC, Spaeth GL, Katz JL, Shoemaker JA, Martin BJ (1994) Color Doppler analysis of ocular vessel blood velocity in normal-tension glaucoma. Am J Ophthalmol 118:642–649
21. Graham SL, Drance SM, Wijsman K, Douglas GR, Mikelberg FS (1995) Ambulatory blood pressure monitoring in glaucoma. The nocturnal dip. Ophthalmology 102:61–69
22. Meyer JH, Brandi-Dohrn J, Funk J (1996) Twenty four hour blood pressure monitoring in normal tension glaucoma. Br J Ophthalmol 80:864–867
23. Ishida K, Yamamoto T, Kitazawa Y (1998) Clinical factors associated with the progression of normal tension glaucoma. J Glaucoma 7:372–377
24. Sawada A, Kitazawa Y, Yamamoto T, Okabe I, Ichien K (1996) Prevention of visual field defect progression with brovincamine in eyes with normal-tension glaucoma. Ophthalmology 103:283–288
25. Drans SM (1989) Disc hemorrhages in the glaucomas. Surv Ophthalmol 331–337
26. Sugiyama K, Tomita G, Kitazawa Y, Onda E, Shinohara H, Park KH (1997) The association of optic disc hemorrhage with retinal nerve fiber layer defect and peripapillary atrophy in normal-tension glaucoma. Ophthalmology 104:1926–1933
27. Drance SM, Douglas GR, Wijsman K, Schulzer M, Britton RJ (1988) Response of blood flow to warm and cold in normal and low-tension glaucoma patients. Am J Ophthalmol 105:35–39
28. Gasser P, Flammer J (1991) Blood-cell velocity in the nailfold capillaries of patients with normal-tension and high-tension glaucoma. Am J Ophthalmol 111:585–588
29. Usui T, Iwata K (1992) Finger blood flow in patients with low tension glaucoma and primary open-angle glaucoma. Br J Ophthalmol 76:2–4
30. Okabe I, Kitazawa Y (1994) Glaucoma secondary to vascular insufficiency: should more attention be focused on microcirculatory factors? J Glaucoma 3:181–183
31. Cartwright MJ, Grajewski AL, Friedberg ML, Anderson DR, Richards DW (1992) Immune-related disease and normal tension glaucoma. A case-control study. Arch Ophthalmol 110:500–502
32. Hayakawa T, Sugiyama K, Tomita G, Kawase K, Onda E, Shinohara H, Tsuji A, Kitazawa Y (1999) Correlation of the peripapillary atrophy area with optic disc cupping and disc hemorrhage. J Glaucoma (in press)
33. Furchgott RF, Martin W, Cherry PD (1985) Blockage of endothelium-dependent vasodilation by hemoglobin: a possible factor in vasospasm associated with hemorrhage. Throb Leuk Res 15:488–502

CHAPTER 18

What is the Potential for Optic Disc Imaging in the Management of POAG?

R. A. Hitchings

Introduction

The management of chronic glaucoma has to be directed towards the prevention of further visual loss. Although it has been traditional to lower intraocular pressure, this approach can only be seen as manipulation of a risk factor for progression. The true outcomes for management are both the halting/slowing of the rate of visual loss and glaucomatous cupping of the optic disc. Here, I discuss whether there is a role at the present time for optic disc imaging in management of POAG. Can sequential imaging of the optic disc demonstrate changes which indicate progression, and can these changes be seen to predate changes in the visual field?

I have used data from a prospective longitudinal study of patients with ocular hypertension to address this question.

Material and Methods

Patients with ocular hypertension were entered into a treatment/no treatment study at Moorfields Eye Hospital. They were followed for a minimum of 2 years together with a group of age matched normals. During that period each subject underwent sequential imaging of the optic disc with the scanning laser ophthalmoscope (Heidelberg Instruments, Heidelberg, Germany), the images being obtained 12 months apart. For analysis each image was divided into six segments (superotemporal, temporal, inferotemporal, inferonasal, nasal, and superonasal) and the area of the neuroretinal rim and optic cup within each segment was measured (Software version 2.01). For each subject the contour line was exported to sequential images to ensure continuity between measurements. Two images were analysed for each study eye and are known for the purposes of comparison as SLO 1 and SLO 2.

The normal subjects were age matched with the patient group. Each subject had in addition to a normal intraocular pressures a normal visual field when tested with threshold perimetry (Humphrey Instruments, Palo Alto, CA, 24-2 program) scoring zero on the AGIS template. Each ocular hypertensive patient also had a zero score on entry into the study; conversion of the visual field was considered to have occurred when a reproducible visual field defect developed.

Optic disc appearances were not included as entry criteria for the study.

Patients with ocular hypertension who developed a visual field defect were known as 'converters'; the optic disc characteristics on sequential testing were compared in this group with the remaining ocular hypertensives, who were known as 'nonconverters', and the control group.

Results

Twenty-one patients 'converted'. The optic disc characteristics developing between their sequential SLO images were compared with those ocular hypertensives who did not convert (165 patients) and with the normal group (21 subjects).

Those optic disc parameters that showed significant differences between SLO 1 and SLO 2 in the converter group were global cup volume, supero- and inferotemporal and infero-nasal cup volume. These changes were seen before visual field conversion developed, and in each case were seen as an enlargement of the optic cup.

None of the normal group showed significant change between SLO 1 and SLO 2.

Forty seven of the 165 eyes in the nonconverter ocular hypertensive group showed significant enlargement of the same parameters of cup volume as had been seen in the converter group.

Discussion

The study demonstrated that sequential images obtained 12 months apart in a group of normal subjects exhibit a uniform appearance, with no significant change between the images of the two eyes. In contrast significant enlargement of the optic cup developed in 21 eyes that subsequently showed visual field changes. Twenty-five percent of a 'nonconverter' group of ocular hypertensives also showed similar, albeit smaller, changes on optic cup colume, suggesting that with continued enlargement of the optic cup, visual field defects could develop in these eyes too.

The results obtained in this study would suggest that, for eyes in which good images of the optic nerve can be obtained, significant and measurable changes at the optic nerve could be seen before white on white changes in the visual field. This finding offers the possibility for the scanning laser ophthalmoscope to be used in the identification of early change at the optic disc in chronic glaucoma.

CHAPTER 19

Early Detection of Paracentral Defects: Implications for Neuroprotection in Primary Open-Angle Glaucoma

I. Bodis-Wollner

Introduction

Over the last decades the concept of "neurodegenerative" diseases, such as Parkinson's disease (PD), Huntingtons's disease and Alzheimer's disease, has undergone significant changes. These conceptual changes result from an explosion of research in cellular biology and from advances in clinical pathophysiological studies.

A more thorough understanding of diverse mechanisms of cell has led to an investigation of the specifics of neuronal loss in several neurodegenerative diseases. For instance, distinguishing necrotic cell death with secondary inflammatory reactions from apoptosis is important not only for biology but also from a clinical point of view. One key issue of protective therapy is early diagnosis, since by the time a neurodegenerative disease is diagnosed by common clinical criteria, about 60 %–70 % of the neurons are lost. The second key issue is related to the ultimate failure of symptomatic therapy. The progression of neurodegenerative diseases is known to occur irrespective of most forms of current symptomatic and or replacement therapy. In fact, in some diseases, such as PD, it is known that symptomatic levodopa therapy in itself may contribute to the progressive cell death of specific and vulnerable neurons. It hardly needs to be stated, thet therefore early diagnosis is essential for effective neuroprotection.

Some of these conceptual changes which guide current research in neurodegenerative diseases are also applicable to the understanding and clinical management of primary open-angle glaucoma (POAG). In many ways glaucomatous optic neuropathy is a typical neurodegenerative disease. POAG is often diagnosed by the presence of two of three cardinal signs: elevated intraocular pressure, optic nerve damage and characteristic visual loss. Therefore it is important to detect early visual loss in POAG. Unfortunately, by best estimates of Quigely and colleagues (Quigley et al. 1982, 1987, 1989), cellular loss is above 60 % (i.e. six out of ten neurons are lost) when routine clinical perimetry identifies a visual loss. Contrast sensitivity measurements introduced into clinical medicine (Bodis-Wollner 1972), and specifically for the early detection of glaucoma (Aktin et al. 1979), have only addressed visual deficits of the very central area of the visual field (Bodis-Wollner et al. 1984; Storch and Bodis-Wollner 1990; Bodis-Wollner and Brannan 1994). We have been interested in new methods which target the earliest specific neuronal losses of POAG outside the fovea.

Here, I will describe some results obtained with a relatively new method of vision testing combining the advantages of visual field *and* contrast sensitivity analysis. The method relies on measuring spatial pooling of retinal signals (Sloan and Brown 1962;

Wilson 1967; Findlay 1969; Koenderink and van Doorn 1978; Mc Call et al. 1978; Robson and Graham 1981; Bodis-Wollner and Brannan 1991). The results will be discussed in reference to normal physiology and in reference to the question of which types of retinal ganglion cells or possibly their interconnections suffer first in POAG.

Methods

Stimuli

The detailed description of the stimuli and the relevant literature references can be found in Bodis-Wollner and Brannan (1997). Briefly the growth of contrast sensitivity (CS) as a function of the area of a sinusoidal grating of a fixed spatial frequency (1 cpd) was explored in four quadrants of the visual field (Fig. 1). The stimuli were presented on a Joyce VM 1 monitor under Venus software control. Mean luminance was 100 cd/m^2. Details of calibration of luminance and contrast followed procedures described in detail by Bodis-Wollner and Hendley (1979). We used aperture limited sinusoidal grating using stimuli based on signals orginally proposed by Gabor (1946) and applied to vision by Marcelja (1980). The luminance distribution of the spatial "parch" stimulus we use may be described as:

$$L(x,y,t)+L[1+cw(x,y)\cos (2\pi Fx)\cos(2\omega t)$$

where y is vertical distance and t is time, while W is the spatial (x and y) window function:

$$w(x,y)-\exp[x/Sx)^2-y/Sy)^2]$$

where S is the space constant which determines aperture size. A measure of S we adopted is the distance over which the Gaussian falls from 1 to $1/e^4$. We call a stimulus narrow-band (see Discussion) when over S the spectral spread around F_c is less then $1/3$ octave. In the present study, F_c was always 1 cpd.

The reasons for selecting a smoothly contoured stimulus is to avoid edges. When contrast abruptly rises at the edge of an extended grating pattern, then the observer's detection threshold may rely less on *pooling* of contrast signals, than on abrupt local luminance variations. Depending in various factors, such as spatial frequency and field size, an observer may detect a grating pattern easier by judging its edge. When a pattern is eccentically presented the advantage of edge detection is further enhanced by the inverse relationship between eccentricity and the spatial grain of the retina (Westheimer 1982). This means that the edge closest to the fovea has a higher weight in the detection process than, e.g., the center of the pattern which is further from fixation. Hence, patterns which do not squarely emerge from the background, but do so gradually are better suited to explore spatial summation of contrast signals as opposed to edge detection in paracentral vision.

To produce the stimulus the vertical grating was multiplied by a 2-dimensional Gaussian aperture so that maximum contrast was localized to a point 4° along the diagonal from fixation, presented without crossing the midline. Diameter in these studies was defined as the width of the Gaussian aperture measured where contrast was $1/e^4$ of the peak amplitude (contrast). The numerical value of $1/e^4$ is 0.01831, hence when the observer's peak contrast threshold is, e.g., 10 % the contrast t, the "edge" contrast of the 8-diameter pattern, is 0.001831 or 0.18 % (less than 1 %). Similarly, for a contrast threshold of, e.g., 20 % peak contrast at the "edge" is 0.36 % contrast. For a patch of half this size, the same is true at 4° diameter. We tested the central 16° of the field. While many VF studies suggest that more peripheral visual field (VF) defects occur early in glaucoma, those results are based on predominantly luminance

Fig. 1A,B. This sketch represents the stimulus arrangement of the present study. Gabor patch stimuli are symbolized by *large circles* in each quadrant of the central 20° (10° to each side) of the visual field. *Small circles* represent the fixed loci for the luminance stimuli used in the Humphrey 30-2 perimetry program. B A photograph of a medium-sized Gabor patch stimulus used for contrast perimetry. (From: Bodis-Wollner and Brannan 1997 by permission)

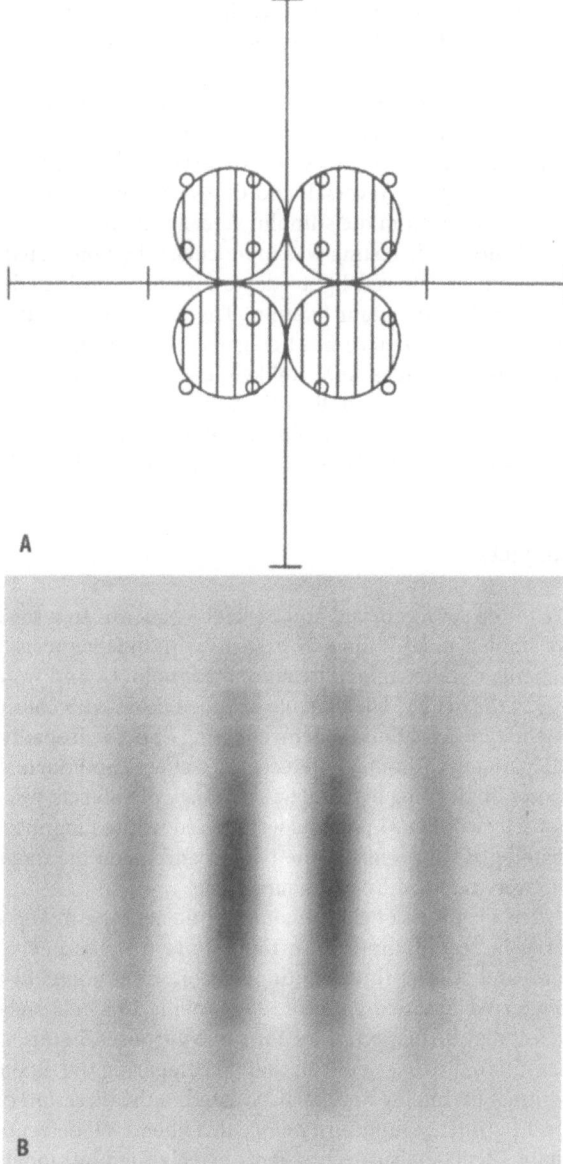

target perimetry. In contrast, many foveal CS studies (Lustgarten et al. 1990) suggested that a relatively large (10°–16°) central retinal area is vulnerable when using patterned stimuli. In our study we wished to bridge the two techniques. As the results show, the central 16° of the VF shows significant defects even when routine perimetry, covering a much larger area, is normal.

CS was obtained in each of the four quadrants to ten different stimulus sizes. On each block of trials, the stimulus first appeared at 90 % contrast. After assuring that the observer could see the stimulus, contrast was reduced to 50 % and threshold determination began. Before each presentation, the investigator verbally instructed the subject. If the observer responded they saw the stimulus, its contrast was reduced by 1 dB. If the observer did not detect the stimulus, contrast was increased by 1 dB. Each stimulus presentation was linearly and slowly (600 ms) ramped on/off to reduce transient temporal stimulation. Duration was at least 2 s but less than 5 s. Offset was sharp (square wave) once the observer responded. Contrast threshold was determined after three reversal, and CS was calculated as 1/threshold. The observer's distance was 2 m from the stimulus screen, which was surrounded with an evenly illuminated surround. Testing was monocular; the non-tested eye was covered with a light patch which allowed light adaptation, but eliminated spatial detail. Subjects were instructed to maintain fixation. The experimeter watched the corneal reflection to ensure that the pattern was being observed. Eye movements were not measured: however, microsaccades were unlikely to confound the results due to the lack of sharp edges in a Gabor patch. Foveal CS was tested with the Pelli-Robson chart. The results were analyzed by manual plotting of the data and entered into a Macintosh computer for numerical analysis and to compare empirically with predicted results.

Subjects

We tested seven normal and 22 POAG patients. In a separate study (Antal et al. 1998) we studied an additional 31 patients with the diagnosis of multiple sclerosis (MS). All patients were examined by an ophthalmologist and were free of cataract and pathology of the media. The patients included those with complete or incomplete VF defects due to glaucomatous or demyelinating optic neuropathy, and glaucoma suspects and MS patients without VF defects. All patients and normals had a best corrected visual acuity of 20/30 or better. The age range of subjects was from 27 to 69. Patients were not selected: POAG patients were tested whose diagnosis was established by a glaucomatologist who referred the patient and made the diagnosis of POAG. Patients with MS were referred by two neurologists.

The diagnosis of glaucomatous optic neuropathy was established using routine criteria: increased cup-to disc ratio above 0.6, elevated interocular pressure above 22 mm, and at least three contiguous abnormal points in the VF defined by perimetry (Preferred Practice Pattern 1989). While this relatively routine definition of a VF defect may be inappropriate for some purposes, in this study it served well as a liberal definition. By that we mean that, in comparing the diagnostic yield of routine VF and contrast perimetry we may have erred in the direction of not being able to show contrast perimetry superiority since this liberal VF defect definition increased VF sensitivity. Glaucoma suspect patients had elevated intraocular pressure and a cup-to-disc ratio larger than 0.6 but not VF defects (using the criteria of three adjacent contiguous points as representing a VF defect). Abnormal points were defined by their deviation (2 SD) from normal. Glaucoma patients were on various treatments while glaucoma "suspects" were on no medication. Glaucoma suspects (without VF defects) were defined according to the criteria laid down by the American Academy of Ophthalmology (Preferred Practice Pattern 1989).

The diagnosis of demyelinating optic neuropathy was based on accepted clinical and laboratory criteria (Poser 1984). These include two or more different clinical signs consistent with different anatomical regions and laboratory criteria. However, any subject showing active or exacerbated disease at the time of the study was excluded. Other exclusionary criteria for all subjects were best corrected acuity of 20/50 or worse, ocular pathology, cataract or any other medial opacity, a pupil smaller than 3 mm, or CNS disease of any kind. Their diagnosis of MS was supported by MRI electrophysiological and/or spinal fluid studies. Patients with past history of unilateral optic neuropathy or bilateral optic neuropathy were included. However, their results will be only summarized here, in contrast to the results obtained in POAG patients.

Results

Normals

Since the stimulus was presented in single VF quadrants without crossing either the horizontal or vertical midline, we avoided spatial summation involving both cerebral hemispheres. Maximum sensitivity (S-max) of the function can be defined as CS for the largest area possible for a given point in a single VF quadrant. S-max roughly corresponds to "conventional" CS using extended patterns except, as noted before, the stimulus is located in one quadrant of the VE. The summation function of CS in normals can be described as an S-shaped curve (Fig. 2). There was remarkable consistency of the functions between the four quadrants in each observer and between observers. The mean normal S-max was 26.57 (SD 4.4; range 20-31). Half-max, defined as the Gaussian aperture size for which the function reaches half of the maximum value, was 4.50° for normals (SD 0.28; range 4.00–4.75). Sensitivity for the smallest stimulus (S-min) was 5.64 (SD 1.18; range 4-7). The slope of the function, fit by the Quick psychometric function (Quick 1974) Was 3.97. The slope represents the strength of spatial summation among different units or mechanisms. In many psychophysical experiments, its value is typically between 3 and 8.

POAG patients

The VF was tested using the Humphrey 30-2 automated perimeter in eight glaucoma patients (group I), and in 14 patients suspected of having glaucoma (group II). Patients in either of the two groups (with or without perimetric losses) did show decreased maximum sensitivity and inefficient summation (higher half-max) as well as decreased minimum sensitivity. In order to visualize losses, we first established normal values by taking the mean sensitivity value for corresponding stimulus sizes

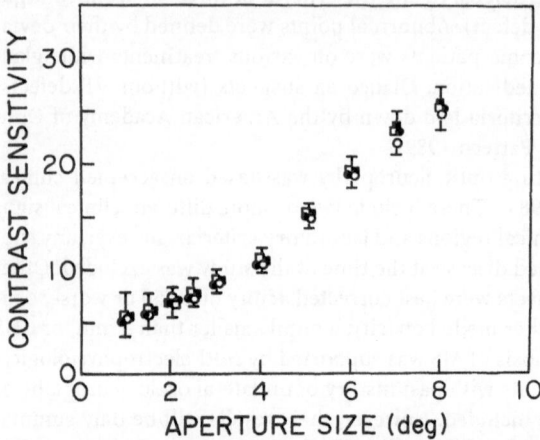

Fig. 2. Mean contrast sensitivity as a function of size of the gaussian aperture in seven normal observers, age 22-53. *Bars* represent one standard deviation. *Open circles* represent the sensitivity to stimuli localized in the inferior nasal quadrant while *solid circles, open squares,* and *solid squares* represent the superior nasal, inferior temporal, and superior temporal quadrants, respectively. Each contrast summation function approximates a sigmoid, with highest contrast sensitivity occurring to the 8° stimulus which is centered 4° from the fovea. As indicated in the text, aperture size refers to $1/e^4$ diameter for the gaussian. (From: Bodis-Wollner and Brannan 1997 by permission)

in all four quadrants of both eyes (64 measures per point). We then set a limit of 2.5 SD for each mean value for the composite curve. Then we took the ratio of the abnormal to normal CS for each stimulus size and plotted „loss" as a function of stimulus size. We define a loss when a given value is more than 2.5 SD from the normal mean and we define a loss function as "flat" when it shows less than 6 dB per octave of stimulus size, and as "sloping" when the loss function has a steeper slope. The slopes we found in this study were either flat or negative, i.e. less loss with increasing stimulus size. In the POAG patient population we studied, there were no deficits which were evident for large but not for small stimuli. We then evaluated the results of each POAG patient in each group for answering the following questions. How many *patients* had abnormal VF on the Humphrey perimeter vs contrast perimetry (CP)? How many *eyes*? How many *quadrants*? What was the correlation matrix between VF and CP in each quadrant? Finally, what kind of (flat vs sloping)/loss occurred in each quadrant?

All eight glaucoma patients (two with monocular VF defects) had abnormal results on CP. The correlation of the number of eyes with normal vs abnormal results of CP vs VF is shown in Fig. 3, revealing high concordance in this group, with CP showing higher sensitivity than VF. Of the 14 glaucoma suspect patients, none of whom had a VF defect, six patients had abnormal CP in both eyes, three in one eye only, and five were normal. Of all 112 quadrants, 54 were normal and 58 abnormal on CP. (Over 80 % of patients with demyelinating monocular optic neuropathy were abnormal in *both eyes* on CP.) The correlation matrix against the VF is shown in Fig. 3. Then we examined the *kind* of loss which occurred in each group (Fig. 4). We tested for the difference between two bionominal probabilities for each patients group, which is a variation on the χ^2 test (Pollard 1977). The results were significant for each group at the

Fig. 3. The Correlation of visual field (*VF*) and contrast perimetry (*CP*) results in patients with glaucomatous visual field defects and in glaucoma suspects. *N* stands for normal, *A* for abnormal result. The difference between VF and CP yield was significant (see text), indicating that CP is more sensitive than VF. The kind of CP loss (flat versus sloping) is significantly different in each group (see text and Fig. 4)

I. Glaucoma

CP \ VF	N	A
N	18	5
A	15	26

II. Glaucoma suspects (no field defect)

CP \ VF	N	A
N	54	0
A	58	0

0.05 level. Therefore, there is a significant difference between CP and VF testing with CP showing more abnormalities. In glaucoma patients, 49 quadrants were abnormal on CP and 31 on VF. Flat loss occurred in 15 quadrants, *all* of which showed a VF loss. Sloping loss was concordant with VF in 11 quadrants, while in 13 abnormal CP quadrants VF was normal in the definite glaucoma group. Comparing the POAG and MS (Antal, Aita and Bodis-Wollner, submitted) results raises some thoughts concerning

Fig. 4. A comparison of visual field and contrast perimetry results in each quadrant of each eye of patients with glaucomatous optic neuropathy. A *heavy dot* represents an abnormal VF quadrant on the Humphrey 30-2 program, while *lining* represents abnormal CP results. Of the lining in horizontal, the loss was "flat" (see "Methods"), while slanted lining represents a sloping loss. Note the presence of more "lined" than "dotted" quadrants, suggesting the greater sensitivity of CP in patients with definite optic neuropathy, but supposedly normal VF quadrants

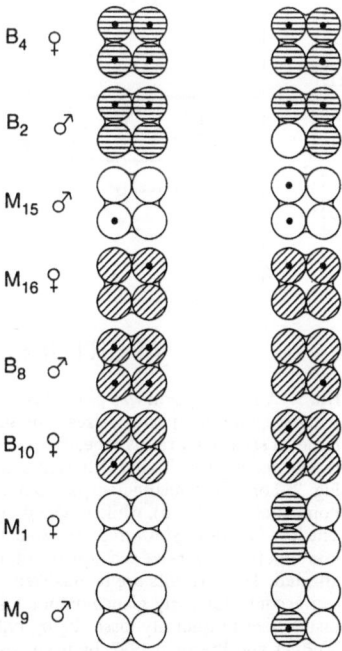

the differences between flat and sloping losses. While the overall ratio of the two different types of abnormalities was 40 % flat and 60 % sloping in the glaucoma group, in the suspects it was 20 % vs 80 %. In MS and demyelinating optic neuropathy patients, we found a flat loss exceedingly rare. We tested these ratios using the differences between two binominal probability statistics. These differences were statistically significant and raise the possibility that with *advancing* glaucoma, and with perhaps more generalized ganglion cell loss, a flat loss becomes more dominant. It is therefore noteworthy that in demyelinating disease with little primary neuronal damage, a deficit is not apparent for small targets, and in roughly half of the glaucoma suspect eyes, spatial summation was only abnormal for small stimuli. In several eyes, a sloping type of loss resulted from the abnormal shape of the summation curve, while S-max remained entirely normal (Fig. 4), suggesting that CS to extended gratings is only an endpoint mesaure of spatial summation and may be insufficient to detect the earlier visual defects.

Taking all the data together, of the 176 quadrants (44 eyes), only 17, or 10 % of the POAG group showed a result consistent with a flat loss. The results in POAG therefore do not represent a simple downscaling of normal sensitivity. Figure 5 shows loss functions which cannot be interpreted either by assuming a simple down-scaling of sensitivity, nor by assuming a shift of the spatial summation curve to the right. In fact, if a patients' data resulted from a shift of the normal summation curve to the right, based on the shape of the normal curve the greatest loss should occur for stimuli with larger diameters, a pattern not observed in any of the 22 glaucoma patients.

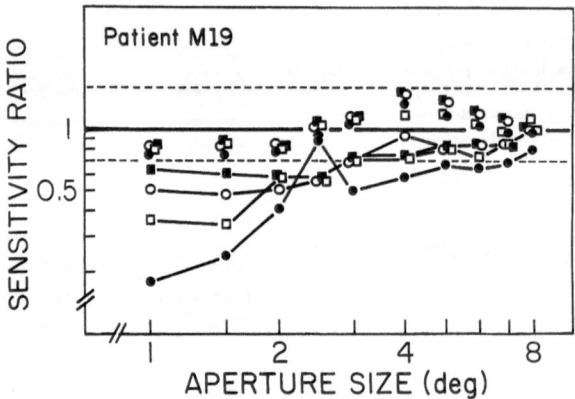

Fig. 5. A loss function was plotted by taking the contrast sensitivity ratios of a patient to the normal at corresponding aperture sizes. The interrupted lines represent the mean ± 2.5 SD for the normal range of sensitivity ratios for each aperture size. Data points falling between the interrupted lines represent normal sensitivity. Different symbols represent different VF quadrants and are described in Fig. 2. For this glaucoma-suspect patient, all data points are within the normal range for OS (date points not connected), while in OD there is a profound loss at small apertures but not at larger ones. The loss functions show impaired sensitivity to all except the largest stimulus sizes. Furthermore, the loss function separates each quadrant; the superior nasal is worst and the superior temporal is little affected. These results are inconsistent with the possibility that simple scaling of normal sensitivity can account for early glaucomatous losses and furthermore reveal that CS to extended gratings is insufficient to quantify losses being only an endpoint measure of spatial summation. (From Bodis-Wollner and Brannan 1997, by permission)

Discussion

The current data suggest an improved technique for evaluating the early and perhaps earliest visual dysfunction in the central 16° visual field of glaucoma suspect patients. The traditional view is that in POAG visual field defects occur outside the 16° -however this interpretation, as our data show, may be dependent on technique rather than specific to the pathological process of glaucoma. CP is more sensitive for the initial visual deficit in POAG, than routine automated perimetry. It has been also recently reported (Harwerth and Smith 1996) in the monkey model of glaucoma that Gabor patch test targets, as we have used, are more sensitive than Goldmann perimetry.

 . The kind of sensitivity losses we have observed show that a "seemingly" unitary spatial summation function in normals (Bodis-Wollner and Brannan 1997) falls apart in early glaucoma. The spatial energy spectrum of the stimuli we used is such that with *small* area stimuli one may expect to stimulate a large variety of ganglion cells, with different receptive field center sizes, all centered on a relatively small area. Alternatively, a single type of neuron, but spatially unselective or "broad-band" is affected. Each explanation is plausible, however the second explanation is more consistent with pathological studies of ganglion cell vulnerability in glaucoma. Studies both in humans (Quigley et al. 1987, 1988; Marx et al. 1998a) and the monkey model of glaucoma (Marx et al, 1998b); Glovinsky et al. 1991) suggest that large ganglion cells are primarily affected.

If one puts therefore the properties of the initially vulnerable ganglion cells in the perspective of CP data, the following emerges. In POAG the initially vulnerable ganglion cells may be: (a) in any quadrant of the central 16° field; (b) and have spatially broad-band profiles. Whether such cells belong to the α or β type ("magno", vs "parvo") awaits a more definite test. The suggested selective vulnerability of the magno vs parvo pathway in the monkey model of glaucoma (Marx et al. 1988b; Glovinsky et al. 1991) is currently controversial (Vickers et al. 1997). Indeed, both luminance and colour contrast deficiences are reported in POAG patients (Hart et al. 1990). Whether or not the initially affected, large, spatially broad-band neurons belong to one functional subclass, or represent both classes of cells, we suggest that they are vulnerable because of their high energy demands.

It is well known that different neurons of the retina have differing energy demands. It was originally reported that, unlike in lower species, in macaque monkeys large retinal (and LGN) ganglion cells show higher metabolic activity (Kageyama et al. 1984). It has been shown (Dreyer et al. 1994) that large ganglion cells are especically sensitive to NMDA (n-methyl-d-aspartate) mediated cell death. Recent studies of the macaque retina (Wong-Riley et al. 1998) suggest a functional link between glutamate related postsynaptic mechanisms (NMDAR-1 and nitric oxide synthase, nNOS) and high energy requirements (cytochrome oxidase and Na+K+ ATPase) in several layers of the retina. The most conspicuous assiciation between NMDAR-1 and NOS immunoreactivity is in the ganglion cell layer. One is therefore tempted to speculate that the death of ganglion cells, which show this association, may be related to glutamate activals and calcium influx, i.e. excitoxicity. This mode of death of large cells with high metabolic demand may be especially promoted by a postulated feedforward link between NMDA receptors and nNOS via calcium influx (Garthwaite 1991). Excitoxicity is frequently implicated as a cause of neuronal death in PD, an archetypical neurodegenerative disease (Meldrum and Garthwaite 1990). It has been shown over 40 years ago already that glutamate is toxic to the inner layers of the retina (Lucas and Newhouse 1957). One theory is that excitoxicity is due to increased endogenous formation of glutamate. The vitreous contains elevated glutamate levels in humans and monkeys with glaucoma (Dryer et al. 1996). Is it a reflection of dying cells or is it a cause of neuronal death? One theory linking glutamate excitoxicity and intrinsic ganglion cell mechanisms postulates that a reduced energy supply, caused by a mitochrondrial defect, weakens the ATP-dependent MG-blockade of NMDA receptors and allows physiological concentration of glutamate to mediate calcium influx.

Based on these considerations, several new thoughts emerged in recent years concerning neuro-protective therapy in POAG. One approach is to block NMDA receptors and attenuate glutamate induced calcium reflux. Currently it is accepted that NMDA antagonists should protect the vulnerable neurons. Present studies with clinically stable NMDA blockers, such as amantidine hydrochloride and sulfate, have not yet been shown to exert a protective effect on vision in POAG. There is a need for such studies using sensitive and reliable short term markers of VF changes.

A second important concept is that excitoxic-apoptotic damage may be directly linked to nitric oxid (Dawson et al. 1991) as a cause of cell loss in PD and possibly in POAG. Nitric oxide (NO) itself may lead to excitoxicity. NO may be generated from NO donors and it can be also synthesized endogeneously following NMDA receptor activation. However, NO itself may block NMDA receptors, via a postulated feedback mechanism (Manzoni et al. 1992; Lei et al. 1992). Thus NO itself could also prevent excitoxity. It is clear that NO's effect is bimodal and may be under complex modulatory effects of redox mechanisms (Aizenman et al. 1989; Levy et al. 1990; Lei et al. 1992; Lipton et al. 1993). In fact, is has been recently suggested (Zurakowski et al. 1998) that nitrate therapy, promoting NO generation, may limit excitroxic damage in POAG by modulating glutamate receptors.

Finally, several mechanisms are interlinked to create cell death, but it appears that the mitochondrial membrane and respiratory chain represent the final common pathway (Beal et al. 1997). A mitochondrial defect itself may be linked to apoptosis. A change in the mitochondrial membrane potential is thought to occur initially in apoptosis (Tatton 1998). In PD a mitochondrial defect, causing a seemingly unbridgeable gap in the respiratory chain (complex I), may be the reason for energy failure. It has been, however, recently shown that mitochondrial complex I defect may become only symptomatic, i.e. lead to respiratory chain block, when the nuclear milieu of the cell is altered (Gu et al. 1998). These considerations raise possibilities of protecting vulnerable neurons by mitochondrially effective therapies. Bodis-Wollner et al. (1991) have shown in the monkey that MPTP toxicity is prevented by actyl-levo-carnitine (ALC) and suggested that ALC, which equilibrates across the mitochondrial membrane, may allow partially affected cells to survive by bypassing a respiratory chain (complex I) defect. More recently Tatton et al. (1996) have shown ALC's protective effect in vivo. ALC has not been used to our knowledge in POAG. Since MPTP is selectively taken up by DA neurons and its final "cytotoxic" effect is on the mitochondria (see Mari and Bodis-Wollner 1997), it appears relevant to neuro-protective therapy in POAG that the neuronal NOS inhibitor 7-nitroindazol (7NI) protects dopaminergic neurons in the MPTP model of PD (Schulz et al. 1995; Hantraye et al. 1996). Apparently 7NI may be effective in directly attenuating the mitochondrial damage caused by MPP+ (the toxic product of MPTP). In view of the results of Wong-Riley et al. (1998) it seems therefore reasonable to investigate the effect of 7-NI and similar agents protecting large retinal ganglion cells which contain NMDAR-1 receptors and NOS.

In summary, based on the new contrast VF testing results, we suggest that in POAG "large" neurons which have a physiologically broad-band spatial profile may be candidates for the earliest cellular damage in POAG. These neurons may belong to a subclass with NMDAR-1 receptors and high NOS immunoreactivity.

References

Aizenman E, Lipton SA, Loring RG (1989) Selective modulation of NMDA responses by reduction and oxidation. Neuron 2:1257–1263

Atkin A, Bodis-Wollner I, Wolkstein M, Moss A, Podos S (1979). Abnormalities of central contrast sensitivity in glaucoma. Am J Ophthalmol 88:205–211

Beal MF, Howell N, Bodis-Wollner I (1997) Perface. Mitochondria and Free Radicals in Neurodegenerative Diseases. New York, Wiley Liss

Bodis-Wollner I (1972) Visual acuity and contrast sensitivity in patients with cerebral lesions. Science 178:769–771

Bodis-Wollner, Brannan J (1991) Hidden paracentral contrast sensitivity loss in optic neuropathy. Invest Ophthalmol Vis Sci 32:4, 948

Bodis-Wollner I, Brannan JR (1994) Assessment of current visual psychophysical testing methods with special reference to primary open angle glaucomatous disease (POAGD). Neuro-ophthalmol 14:61–71

Bodis-Wollner I, Brannan J (1997) Hidden visual loss in optic neuropathy is revealed using Gabor patch Contrast Perimetry. Clin Neurosci 4:284–291

Bodis-Wollner I, Chung E, Ghilardi MF, Glover A, Onofrj M, Pasik M, Samson Y (1991) Acetyl-levocarnitine protects against MPTP-induced parkinsonism in primates. J Neural Transm 3:63–72

Bodis-Wollner I, Hendley C (1979) On the separability of two mechanism involved in the detection of grating patterns in humans. J Physiol 291:251–263

Bodis-Wollner I, Podos S, Atkin A, Nitzberg S, Mylin L (1984) Psychophysical studies of spatial contrast defects in glaucoma. In: Ocular Hypertension. Würzburg, Germany, Krieglstein GK, Leydhecker W (eds) Processings of the Symposium of the European Glaucoma Society. Dr. Kaden Verlag, Heidelberg, pp 69–77

Dawson IM, Bredt SS, Fotuhi M, Hwang PM, Snyder SH (1991) Nitric oxide synthase and neuronal NADPH diaphorase are identical in brain and peripheral tissue, Proc Natl Acad Sci USA 88:7797–7801

Dreyer EG, Pan Z-Ph, Storm S, Lipton SA (1994) Greater sensitivity of larger retinal ganglion cells to NMDA-mediated cell death. Neuro Report 5:629–631

Dreyer EG, Zurakowski D, Schumer RA, Podos SM, Lipton SA (1996) Elevated glutamate levels in the vitreous body of humans and monkeys with glaucoma. Arch Ophthalmol 114:299–305

Findlay JM (1969) A spatial integration effect in human vision. Vis Res 9:157–166

Gabor D (1946) A theory of communication. J Inst Elec Eng 93:429–457

Garthwaite J (1991) Glutamate, nitric oxide and cell-cell signalling in the nervous system. Trends Neurosci 14, 60–67

Glovinsky Y, Qugley HA, Dunkelberger GR (1991) Retinal ganglion cell loss is size dependent in experimental glaucoma. Invest Ophthalmol Vis Sci 32:484–491

Gu M, Cooper JM, Taanman JW, Schapira AHV (1998) Mitochondrial DNA Transmission of the Mitochondrial defect in Parkinson's Disease. Ann Neurol 44:177–186

Hantraye P, Brouillet E, Ferrante R et al. (1996) Inhibition of neuronal nitric oxide synthase prevents MPTP-induced parkinsonism in baboons. Nature Med 2:1017–1021

Hart WM Jr, Silverman SE, Trick GL, Nesher R, Gordon MO (1990) Glaucomatous visual field demage. Luminance and color-contrast sensitivities. Invest Ophth Vis Sci 31, 2:359–367

Harwerth RS, Smith III EL (1996) Visual field defects in glaucoma: Ganor patch vs. Goldmann III test target. Invest Ophth Vis Sci (Suppl) 8509

Kageyama GH, Wong-Riley MT (1984) The histochemical localization of cytochrome oxidase in the retina and lateral geniculate nucleus of the ferret, cat, and monkey, with particular reference to retinal mosaics and ON/OFF-center visual channels. J Neurosci 4:2445–2459

Koenderink JJ, van Doorn AJ (1978) Visual detection of spatial contrast: influence of location in the visual field, target extent and illuminance level. Biol Cybernetics 30:157–167

Lei SZ, Pan Z-H, Aggarwal SK, Chen H-S V, Hartman J, Sucher NJ, Lipton SA (1992) Effect of nitric oxide production on the redox modulatory site of the NMDA receptor-channel complex. Neuron 8:1087–1099

Levy DI, Sucher NJ, Lipton SA (1990) Redox modulation of NMDA receptor-mediated toxicity in mammalian central nervous. Neurosci Letters 110:291–196

Lipton S, Choi Y-/B, Pan Z-H, Lel SZ, Chen H-S V, Sucher NJ, Loscalzo J, Singel DJ, Stamler JS (1993) A redox-based mechanism for the neuroprotective and neurodestructive effects of nitric oxide and related nitrosocompunds. Nature 364:626–628

Lucas DR, Newhouse JP (1957) The toxic effect of sodium L-Glutamate on the inner layers of the retina. Arch Ophthalmol 58:193–201

Lustgarten JS, Marx MS, Podos SM, Bodis-Wollner I, Campeas D, Serle JB (1990). Contast sensitivity and computerized perimetry in early detection of glaucomatous change. Clin Vis Sci 5:407–413

Marcelja S (1980) Mathematical description of the responses of simple cortical cells. J Opt Soc Amer 70:1297–1300

Manzoni O, Prezeau L, Marin P, Deshager S, Bockaert J, Fagni L (1992) Nitric Oxide-induced blockade of NMDA receptors. Neuron 8:653–662

Mari Z, Bodis-Wollner I (1997) MPTP-induced Parkinsonian syndrome in humans and animals: How good is the model? In: Beal MF, Howell N, Bodis-Wollner I (eds) Mitochondria and free radicals in neurodegenerative diseases. Wiley-Liss, New York Ch 9: 189–228

McCann JJ, Savoy RL, Hall JA (1978) Visibility of low frequency sine warve targets: dependence on number of cycles and surround parameters. Vis Res 18:891–894

Marx MS, Bodis-Wollner I, Lustgarten JS, Podos SM (1988a) Electrophysiological evidence that early glaucoma affects foveal vision. Documenta Ophthalmologica 67:281–301

Marx MS, Podos SM, Bodis-Wollner I, Lee P-Y, Wang R-F, Severin C (1988b) Signs of early damage in glaucomatous monkey eyes: low spatial frequency losses in the pattern ERG and VEP. Exp Eye Res 46:173–184

Meldrum B, Garthwaite J (1990) Excitatory amino acid neurotoxicity and neuro-degenerative disease. Trends Pharmacol Sci 11:379–387

Pollard JH (1977) A handbook of numerical and statistical techniques. Cambridge University Press, Cambridge UK

Poser CM (1984) The Diagnosis of Multiple Sclerosis. Thieme-Stratton, New York

Preferred Practice Pattern (1989) Glaucoma Suspect, American Academy of Ophthalmology. Quality for Care Committee Glaucoma Panel, San Francisco CA, p 1

Quick RF (1974) A vector-magnitude model of contrast detection. Kybernetik. 16:65–67

Quigley HA, Addicke EM, Green WR (1982) Optic nerve damage in human glaucoma: III. Quantitative correlation of nerve fiber loss and visual field defect in glaucoma, ischemic neuropathy, papilledema, and toxic neuropathy. Arch Ophthalmol 100:135–146

Quigley HA, Sanchez RM, Dunkelberger GR, l'Hernault NL, Baginski TA (1987) Chronic glaucoma selectively damages large optic nerve fibers. Invest Ophth Vis Sci 28:913–920

Quigley HA, Dunkelberger GR, Green WR (1988) Chronic human glaucoma causing selectively greater loss of large optic nerve fibers. Ophth 95:357–363

Quigley HA, Dunkelberger GR, Green WR (1989) Retinal ganglion cell atrophy correlated with automated perimetry in human eyes with glaucoma. Am J Ophth 107:453–464

Robson JD, Graham N (1981) Probability summation and regional variation in contrast sensitivity across the visual field. Vis Res 21:409–418

Schulz JB, Matthews RT, Muqit MMK, Browne SE, Beal MF (1995) Inhibition of neuronal nitric oxide synthase by 7-nitroindazole protects against MPTP-induced neurotoxicity in mice. J Neurochem 64:936–939

Sloan LL, Brown DJ (1962) Area and luminance of test object as variable in projection perimetry. Vis Res 2:527–541

Storch RL, Bodis-Wollner I (1990) Overview of contrast sensitivity and neuro-ophthalmic disease. In: MD Nadler, D Miller, DJ Nadler (eds) Glare and Contrast Sensitivity for Clinicians. New York: Springer-Verlag, 85–112

Tatton WG, Ju WYH, Frase AD, Chalmers-Redman RME, Wadia J, Tatton NA (1996) Treating neurodegeneration by altering genomic and mitochondrial protein synthesis. Abstract of Fourth International Congress of Movement Disorders Vienna vol. 11/suppl. 1/1996 M11

Tatton WG, Olanow CW (1999) Apoptosis in Neurodegenerative Diseases: The Role of Mitochondria. Biochemia and Biophysica Acta (in press)

Vickers JC, Hof PR, Schumer RA, Wang RF, Podos SM, Morrison JH (1997) Magnocellular and parvocellular visual pathways are both affected in a macaque monkey model of glaucoma. Aust NZJ Ophthalmol 25:239–243

Westheimer G (1982) The spatial grain of the perifoveal visual field. Vis Res 22:157–162

Wilson ME (1967) Spatial and temporal summation in impaired regions of the visual field. J Physiol 189: 189–208

Wong-Riley MTT, Huang Z, Liebl W, Nie F, Xu H, Zhang Ch (1998) Neurochemical organization of the macaque retina: effect of TTX on levels and gene expression of cytochrome oxidase and nitric oxide synthase and on the immunoreactivity of Na+K+ ATPase and NMDA receptor subunit I. Vis Res 38:1455–1478

Zurakowski D, Vorwerk Ch, Gorla M, Kanellopoulos J, Chaturredi N, Grosskreutz D, Lipton S, Dreyer E (1998) Nitrate therapy may retard glaucomatous optic neuropathy, perhaps through modulation of glutamate receptors. Vis Res 38:1489–1494

A New Unification Hypothesis of the Pathogenesis of Glaucomas Based on Clinical Studies on Disc Appearance in Relation to the Stage of Visual Field Loss in Different Types of Glaucoma

E. Gramer and G. Gramer

Introduction

Over the last few decades many studies have demonstrated that glaucomatous optic neuropathy (GON) is a multifactorial disease [8, 13–17, 20, 24–26, 28–35, 38, 41–45, 47, 49, 52–56, 60, 63, 66, 84, 85, 91]. Therefore, intraocular pressure (IOP) is not the only "villain" we must deal with in glaucoma.

Risk Factor: Intraocular Pressure

The risks posed by high IOP do not need a spirited defense [13] and are obvious in secondary glaucomas, e.g. pigmentary glaucoma (PG), or in primary congenital glaucoma, or chronic angle-closure glaucoma (CACG), in which pressure elevation alone can probably be responsible for the glaucomatous damage of the disc and visual field.

Not known, however, is the time dynamic of visual field progression caused by elevated IOP alone. We therefore tried to obtain indirect information on IOP-dependent visual field progression from patients with pigmentary glaucoma: From stage of visual field loss (VFL) and age of the patient at the time of diagnosis in 161 patients with so far untreated PG, we judged indirectly the time dynamic of VFL [52], demonstrating the impact of the risk factor IOP. For untreated PG patients with average maximum IOP peaks of 34.9 ± 11.5 mm Hg, we found that the time frame from beginning of VFL to blindness is approximately 8.5 years only. Table 1 shows the

Table 1. Visual field loss and time of diagnosis in patients with untreated PG

| | Patients/eyes (n = 161) | | |
	(n = 88)	(n = 48)	(n = 25)
Visual field loss	Stages *I and II*	Stages *III and IV*	Stage *V*
Mean IOP (max) (mm Hg)	32.5 ± 8.2	35.1 ± 12.9	34.9 ± 11.5
Mean myopia (dpt)	−4.3 ± 3.5	−3.5 ± 3.4	−5.0 ± 5.0
Meag age at the time of diagnosis (years) ($p < 0.05$)	42.5 ± 13.2	46.2 ± 13.8	51.1 ± 17.3
Onset of the disease before the age of 40	3.5 years $\longrightarrow$	5 years $\longrightarrow$	Blindness
	8.5 years $\longrightarrow$		

mean age of the patients with PG at the time of diagnosis, mean maximum IOP and mean myopia for 88 patients/eyes with PG in stages I and II of VFL, 48 eyes/patients with visual field loss stages III and IV, and 25 patients with VFL stage V. Mean maximum IOP and mean myopia were not significantly different in the three groups. For patients with stage I and II of VFL, the mean age at the time of diagnosis was 42.5 ± 13.2 years, for patients with stages III and IV the age at the time of diagnosis was 46.2 ± 13.8 years and for patients with stage V the age at the time of diagnosis was 51.1 ± 17.3 years. The average onset of the disease is before the age of 40 years. In PG the risk factor IOP and the time of diagnosis are important for the prognosis of the disease [52, 53].

In contrast, in primary open-angle glaucoma (POAG) and normal tension glaucoma (NTG), there are, beside IOP-related risk factors, IOP-independent risk factors [49]. The latter are particularly striking in NTG but are also involved in POAG or other types of glaucoma. Risk factors which are IOP-independent can be evaluated more effectively in NTG than in POAG because the degree of visual field defect (VFD), aside from being influenced by systemic risk factors, is influenced more by the various heights of IOP in POAG than in NTG. NTG, therefore, provides the opportunity to evaluate IOP-independent risk factors. Eyes with NTG or POAG and controlled IOP which show a further deterioration of VFD at pressures of 21 mm Hg or less (arbitrary border line) will also allow conclusions to be made as to the risk factors of the more IOP-independent glaucomatous damage. To show the impact of risk factor IOP elevation in POAG, we performed an intra-individual examination of 108 eyes of 54 patients in order to compare the height of the IOP in relation to the asymmetry of VFD between both eyes, calculating the total loss with Program 31/Delta of the Octopus perimeter [32]. We found that only eyes with a four times higher total loss in VF in one eye than in the other had a significantly higher maximum IOP in the fellow eye with the more severe VFD. This highlights the influence of additional IOP-independent risk factors in POAG [32]. The comparison of disc and visual field findings in different types of glaucomas may lead to a better understanding of some of the unanswered questions about differences in the risk factors involved in the pathogenesis of the different types of glaucomas. There may be two groups of glaucoma patients. In one group there is a relationship between IOP and the amount of damage. This is more probable for eyes with CACG, PG and POAG with high IOP. By contrast, there may be a group of glaucoma patients in whom the IOP may be much less or not related to the damage. These patients may be more frequent found in the group of NTG or POAG with less elevated IOP. Although we know that IOP does not separate two diseases, the NTG group may more frequently have additional risk factors such as a low systolic blood pressure and/or risk factors in the morphology of the optic nerve head (ONH). NTG and POAG with less elevated IOP seem to be the same disease and differ only in the height of the risk factor IOP. The results of our perimetric long-term follow-up of patients with POAG and regulated IOP in comparison to patients with NTG support this hypothesis: Within the same observation time we found between eyes with POAG and regulated IOP and eyes with NTG (no significant difference in pre-existing VFL between groups) no significant differences in the frequency and amount of VF deteriorations [20, 30]. NTG and POAG with regulated IOP seem to have the same VF prognosis, and a VF deterioration was found in NTG and POAG in every fifth patient [20]. POAG patients with IOP regulation by trabeculectomy also showed a VF deterioration in every fifth patient [66]. This suggests that all of these patients (NTG, POAG) suffer from only one disease and points out the weakness of the pressure-related definition of NTG. In comparison to IOP-related glaucomas these less IOP-related or not IOP-related glaucomas provide an opportunity to re-examine the fundamental concepts of glaucomatous damage by means of clinical observation. The vasogenic theory supports the hypothesis that hypoperfusion of the papilla is responsible for ONH impairment. There are many systemic factors, e.g. a low blood pressure (BP) [28], increased blood and plasma viscosity, severe anemias and ocular factors, including IOP and retinal vascular sclerosis, acting in different combinations to interfere with ONH circulation in the production of GON and VFL [49]. The incidence of these factors may be different in the different types of glaucoma. In NTG patients, we found, for example, more often a low systolic BP than in patients with POAG at the same stage of VFL (stage II) [42], more often a cardiac disease than in patients with ocular hypertension (OH) (50 % in NTG and POAG vs 11.5 % in eyes with OH) [38], and very often a vasospasm in patients with NTG [49]. However, there are individuals with general risk factors, e.g. low BP, vasospasm, cardiovascular diseases, or patients with elevated IOP over many years who do not develop a GON or glaucomatous VFL. Some ONHs must be more susceptible to risk factors than others. This leads to the question whether there is evidence of a risk factor in the morphology of the optic disc itself which might explain the individual different tolerance of the ONH for elevated IOP and for general risk factors.

Hypothesis of a Further Risk Factor in the Morphology of the Optic Nerve Head Based on Morphological Differences in the Optic Nerve Head Between Different Types of Glaucoma

In several studies, therefore, we compared the appearance of the ONH in different types of glaucoma, comparing eyes with the stame stage of VFL. The results are first briefly summarized in the following and then explained in detail in connection with the introduction of a new hypothesis on the pathogenesis of glaucomas: Given the same stage of VFL, patients with NTG had a larger cup-disc ratio (CDR), a smaller neuroretinal rim area, a significantly steeper slope and flatter bottom of the excavation in stages I and II of VFL than eyes with POAG. Furthermore, comparison of the CDR between eyes with NTG, POAG, PG and CACG was made, and significant differences were found, e.g. larger CDRs in NTG in stages I and II of the disease than in other types of glaucoma. We also evaluated whether there are any differences in disc size between NTG, POAG and healthy eyes; no significant differences were found. Further, we compared disc size in different types of glaucoma between eyes with stages I, II, III and IV of VFL; no significant differences were found. This shows that disc size is not a risk factor and that groups of different types of glaucoma are comparable. For healthy eyes we evaluated the correlation between disc size and CDR, disc size and neuroretinal rim area, and CDR and neuroretinal rim area; a significant correlation was found. We also evaluated the frequency of disc hemorrhages (DH) in NTG, POAG, and PG for eyes with the same mean VFL and regulated IOP during observation time. No differences were found between NTG and POAG but differences were found compared to PG. Differences were also noted in the topography of DH in the quadrants of the optic disc comparing eyes with POAG and anterior ischemic neuropathy (AION) with the same stage of VFL. In further studies we investigated the topography of VFL and the correlation of VFL to disc findings in the different types of glaucoma and found quantitative differences between the different glaucomas using quantitative disc analysis (ONH analyzer, laser tomographic scanner, Heidelberg retina tomograph, etc.). In addition, we evaluated the effect of aging on nerve fiber layer thickness (NFLT) in normal eyes and found that age-related nerve fiber loss occurs predominantly in the inferior temporal quadrant of the ONH. An age-dependent NFLT loss therefore occurs mostly in the inferior temporal nerve fibers which pass through the inferior temporal connective tissue structure of the lamina cribosa. These morphological differences in the appearance of the ONH and the quantitative difference in VFL between the different types of glaucoma cannot result from a difference in the amount of neural substance because the eyes compared were at the same stage of VFL in all of the studies conducted. All of these findings encouraged us in the hypothesis that the amount of connective tissue in the lamina cribosa may explain these morphological and functional differences in the different types of glaucoma. Possible mechanisms for this morphological difference in, e.g. CDR between NTG, POAG, PG and CACG, may be the presence of a preexisting large cup which is more frequent in NTG as a congenital or familiar feature before atrophy developed than in to other types of glaucoma.

The aim of this contribution is to summarize the total results of these studies and to discuss four topics from these results: (1) To discuss the relevance of the differences in the disc/VF correlation between the various types of glaucoma for the pathogenesis of the glaucomas; (2) To discuss the relevances of the differences in mean CDR and stage of mean VFL in the different types of glaucoma for possible differences in the diagnostic sensitivity of disc analysis and perimetry. For the already published results a brief result summary will be given, referring for details to the original publication. The results of four unpublished studies are included here in detail. All these results are comparable to pieces of a mosaic puzzle which fit together. (3) To form a new hypothesis of a further risk factor in the morphology of the optic disc. The possible presence of a genetically determined risk factor in the extracellular matrix of the lamina cribosa of the ONH provides for a unifying hypothesis of the mechanical and vasogenic theories of the pathogenesis of glaucoma. (4) The fourth aim of this contribution is to discuss whether there is a conformity of this new hypothesis with the clinical features of the different types of glaucoma. This review will give, therefore, a brief summary of our opinions taken form our – in parts – unpublished studies combined with a review of only some of the literature of particular interest in this field. This brief report cannot review the extensive disc literature in any great detail and shall, therefore, only focus on some aspects of the correlation of CDR and VFL. The reviewed relation of the CDR, of the rim area, and of DHs to VFL does not mean, of course, that these are the only relevant morphological parameters of glaucomatous alterations in the optic disc. These were just some of the parameters used to compare the optic disc in the different types of glaucoma in order to highlight the relevance of the results for new insights into the pathogenesis of glaucomatous damage and into the diagnostic sensitivity of disc analysis compared to perimetry.

Staging of Visual Field Loss

The precondition of every comparison of different types of glaucoma is that the eyes compared are at the same stage of VFL. For all our studies we used the Octopus perimeter 201 (program 31, 33, 32, or a program combination 4.2° pattern) for the quantification of VFL. Staging of VFL was performed according to the definition of Aulhorn [5] and, in many studies, by calculation of the total loss in VF. This approach summarizes size and depth of the scrotomas in one measurement value, evaluated by means of program Delta of the Octopus perimeter 201 [20, 22, 28, 29, 36, 37, 67].

Cup-Disc Ratio in NTG and POAG in Patients with Visual Field Defects, Stage II

The first study which evaluated differences in the relationship of cup-disc ratio (CDR) and VFL loss between different types of glaucoma was presented by Gramer and Leydhecker in 1984 [43] and 1985 [42, 45]. It compared the mean CDR in eyes with NTG and POAG in a total of 184 eyes with VFD, stage II (Fig. 1).

There were 61 eyes with a maximum IOP of 21 mm Hg. These are the NTGs shown in the black columns of Fig. 1. There were 61 eyes with POAG and a maximum IOP of 22–29 mm Hg (hatched columns) and 62 eyes with POAG and maximum IOP of 30–39 mm Hg (white columns). For the same amount of VFD, we observed larger CDRs much more frequently in NTG (black columns) than in POAG with high IOPs (white columns). The eyes compared were at the same stage of the disease. We there-

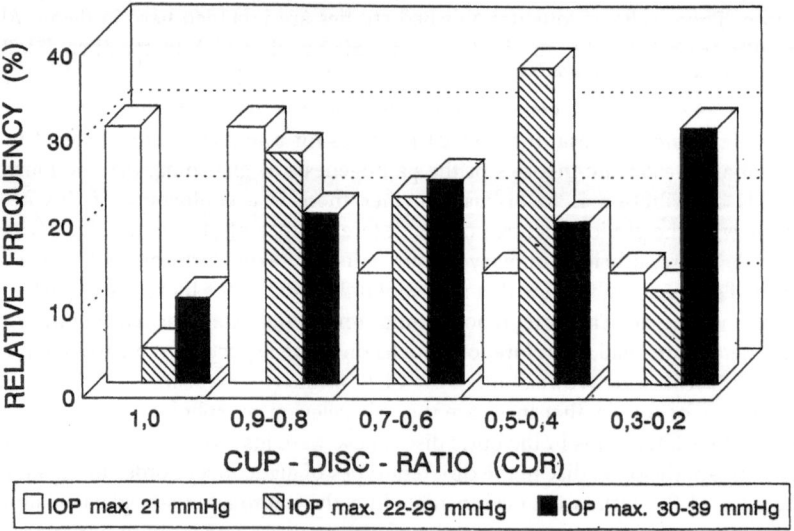

Fig. 1. Cup-disc ratio (CDR) in eyes with normal-tension glaucoma (NTG) and primary open-angle glaucoma (POAG) with two different IOP levels and stage II of VFL. For details, see text

fore speculated that there may be differences in the morphology of the optic disc between different types of glaucoma regarding the amount of connective tissue of the ONH [42, 43, 45]. Caprioli and Spaeth also described disc difference in high and low tension glaucoma in 1985 [9]. They found that the mean of the overall width of the neuroretinal rim in patients with NTG was smaller than that of patients with POAG and that the difference was most pronounced in the inferior and inferotemporal portions of the rim. This is in conformity with our results and our findings with the ONH analyzer [23]. Their groups also showed a considerable overlap. In a recent study we reevaluated the relationship of CDR and VFL comparing four stages of VFL of four different types of glaucoma.

Mean CDR in Stages I, II, III, IV in Patients with CACG, POAG, PG, NTG

Purpose

In this study we were especially interested in two questions: The first purpose was to evaluate whether there are any differences in mean CDR in CACG, POAG, PG and NTG, comparing eyes at the same stage of VFL. The second purpose was to evaluate the relative change in CDR from the onset of the disease, defined as stage I of VFL, and the advanced glaucomatous damage, defined as stage IV, in these four different types of glaucoma [24, 25, 26, 49, 65]. Quantitative differences in the relation between CDR and VFL in these different types of glaucoma will have scientific and clinical relevance. If there is a difference in the CDR between the various types of glaucoma, this may allow conclusions about differences in the pathogenesis of the glaucomatous ONH damage of the various glaucomas. For clinical relevance, it follows that if a difference in CDR exists at a given stage of VFL, conclusions may be made for which type of glaucoma perimetry may be more sensitive than disc analysis with regard to detection and follow-up of the disease.

Methods

Cup-disc ratio was evaluated in patients with glaucomatous VFD of stages I–IV by the same examiner, the author. CDR was determined with the 78 dpt lens in the vertical diameter in 82 eyes of 82 patients with CACG, 139 eyes/patients with POAG, 115 eyes/patients with PG and 81 eyes/patients with NTG. Inclusion criteria were a visual acuity of 0.8 or better, refraction of not more than ± 3 dpts (except for PG patients, who were more myope) and Octopus perimetry with the Octopus perimeter 201, program 31, 33 or 32. Staging of VFL was performed according to the definition of Aulhorn [5].

Results

Figure 2 and Table 2 show the mean CDR in stages I–IV of VFL in patients with CACG, POAG, PG and NTG.

For CACG with VFL stage I in 30 eyes of 30 patients, a mean CDR of 0.17 ± 0.28 was found; for stage II, the mean CDR was 0.44 ± 0.31. Thus, in eyes with CACG, even

Fig. 2. Mean CDR in stage I to stage IV of VFL in NTG, PG, POAG and CACG

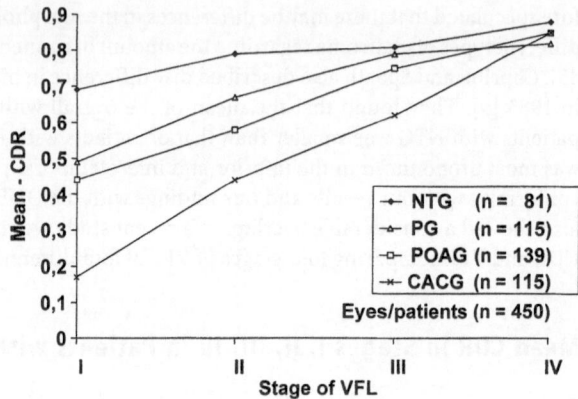

Table 2. Mean CDR in stages I–IV of visual field loss (VFL) in patients with CACG, POAG, PG, and NTG

Stage of VFL	CACG (n = 82) Eyes/patients	m-CDR	Δ-CDRᵃ	POAG (n = 139) Eyes/patients	m-CDR	Δ-CDRᵃ
I	30	0.17 ± 0.28		52	0.44 ± 0.27	
II	26	0.44 ± 0.31	0,68	36	0.58 ± 0.28	0,38
III	12	0.62 ± 0.39	(80 %)	30	0.75 ± 0.21	(43 %)
IV	14	0.85 ± 0.14		21	0.82 ± 0.23	

Stage of VFL	PG (n = 115) Eyes/patients	m-CDR	Δ-CDRᵃ	NTG (n = 81) Eyes/patients	m-CDR	Δ-CDRᵃ
I	35	0.49 ± 0.21		25	0.69 ± 0.12	
II	36	0.67 ± 0.20	0,33	26	0.79 ± 0.14	0,19
III	25	0.79 ± 0.15	(40 %)	18	0.81 ± 0.09	(22 %)
IV	19	0.82 ± 0.19		12	0.88 ± 0.14	

ᵃ Change between stage I and stage IV.

with normal appearing discs with a mean CDR of 0.17, a VFL stage I, or with a mean CDR of 0.44, a VFL stage II can be present. Thus, if only CDR is taken into consideration for early diagnosis, the onset of the disease can easily be missed if perimetry is not performed additionally. Concerning the difference of mean CDR between stage I and stage IV we found the largest difference to be 0.68 in CACG, an 80 % change in CDR (Table 2). For sensitivity of follow-up, this implies that progression of the disease may be detected by disc analysis within the entire follow-up period of the disease.

For POAG (Table 2), we found in stage I of VFL in 52 eyes a mean CDR of 0.44 ± 0.27. As shown before in CACG, at a mean CDR of 0.44 a stage II of VFL was found. In POAG there is, therefore, already a larger CDR at stage I of the disease than in CACG. In POAG the change of mean CDR between stages I and IV was 0.38 (43 %). Quantification of the progression of the disease with disc analysis may already be more difficult in POAG than in CACG.

For PG (Table 2) we found a mean CDR of 0.49 ± 0.21 for 35 patients with VFL stage I. The change of mean CDR between stages I and IV was 0.33, which is a relative change of 40 % and which is similar to POAG.

In patients with NTG (Table 2), we found for 25 patients with VFL stage I a mean CDR of 0.69 ± 0.12. The mean change of CDR between stages I and IV is only 0.19 in NTG, which is a relative change of only 22 % between the onset of disease and the advanced stage. This small change in CDR might not allow quantification of the progression by disc analysis alone. The onset of the disease in NTG at a mean CDR of 0.69 is approximately equal to a stage III VFL in CACG or POAG and to stage II in PG. This signifies that at a given mean CDR there is in NTG a smaller VFD at two stages of the disease than in POAG or CACG, or at one stage when compared to PG. Thus there are remarkable differences in mean CDR at stage I, in other words at the onset of the disease, with 0.17 for CACG, 0.44 for POAG, 0.49 for PG and 0.69 for NTG. This suggests the existence of a number of different, interrelated pathogenetic mechanisms producing the damage which we call glaucoma. The relevance regarding early diagnosis clear, because we may expect differences in the detection probability using disc analysis for discovery of the onset of the disease in the various types of glaucoma. The change in mean CDR between stage I and stage IV of VFL is 80 % for CACG, 43 % for POAG, 40 % for PG and only 22 % for NTG and is significant for selecting the appropriate examination method for follow-up: We can expect differences in the sensitivity between perimetry and disc analysis for follow-up in the different glaucomas. There is a decreasing sensitivity for disc analysis in comparison to perimetry and an increasing sensitivity for perimetry, in comparison to disc analysis from CACG via POAG and PG to NTG. These remarkable differences between morphology and function in the various types of glaucoma are illustrated in Fig. 2.

The upper line in Fig. 2 illustrates the relation between CDR and VFL in NTG. There is only very little change in mean CDR, from 0.69 at the onset of the disease to 0.88 in the advanced stage. Perimetry, therefore, is more sensitive than disc analysis in NTG for quantifying the progression of the glaucomatous damage at all stages of the disease. The lower line illustrates the relation between mean CDR and VFL in CACG. In contrast to NTG the onset of the VFL already appears at a mean CDR of 0.17 and shows a nearly linear relation between CDR and VFL from stage I to IV. This may allow a good follow-up of progression by disc analysis and perimetry, but the onset of glaucomatous disease can easily be missed if only the disc is examined. In between is the relationship of mean CDR and VFL for POAG and PG. The distribution of the CDR values in stage I and stage II of VFL in patients with PG, NTG and POAG are shown in Fig. 3a and 3b. The larger CDRs in NTG are significant, with $p < 0.001$ between NTG and POAG and $p < 0.01$ between NTG and PG. There is also a significant difference between PG and POAG ($p < 0.05$) (Mann-Whitney U test). The comparison of the CDR in stage II of VFL shows larger CDRs in NTG with significant differences between NTG and POAG ($p < 0.01$), and NTG and PG ($p < 0.05$) and also between PG and POAG ($p < 0.05$) (Mann-Whitney U test). In stages III and IV, no significant differences in CDR between the three types of glaucoma are found (Fig. 3c, 3d).

Conclusion

To summarize, the results of this study show that there are significant differences in the appearances of the ONH between NTG and the more IOP-dependent glaucomas. Taking all the types of glaucoma into consideration, a small CDR cannot exclude the

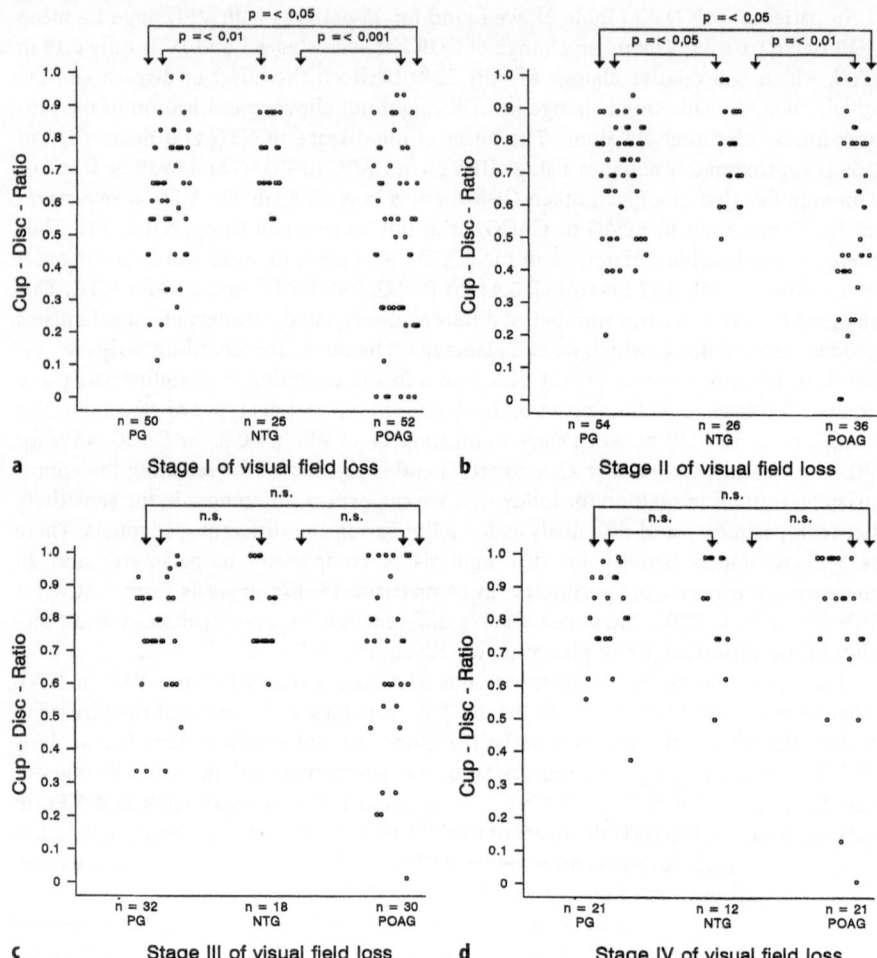

Fig. 3a–d. Comparison of CDR in stages I–IV of VFL between NTG, POAG, PG

existence of a VFD (stage I) in IOP-dependent glaucomas and in NTG we find large CDRs with only small VFD. From the size of the CDR, therefore, no conclusion can be made about the amount of VFL. Thus, CDR on its own is a poor indicator for quantifying glaucomatous damage. Staging of the glaucomas by disc appearance alone is therefore not possible.

Figure 4 summarizes the stage-dependent principle relation between morphology and function in glaucomas in general. In the initial stages of glaucomatous disease, a relatively large change in the optic disc and only a small change in the VFL may be found. In the advanced stages, however, the same change in CDR may result in a much greater change in VFL. This means, for all types of glaucomas, that in the advanced stages of the disease perimetry is the more sensitive method than disc analysis for detecting any deterioration.

Fig. 4. The stage-dependent difference in the relationship of morphology and function in the glaucomas

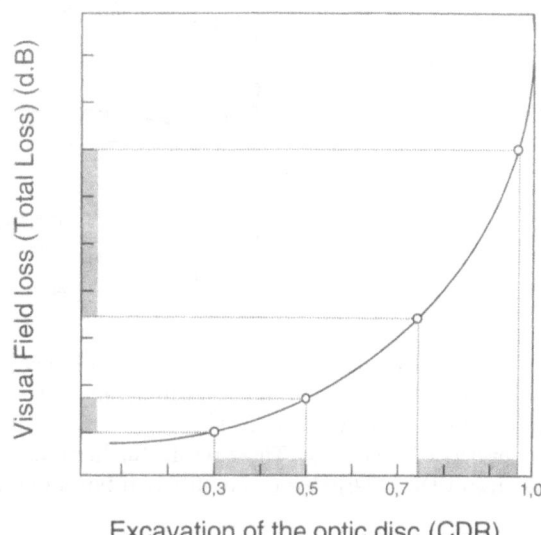

Excavation of the optic disc (CDR)

Disc Area in Different Types of Glaucoma

When comparing disc parameters of different types of glaucoma, the question arises whether there are any differences in disc sizes between NTG, POAG and, for instance, healthy eyes. By means of confocal examination techniques (laser tomographic scanner (LTS), Heidelberg retina tomograph, HRT) we evaluated disc size and disc diameter in eyes with NTG and POAG and in healthy eyes [64]. Using the LTS to examine 153 eyes we found no significant differences in the vertical and horizontal diameter nor, using the HRT and comparing 105 eyes, any significant differences in disc size. Figure 5 shows the HRT results of mean disc area in healthy eyes and eyes with OH, POAG and NTG.

Furthermore, in stages I, II, III and IV of VFL we found no significant differences in disc diameter when examining 53 eyes with POAG and 30 eyes with NTG comparing vertical and horizontal disc diameter using the LTS (Fig. 6). Therefore we con-

Fig. 5. Mean disc size (mean value with standard deviation), evaluated with the HRT in healthy eyes, eyes with OH, POAG and NTG

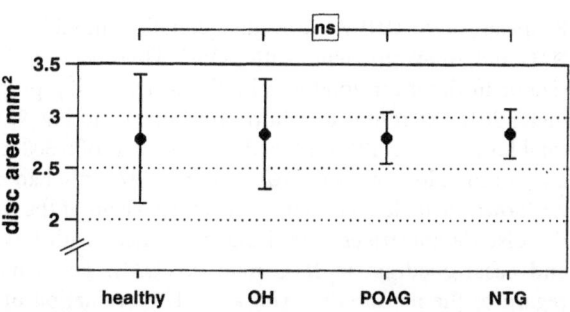

Fig. 6. Mean horizontal and vertical disc diameters in relation to stages I–IV of VFL in POAG (n = 53 eyes/patients) and NTG (n = 30 eyes/patients)

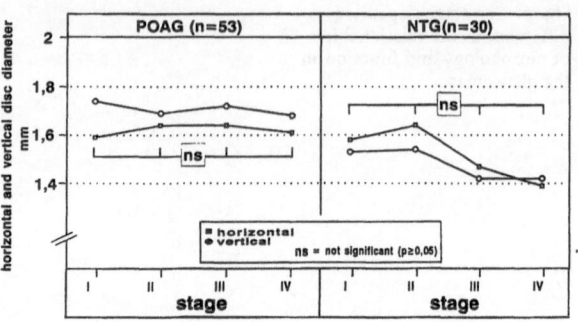

clude, firstly, that patients with NTG have no larger disc size, and, secondly, that in the advanced stages of the disease, compared to the early stages in NTG and POAG, there is no larger disc diameter. Disc size, therefore, seems not to be a risk factor for the severity of the disease. These results further indicate that it is possible to compare the mean CDR of large groups in different types of glaucoma [64].

Correlation of Disc Area and CDR and Rim Area Examined with the Topographic Scanning System

In this unpublished study, we examined the eyes of 199 healthy individuals, with a mean age of 39 ± 10.4 years and an age range from 19 to 76 years, using the topographic scanning system (TopSS). We found a correlation between disc area and CDR (p = 0.0002, R = 0.26) (Fig. 7) and a correlation between disc area and neuroretinal rim area (p = 0.0001, R = 0.63) (Fig. 8) and between CDR and the size of the neuro-retinal rim area (p = 0.0001, R = 0.57).

This means that larger discs have larger CDRs and larger neuroretinal rim areas. Comparison of disc parameters between different types of glaucomas should therefore be matched for disc size. This is possible using automatic disc analysis and was done for the evaluation of CDR and VFL in LTG and POAG using the optic nerve head analyzer (ONHA) and laser tomographic scanner (LTS) [23, 70, 71].

Mean CDR in Eyes with LTG and POAG Examined with the ONHA

By means of the ONHA we evaluated, in this unpublished study, 18 eyes/patients with NTG and 16 eyes/patients with POAG. There were no significant differences in disc size or in the mean total loss in visual field using program 31 of the Octopus perimeter 201. The results are shown in Table 3 and Fig. 9. The NTG group, with a mean total loss of 733 ± 124.5 dB, had a mean CDR of 0.800 ± 0.017; the POAG group, with a mean total loss of visual field of 678 ± 137.0 dB, had a mean CDR of 0.731 ± 0.027. As shown in Table 3 and Fig. 9 the comparison of the mean CDR in the quadrants of the disc demonstrates significant differences with larger CDRs in the upper, lower and nasal quadrant in NTG than in POAG. The same differences are found with regard to the neuroretinal rim area. The evaluation of seven eyes of seven patients

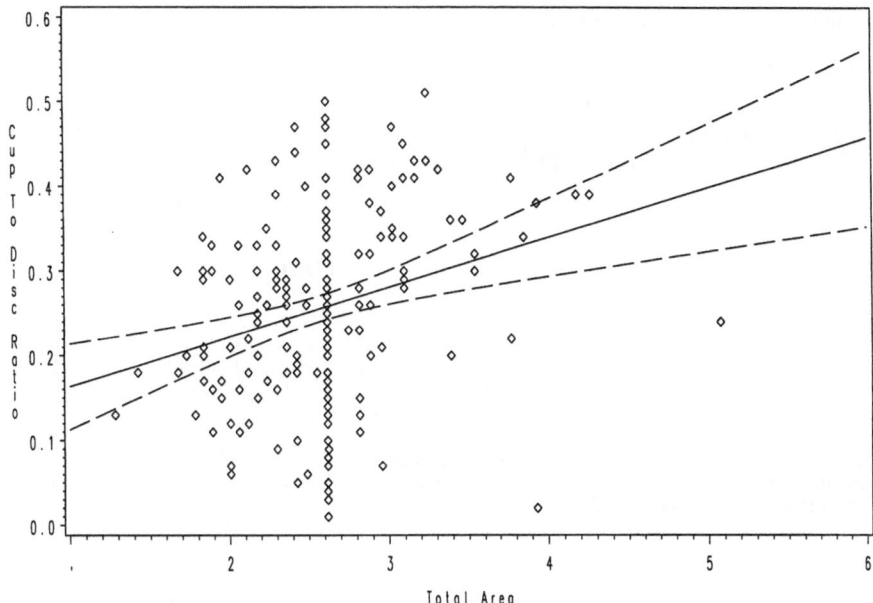

Fig. 7. Correlation of disc area and CDR

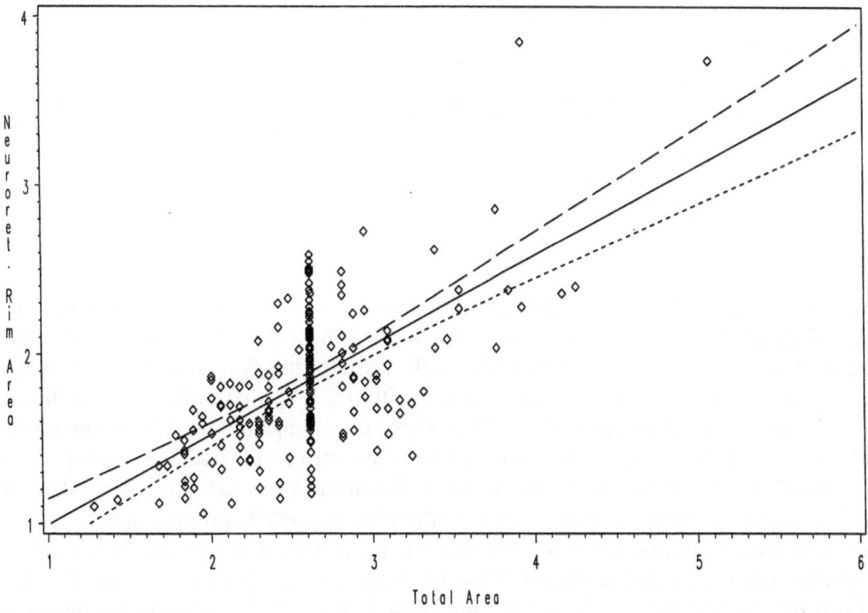

Fig. 8. Correlation of disc area and neuroretinal rim area

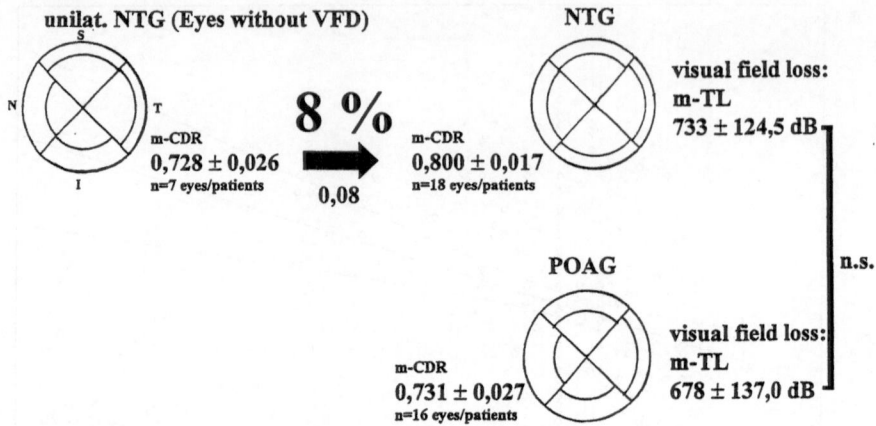

Fig. 9. Mean CDR in eyes with NTG and POAG and in the fellow eye with normal visual field in patients with unilateral NTG. The CDR in the quadrants is illustrated true-to-scale for the three groups from the data shown in Table 3

Table 3. Mean CDR in relation to mean VFL in patients with NTG and POAG

Diagnosis	m-TL ± SD [dB]	m-CDR ± SD	Nasal	Supe-rior	Infe-rior	Tempo-ral	m-IOP max. ± SD[a] (mm Hg)	eyes/ patients (n)	m-age ± SD (years)
Fellow eye without VFL in unilateral normal tension glaucoma (NTG)	0	0.728 0.026	0.62 ± 0.08	0.81 ± 0.01	0.64 ± 0.02	0.84 ± 0.02	17.0 ± 0.84	7	49.2 ± 14.6
Normal tension glaucoma (NTG)	733 ± 124.5	0.800 ± 0.017	0.76 ± 0.03	0.77 ± 0.04	0.80 ± 0.02	0.84 ± 0.02	17.5 ± 0.60	18	60.3 ± 12.7
Primary open-angle glaucoma (POAG)	678 ± 137.0	0.731 ± 0.027	0.69 ± 0.04	0.78 ± 0.03	0.71 ± 0.03	0.79 ± 0.03	35.8 ± 1.40	16	62.8 ± 9.9

with unilateral NTG and no significant difference in disc size compared to NTG and POAG group revealed a mean CDR of 0.728 ± 0.026 in the eye without VFD. This shows that there are already large CDRs at the onset of the disease in NTG, and confirms quantitatively the observation made by Drance [15], that unilateral NTG has a large CDR in the fellow eye with no VFD. There is a change of only 0.08 in the mean CRD, i.e. a relative change of 8 %, which results in a mean VFD with a mean total loss of 733 dB. The mean CDR of the fellow eye with normal VF in patients with unilateral NTG, with the same mean disc sizes as in the NTG and POAG groups, showed a pre-existing large CDR of 0.728 ± 0.026 before the development of atrophy. This value is approximately equal to the mean CDR of the POAG group, with a mean VFL of 678 ± 137.0 dB. In addition to the results mentioned above, this demonstrates, using a quantitative examination technique comparing eyes with the same disc diameter, that patients with NTG, more often than with other types of glaucoma, may have a further risk factor in the morphology of the optic disc. The evaluation of the mean CDR in the disc quadrants (Table 3), illustrated in Fig. 9 true-to-scale, shows further significant differences in the configuration of the optic disc excavation between the three groups.

Configuration of the Optic Disc in NTG, POAG, OH and Healthy Eyes Examined with the LTS

By means of the confocal examination technique of the LTS we evaluated whether there are any quantitative differences in the configuration of the optic disc excavation in healthy eyes and eyes with POAG, NTG and OH with same mean disc sizes and the same stage of VFL. In 82 eyes of 82 patients the configuration of the optic disc excavation was calculated using the ratio of mean excavation depth to the maximal excavation depth and the third moment. (For details of methods, refer to the original paper [46, 70].)

The results are illustrated schematically in Fig. 10. In eyes with NTG in stage I and II we found a significant difference in the steepness of the slope of the excavation and in the configuration of the bottom of the optic disc excavation. Eyes with NTG demonstrate a steeper slope and flatter bottom of excavation in stages I and II than eyes with POAG. In stages III and IV no significant differences in the configuration of the optic disc were found. No significant differences in the configuration of the optic disc excavation could be found in healthy eyes compared to eyes with OH and POAG, stage I (Mann-Whitney U test). However, a significant difference in the steepness of the slope of the excavation for eyes with NTG stage I was found compared to healthy eyes and eyes with OH and POAG, stage I. The change in configuration of the excavation therefore occurs one stage of the disease later (stage defined as the total loss in the VF in dB) in POAG than in NTG. A significant difference exists in the configuration of the excavation between NTG stage I and healthy eyes, eyes with OH and POAG, stage I. Eyes with NTG already demonstrate a steeper slope and flatter bottom of the excavation of optic disc in stage I. Eyes with POAG show only a slight change in the configuration of the excavation between stages I and II. A distinct increase in the steepness

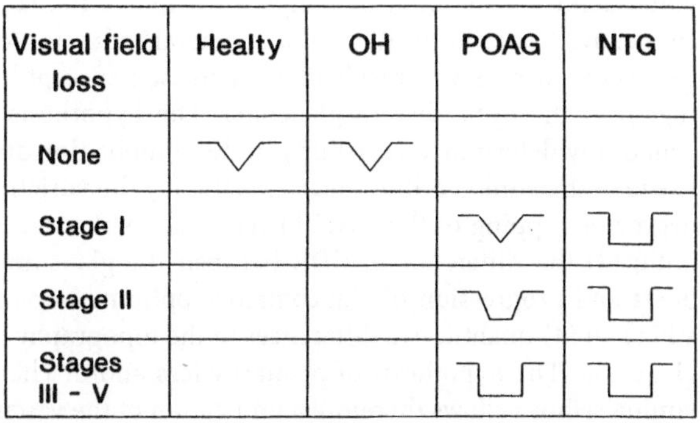

Fig. 10. Configuration of the excavation in healthy eyes and eyes with OH, POAG, NTG

Visual field loss	Healty	OH	POAG	NTG
None	∖∨⌐	∖∨⌐		
Stage I			∖∨⌐	⎍⌐
Stage II			∖∨⌐	⎍⌐
Stages III – V			⎍⌐	⎍⌐

of the slope of the excavation is not evident in POAG before the advanced stages III–V. In contrast, eyes with NTG already demonstrate a steep slope and flat bottom of the excavation at the onset of the disease, which changes only insignificantly in the advanced stages III–V of the glaucomatous disease. This indicates differences between glaucomas in the pathogenesis of the glaucomatous damage in the initial stages. The results described above evaluated with ONHA were with this study confirmed by a quantitative confocal examination of the optic nerve head.

Hypothesis: Genetic Disposition to Primary Less Connective Tissue of the Lamina Cribosa – A Further Risk Factor and More Frequent in NTG?

The differences in the appearance of the ONH between the glaucomas (NTG, POAG and, included as controls, PG and CACG) summarized above may have relevance for new insights into their pathogenesis. The morphological difference in the appearance of the ONH between the different types of glaucoma cannot result from a difference in neural substance because the eyes compared were at the same stage of VFL. These biomorphometric differences [24–26, 42, 43, 46, 49, 65, 70], together with differences found in the topography and progression of VFD in different types of glaucoma [22, 29, 36, 37, 47, 49] and the findings on disc hemorrhages [41], which will be mentioned below, encouraged us in our hypothesis that the amount of connective tissue of the lamina cribosa may explain the morphological differences in the ONH between the glaucomas. Possible mechanisms for this morphological differences in CDR in NTG compared to POAG, PG and CACG may be the presence of a pre-existing large cup in NTG as a congenital or familiar feature, before development of atrophy. The hypothesis is that there are patients with a genetic disposition to primarily less connective tissue of the lamina cribosa and that this disposition is found more frequently in patients with NTG than in other types of glaucoma. Within the sheets of the lamina cribosa, vessels are wrapped. Histological studies suggest that in the inferior temporal region of the lamina cribosa in healthy eyes there is the least amount of connective tissue support of the vessels. Figure 11 shows the vessels structure of the optic disc of a monkey eye.

Axon bundles which are surrounded by less connective tissue beams and vessels within the weaker connective tissue sheets of the lamina cribosa may show increased vulnerability. If the inferior temporal region of the lamina cribosa already has less connective tissue in healthy eyes, a general reduction or changed elasticity of these connective tissues will result in an increased susceptibility of the inferior temporal region of the optic disc in glaucoma. The hypothesis of an individually different, genetically determined variability in the composition and structure of the connective tissue of the lamina cribosa may explain: (1) the variation in both the nature and the degree of cupping of the ONH in response to elevated IOP, systemic risk factors, or both; (2) the difference in CDR between the glaucomas; (3) the differences in the onset and progression of glaucomatous optic neuropathy in relation to the stage of VFL; and (4) quantitative differences in the topography of VFL in the various types of glaucoma. The hypothesis of primarily less and/or changed connective tissue of the lamina cribosa allows therefore a unification of the vascular and mechanical theory of

Fig. 11. Vessel structure of the optic disc of a monkey. If the vessels of the lamina cribrosa are wrapped by primarily less or changed connective tissue, a secondary ischemic glaucomatous damage occurs. This will happen with higher probability if general risk factors are present. (Permission for publication kindly given by K. Sugiyama, Gifu University, Japan)

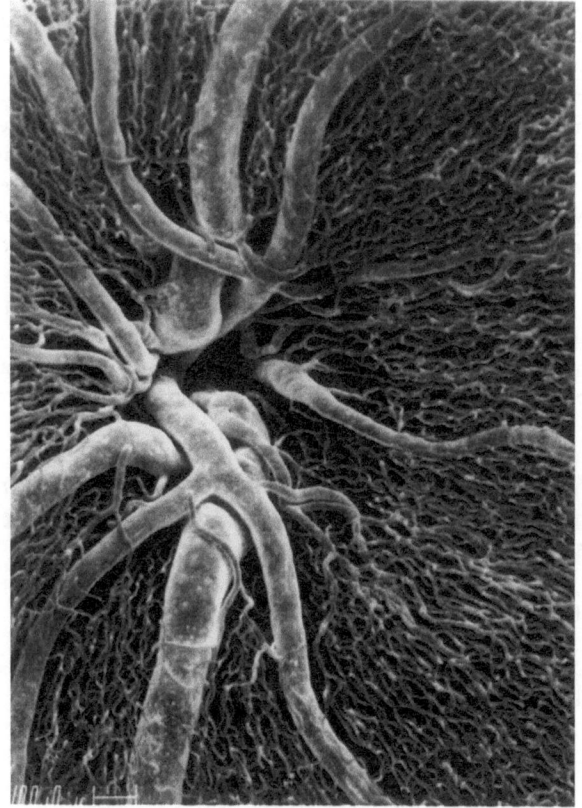

glaucoma damage and explains the individual tolerance of the ONH to IOP-related or IOP-independent risk factors and the genetic disposition of glaucomatous disease. This unification hypothesis also conforms with the clinical features of the disease: If there is a genetic disposition to primarily less connective tissue in the lamina cribrosa, there will first be a loss of capillary support of the laminal cribosa inferior temporally in the optic disc. Elevated IOP and/or general risk factors, e.g. a low BP [25, 34, 35, 49], can lead to capillary compression or capillary collapse, which may result in a higher incidence of DHs in the inferior temporal quadrant. The resulting localized ischemia will then lead to nerve fiber bundle defects inferior temporally in the ONH [1, 69, 86, 90], resulting in more frequent, localized VFD in the nasal upper quadrant of the VF [29, 31, 49]. This is in accordance with the clinical findings in NTG and POAG [25, 29, 31, 34, 35, 41, 49].

Higher Susceptibility of the Inferior Temporal Disc Quadrant

In the inferior temporal region of the optic disc, pallor and thinning of the neuroretinal rim area are found more frequently [73, 80, 83, 84, 88] in early glaucoma. Here we also found a higher incidence of DHs, 52 % in stage II of VFL [41], than in other quadrants, as described below in detail. The higher incidence of DHs inferior temporally is confirmed by many other studies [1, 86, 89] and fits the topography of VFL in NTG and POAG, with a higher incidence of VFL in the upper nasal quadrant [21, 31, 37]. Fluorescence angiographic filling defects are found particularly frequently in the inferior temporal quadrant of the optic disc [84]. Increased blockage of axoplasmatic transport in the temporal sector of the optic disc was found in eyes with experimentally increased IOP [72, 74]. We found nerve fiber bundle defects more frequently in NTG than in POAG using HRT [69]. Central retinal vein occlusions are more frequent in NTG and POAG than in PG, and DHs in NTG are more frequent than in POAG, according to the literature.

In a recent study we examined the age-related loss in nerve fiber layer thickness (NFLT) in 104 healthy eyes of 104 normal subjects using optical coherence tomography (OCT) and found that the age-related loss of NFLT was larger in the inferior temporal quadrant than in other quadrants (unpublished data) [39], as described below.

Age-Related Nerve Fiber Loss Occurs Predominantly in the Inferior Temporal Quadrant of the Optic Nerve Head: A Clinical Study Using OCT

Introduction

Direct nerve fiber layer thickness (NFLT) measurements can be performed with two different techniques:
1. With laser polarimetry, using the nerve fiber analyzer (NFA). The NFA uses the principle of NFL birefringence to rotate polarized light and from this rotation derives a measurement value of NFL thickness [27, 50, 81, 92].
2. With optical coherence tomography (OCT), a measuring technique for high resolution, non-invasive, cross-sectional, morphometric imaging, e.g. of the layered structure of the retina. Cross-sectional information concerning retinal topography and internal tissue structure is obtained with approximately 10 µm of depth resolution from the time delay of reflected light using low-coherence interferometry. It is similar to B-scan ultrasound except that image formation depends on differences in light back-scattering rather than acoustic back-scattering properties of tissue. One possible use of OCT is to image the peripapillary retina cross-sectionally in cylindrical sections of tissue surrounding the ONH. Evaluation of the reproducibility of NFLT measurements showed a standard deviation of 10–20 µm for mean overall NFLT measurements and 15–20 µm for measurements of each hour. From these cross-sectional images and automated computer algorithm quantitates NFLT and total retinal thickness, summarized in four sectors, hour and overall [50]. Two software versions are available; data calculated with the new software are presented here.

NFA and OCT measurements record the typical double-hump configuration of the peripapillary retina in normals. Our previous results of the height contour measurement with HRT [82] or the NFLT measurements with NFA showed that the clinical validity of the results are dependent on the distance of the measurement circle to the papilla.

We showed that, e.g. the height contour and NFLT of the peripapillary retina could be measured all the more accurately the nearer the measurement circle is to the papilla [82]. For this study with the OCT we therefore defined a measurement circle of 1.5-fold of the optic disc diameter concentrically around the papilla. A relative distance related to the disc size seems advantageous due to the large disc diameter variations [48] in normals.

Using the NFA, we discovered in an earlier study that in the lower retinal half – compared to the upper retinal half – a 6.9 % thicker NFL in the lower half was evident when we examined the peripapillary NFLT of 62 healthy persons by means of laser polarimetry. Thus in the lower retinal half there was a significantly greater mean measurement value of the NFLT, with 0.306 ± 0.075, than in the upper retinal half, with 0.286 ± 0.072 ($p = 0.00022$) [50, 81]. Therefore, NFLT asymmetry was reevaluated with OCT.

Purpose

I.   To evaluate with OCT whether there is any asymmetry in NFLT between sectors, between quadrants and between the upper and lower retinal half.
II. To evaluate the effect of aging on the NFLT with the following questions: (a) Is NFLT age-dependent? (b) Is there any difference in age-dependent loss of peripapillary NFLT between quadrants?
III. Is the retinal asymmetry index (RAI) age-independent? The RAI is the quotient of the mean peripapillary NFLT of the upper half to the NFLT in the lower retinal half.

Methods

We examined 104 eyes of 104 normal subjects (59 male, 45 female, mean age 48.2 ± 17.6 years, range: 16–78 years) with the OCT using a circle scan around the optic disc in a distance of 1.5 disc diameters. A total of 48 right eyes and 56 left eyes were examined. Inclusion criteria were a visual acuity of 1.0 [20/20], a refractive error of not more than ± 3 diopters (D), normal VF and normal biomicroscopical findings. These eyes were, e.g. the second healthy eyes of patients with perforating injury in the other eye. The NFLT examination was carried out by the same examiner in all eyes.

From the OCT printout the NFLT-hour values A–L (compare Fig. 12, top) were used to calculate average NFLT values for retinal halves (left), for retinal sectors (middle) and for retinal quadrants (right), as shown in Fig. 12.

Results

I. NFLT. The mean overall NFLT was 84.2 ± 21.5 μm. The mean NFLT between the upper half of the peripapillary retina (85.2 ± 23.4 μm) and the lower half (83.8 ± 22.4 μm) and between quadrants was not significantly different. Figure 13 shows the mean NFLT in retinal sectors. A significantly larger NFLT was found in the lower sector, with $110,1 \pm 26,4$ μm, than in the upper sector, with 104.3 ± 26.9 μm ($p = 0.039$, Wilcoxon test).

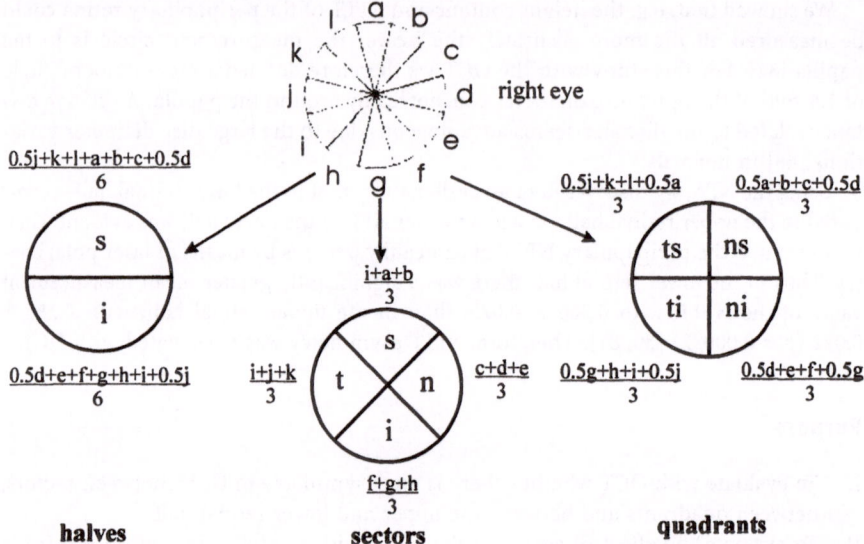

halves   sectors   quadrants

s = superior, i = inferior, n = nasal, t = temporal, ns = nasal superior, ni = nasal inferior, ts = temporal superior, ti = temporal inferior

Fig. 12. Calculation of mean NFLT in retinal halves, sectors and quadrants

II. Effect of Aging on NFLT. A decreasing NFLT with increasing age was found ($r = 0.303$, $p = 0.002$) (Fig. 14) with the highest correlation in the inferior temporal quadrant (Figs. 15, 16) ($p = 0.0003$). Age-related nerve fiber loss occurs predominantly in the inferior temporal quadrant, as shown in Fig. 16 (left).

Fig. 13. Mean NFLT (mm) in retinal sectors in 104 normal eyes (OCT)

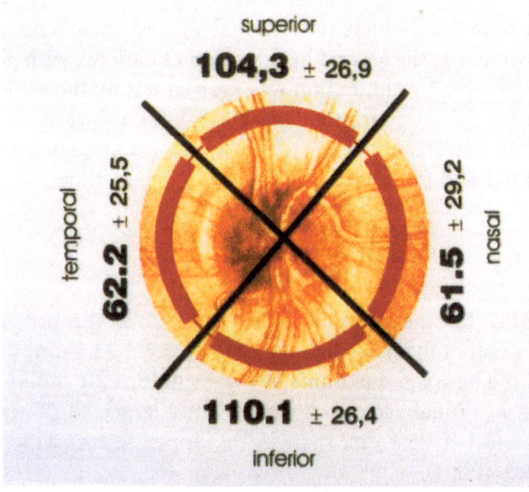

Fig. 14. Correlation of overall NFLT and age

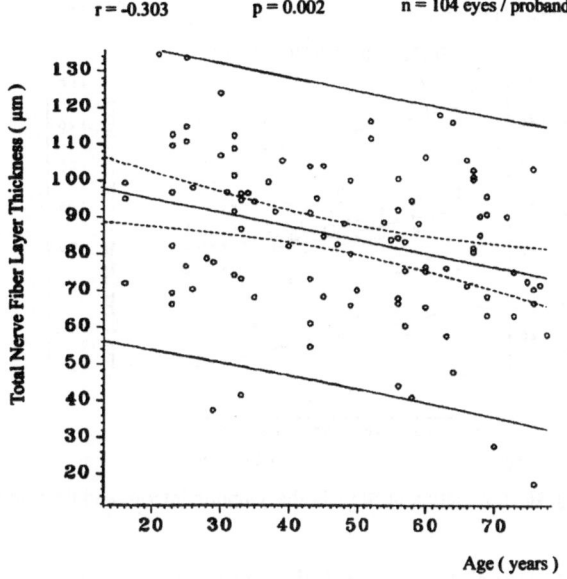

Temporal superior

Nasal superior

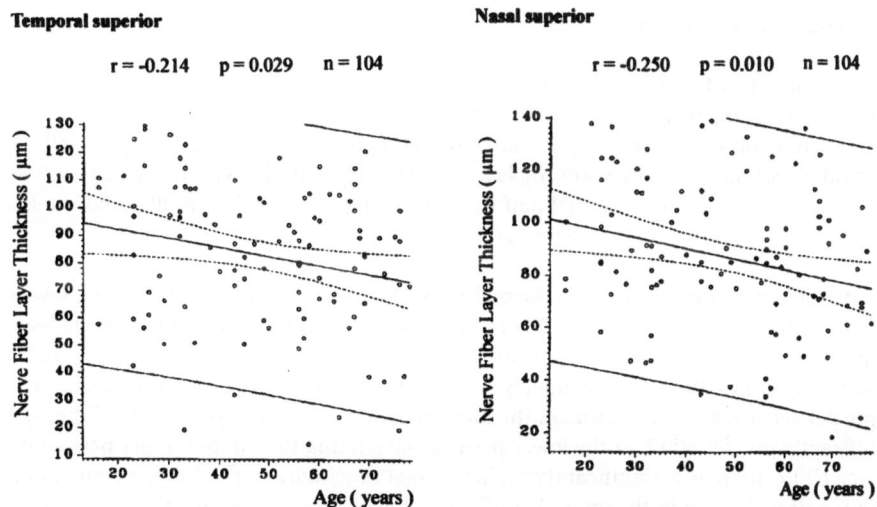

Fig. 15. Correlation of NFLT in the temporal superior and nasal superior quandrant and age

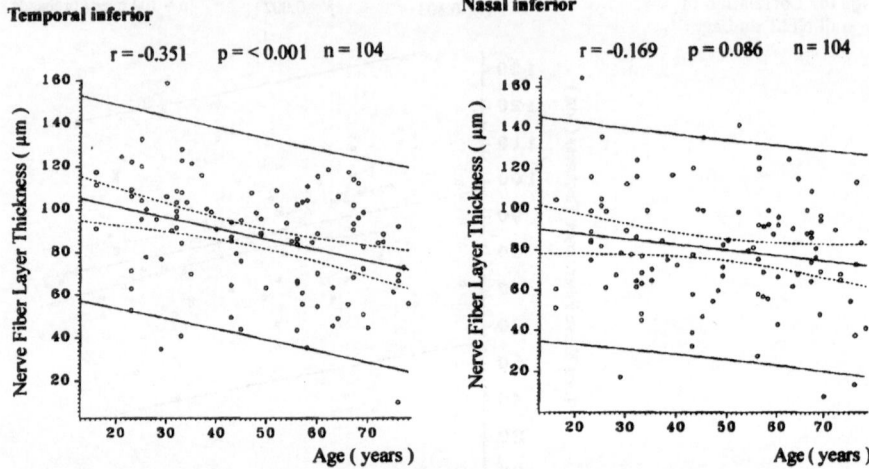

Fig. 16. Correlation of NFLT in the temporal inferior and nasal inferior quadrant and age

III. Retinal Asymmetry Index. The quotient of mean NFLT of the upper half to the lower half (RAI) was 1.046 ± 0.256 and was age-independent (Fig. 17).

Discussion/Conclusion

I. Asymmetry of NFLT. The larger NFLT found with OCT in the lower sector confirms that, comparing sectors in normals, there is a physiological asymmetry of the NFLT, in contrast to the comparison of retinal halves. Of 62 control subjects, all 62 healthy eyes measured by scanning laser polarimetry with the NFA I, showed a 6.9 % larger NFLT in the lower retinal half than in the upper half. This result could not be confirmed for retinal halves using OCT.

Asymmetry of Visual Field in Normal Eyes. The greater NFLT found in the lower peripapillary retinal half with NFA or in the lower retinal sector with OCT would lead us to expect increased retinal sensitivity in the upper visual field in normals. This, however, is not the case. Perimetry tests of healthy persons prove that there is a greater sensitivity of the retina in the lower half of the VF [50, 93]. In spite of the significantly greater NFLT in the lower peripapillary retina than in the upper peripapillary NFLT, there is a significantly higher retinal sensitivity in the lower hemifield of the central VF than in the upper hemifield. In healthy eyes, therefore, there is no conformity between the asymmetry of retinal sensitivity and the asymmetry of the NFLT, which was, however, only found in the OCT with the upper and lower sector. Further investigations are necessary regarding the question whether the physiological asymmetry of the NFLT can be explained by the frequently found thicker axons of the lower nerve fiber bundle in comparison to those of the upper nerve fiber bundle [75].

Fig. 17. Correlation of RAI and age

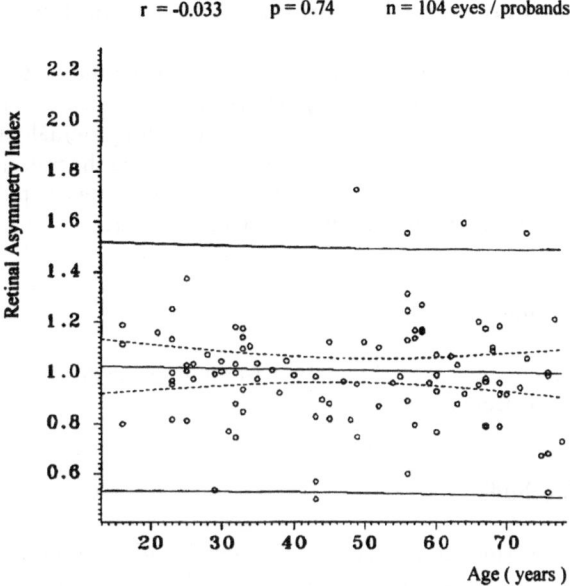

r = -0.033   p = 0.74   n = 104 eyes / probands

II. Effect of Aging on NFLT. NFLT is age-dependent in contrast to RAI. This confirms our earlier results with the LTS [46] and NFA [81]. A new and interesting observation is that age-related nerve fiber loss occurs predominantly in the inferior temporal quadrant of the ONH. An age-dependent NFLT loss therefore occurred mostly in the inferotemporal nerve fibers, which are located in the inferotemporal, weaker connective tissue in the lamina cribosa [78]. Blood vessels, wrapped with the connective tissue sheets of the lamina cribosa, may obliterate first in these weaker areas, producing are-released secondary ischemic damage of nerve fibers.

III. Retinal Asymmetry Index. The age-independent RAI may be useful in a retinal hemifield test (RHT) for glaucoma screening and for individual follow-up of people at risk for glaucoma. This relative NFLT measurement value was found to be independent of age using OCT (compare Fig. 17) and NFA [50] and independent of reference plane and disc size using HRT measurements [82]. The RAI reduces the interindividual variation of NFLT measurements due to age and disc size [50] and may improve screening possibilities for glaucoma. RHT has a further advantage over the glaucoma hemifield test using perimetry, since the measured value obtained is not dependent on patient cooperation. Furthermore, the measured RAI value [50] can be calculated and printed our from peripapillary retinal surface heigh measurements from the respective equipment for automated disc analysis (HRT, TopSS, ONHA) or for measurements on NFLT (OCT, NFA) and may give comparable RAI or retinal asymmetry difference (RAD) values.

Incidence and Topography of Disc Hemorrhages

The cause of DHs in glaucoma is unknown. Microinfarction, mechanical rupture of capillaries or a venous origin have been suggested. It is known, however, that DHs do not occur in disc sectors with no remaining retinal rim or in eyes with end-stage glaucomatous damage. This may indicate that the prevalence and location of DHs are dependent on the stage of the disease. In a recent unpublished study [41], we evaluated DHs with interest in two main purposes.

Purpose I

The first purpose of this study was to evaluate the incidence of DHs in different types of glaucoma.

Methods

We performed a stage-related evaluation of quantitative differences in the prevalence of DHs between PG with regulated IOP, POAG with regulated IOP and NTG with IOP-lowering therapy, comparing eyes with the same stages of VFL in these three types of glaucoma. We evaluated the occurrence of DHs in 431 eyes of 431 glaucoma patients, comprising 44 eyes with NTG, 301 eyes with POAG and 86 eyes with PG. Evaluation periods for DHs were defined as a time period of regulated IOP, which in turn was defined as a pressure lower than 22 mm Hg within the evaluated total follow-up time of the VF. Patients were seen in 6-monthly routine intervals in the out-patient glaucoma department at the Würzburg University Eye Hospital. We recorded IOP, disc appearance, CDR, presence of DH and VF using Octopus perimeter 201 program 31 or 33. VFD was staged by the Aulhorn classification. To be included in the retrospective DH study the following criteria had to be met: A visual acuity of 0.8 or better, refraction within ± 3 dpt (except for PG patients who were more myopic). The IOP had to be controlled, defined as an IOP lower than 22 mm Hg with medical or surgical therapy during the observation period, which was a minimal time of 1 year, equivalent to three consecutive examinations. All patients had reproducible VFDs at baseline examination, and no other known disease such as visible optic disc drusen, diabetic retinopathy, branch vein occlusion or AION. From the charts of the 431 qualifying patients, it was recorded whether a DH was present at the time of VF testing. All patients were seen by the same examiner. Only the first-noted DH in each patient during the observation interval of regulated IOP was included. A DH was defined as an isolated hemorrhage seen within the ONH tissue and/or in the peripapillary retina connected to the disc rim. The mean observation time was 4.3 years and not significantly different between groups, with a range of 1–15 years in NTG, 1–14 years in PG and 1–8 years in POAG. The mean VFL was stage II by Aulhorn classification in all three groups, ranging from stage I to stage III. Within the three groups of glaucoma with no significant difference in the mean stage of VFL, no significant difference in the mean observation time and no significant difference in the number of evaluated examinations, we found the following results.

Results

In POAG, 19 of 301 eyes were bleeders, representing 6.2 %. In NTG, three of 44 eyes bled, representing 6.8 %; and in PG, one of 86 eyes was a bleeder, representing 1.2 %. This difference between groups was not significant, with a 5 % error level.

Conclusions

The results suggest that in NTG and POAG with regulated IOP the incidence of DHs was six times higher than in PG with regulated IOP.

Purpose II

The second purpose of this study was the evaluation of DH location in eyes with POAG compared to eyes with non-glaucomatous, non-arteriitic AION.

Methods

Location of DHs was recorded in each of the four optic disc quadrants from disc photos or disc drawings. Since VFL was on average a stage II in the POAG group, the AION patients had to have less than 500 dB total VFL (total loss in program Delta of the Octopus 201) at the initial presentation. Thus only patients in the initial stages of AION disease were included, defining a comparable group with similar VFL.

Results

In POAG stage II, we found more frequent DHs in the inferior temporal quadrant, with 52 %, followed by the superiortemporal quadrant, with 26 %. In AION, the 59 recorded DHs observed in 24 eyes showed no significant differences between quadrants. The topography of DHs is shown in Fig. 18, top for POAG, bottom for AION.

Conclusion

Glaucomatous DHs may represent an acute ischemic event of the ONH and precede retinal nerve fiber layer defects and optic disc changes such as notching of the neuroretinal rim. The topography of DHs in glaucoma suggests that DHs may be a sign of secondary vascular damage due to changes in the collagenous structure of the lamina cribrosa or less connective tissue of the lamina cribosa with loss of elasticity and vessel support. The assumption of a primary generalized reduction of the collagenous structures could provide an explanation for why vessels are more prone to collapse or obliterate even at normal IOP levels. This would be expected to happen in POAG more frequently inferior temporally. In AION, a primary vascular damage without a

Fig. 18. Topography of 19 DHs in 19 eyes/patients with POAG stage II of VFL: 52.6 % are located in the inferior temporal disc quadrant (top). Topography of 59 DHs in 24 eyes/patients with AION and equal VFL compared to the POAG group; 20 % are located in the inferior temporal disc quadrant (bottom)

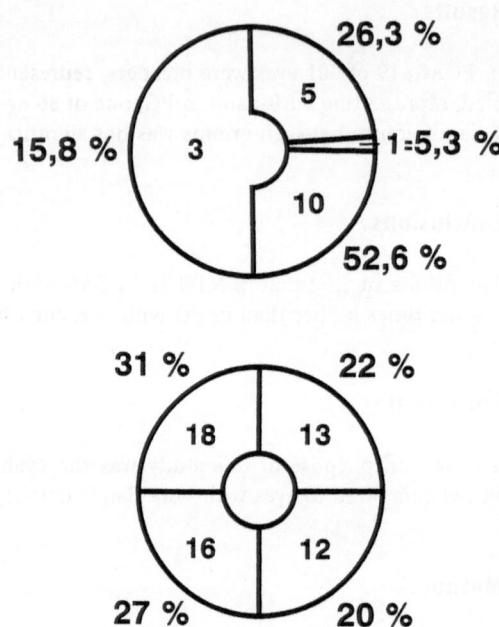

genetic disposition to less connective tissue of the lamina cribosa may be present leading to equal distribution of hemorrhages among disc quadrants. DHs in glaucoma patients, therefore, may be nothing more than a sign that the discs of such patients are made of "poor stuff" due to a genetic dispostion of less or altered connective tissue of the lamina cribosa: DHs in glaucoma patients are a prognostic sign of further VF deterioration, and they are an indicator that these eyes may deteriorate at a pressure level which would not ordinarily cause disease.

Quantitative Differences in Topography and Progression of VFL in NTG, POAG and PG

All the disc findings mentioned above are in accordance with the topography of VFL. We examined the topography of VFL in 83 eyes with NTG, 316 eyes with POAG and 52 eyes with PG with program 31 of the Octopus perimeter 201, comparing the same stages of the disease. Staging was performed according to the total loss in VF, calculated using the program Delta. Mean VFs were calculated from NTG, POAG and PG for stages I, II, III and IV. These mean VFs are comparable because there is no statistical difference in mean total loss for the three types of glaucoma within the same stage of the disease [29, 37, 49]. As shown in Fig. 19, differences in the topography of VF between the three types of glaucoma are obvious.

In POAG and NTG we found more often damage in the upper hemifield, especially in the nasal upper visual field quadrant. In PG the scotomas are distributed equally in the upper and lower hemifield and demonstrated no significant differences

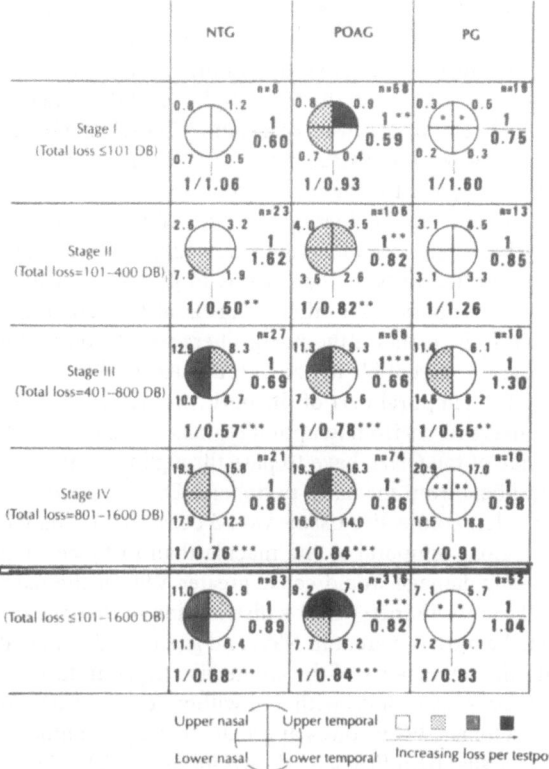

Fig. 19. Topography of VFL in NTG, POAG and PG in stages I–IV of VFL. For 451 eyes/patients a mean visual field is calculated for disease stages I–IV using the average of the mean loss per test point in the quadrants of the central visual field. The number of visual field findings included in each group is shown at the *upper right*. The last three pictures (bottom) illustrate a mean visual field of all stages together for 83 eyes with NTG, 316 eyes with POAG and 52 eyes with PG. Significant differences ($p < 5\%$) of the average loss per test point between several visual field quadrants were hatched, and marked with an *asterisk* when there was a significant difference between two quadrants. The ratio of the mean loss per test point in the two upper quadrants and the mean loss per test point in the two lower quadrants was calculated for each eye examined. The means of these individual values are reported as quotients to the *right of the circles*. For this purpose the loss per test point in the upper visual hemifield was set = 1. Thus the nominator of the fraction reports the mean loss per test point in the lower visual hemifield as a percentage of the damage in the upper visual hemifield. *Asterisks* show significant differences which either occur between two visual field quadrants or between two visual hemifields. * $p < 5\%$; ** $p < 1\%$; *** $p < 0.1\%$. (From [22, 29, 37, 49])

in the amount of damage between quadrants. Compared to PG, with its uniform distribution of field loss, the asymmetry of field loss in POAG and NTG must be caused by factors other than IOP. The topography of DHs inferior temporally is in accordance with the more common VFL in the nasal upper quadrant of NTG and POAG. Quigley hypothesized that the peripheral poles of the ONH are more likely to suffer injury in glaucoma because the connective tissue support for the nerve fiber bundles is spaser [76–78]. In the inferior temporal region of the lamina cribosa there is the least amount of connective tissue support, which again corresponds with the topography of VFDs. The connective tissue of the lamina cribosa contains the vessels, and the weakest connective tissue support is in the inferior temporal region. The blood flow should, according to our hypothesis, be reduced earlier and stronger in this area. This corresponds with the topography of VFDs, which are more frequent in the upper hemifield and upper nasal quadrant. NTG and POAG show more damage in the nasal than in the temporal visual hemifields compared to PG. In stages II–IV of the various glaucoma types, the inequality of occurrence of damage between the nasal and temporal visual hemifield was greater for NTG than for POAG and also greater than for PG. The differences were significant [29]. Thus the nasal half of the visual field was more affected in NTG than it was in glaucomas with elevated IOP. The probability that nerve fibers from different areas of the retina are damaged is directly proportional to the distance the nerve fibers pass through the ONH tissue and lamina cribosa areas susceptible to damage, as suggested by the results of our topography study [29]. The temporal part of the optic disc is penetrated by macular fibers, and this is why nerve fibers from temporal regions of the retina, which also pass over the temporal side of the ONH, have to pass through the optic disc tissue for a greater distance than fibers from the nasal periphery. Thus, randomly occurring local ischemias, e.g. due to less connective tissue, would cause greater damage to nerve fibers for the retinal regions temporal to the macula than to those from the nasal periphery. Hence, ischemic damage would cause greater VFL in the nasal visual hemifield. We found this lack of symmetry in the distribution of damage in the two vertical halves of the VF to be most apparent in NTG and less marked in POAG and PG. This speaks for the differing importance of the connective tissue-induced vascular origin in the etiology of VFDs in glaucomas with and without elevated IOP. With respect to the location of the scotomas, PG involves approximately equal amounts of damage in the upper and lower visual hemifields, as shown in Fig. 19. The damage factor IOP thus affects the upper and lower portions of the ONH to an equal extent if there is no genetic disposition to less or changed connective tissue of the lamina cribosa. In contrast, with POAG and NTG there was more frequent damage in the upper and nasal half of the VF. This non-symmetrical distribution of damage may be due to the presence of less connective tissue of the lamina cribosa in the inferior temporal quadrant of the ONH. This could explain the lower tension tolerance of these parts of the optic disc in NTG and POAG corresponding to the topography of VFD. The differences in the topography of VFD as well as the demonstrated differences in CDR, DHs, etc., between glaucomas suggest that less connective tissue of the ONH is more often a risk factor in NTG and POAG than in PG because of the uniform and symmetrical distribution of VFD in the quadrants in PG. Based on our findings of larger CDRs in NTG, we speculate that there are more often patients in the NTG group with less connective tissue, which is why high IOPs are not necessary to cause collapse or obliteration of the vessels in the lamina cribosa. Localized breakdown of the connective tissue leads to localized loss of capillary support and to collapse or obliteration of these vessels by raised IOP, even within a normal statistical range which would not normally have affected blood flow. Measurements show that blood flow is reduced in eyes with glaucomatous optic neuropathy compared to healthy eyes [13, 55–57, 79]. All our findings suggest that this reduction must not be a primary cause, but that it may be, in many patients, also a secondary cause of the genetically determined glaucomatous optic neuropathy at the level of the lamina cribosa within the extracellular matrix. In the glaucomatous ONH, progressive cupping of the optic disc results from compression, stretching and remodeling of the connective tissue (extracellular matrix) of the lamina cribosa, as demonstrated by Hernandez [58, 59]. Our hypothesis suggests that there may be an individual, possibly genetically determined variability in the composition, structure or reactive processes of the tissue supporting the axons and vessels in the optic nerve. This variability may explain the differences in the nature and degree of cupping and nerve fiber loss in response to IOP and/or general age-related risk factors, with an effect on aging of NFLT and on progression of the glaucomatous neuropathy. Structural and functional variations, e.g. loss of elasticity, in the extracellular matrix of the lamina cribosa may be one of several factors influencing the regional susceptibility for glaucomatous nerve fiber loss within the ONH, which is predominantly damaged in the initial stages of the disease in the inferior temporal disc quadrant. The observation that the pores of the lamina cribosa are small and round in eyes in the early stages of VFL, and bigger and oval in the advanced stages can be explained again by the deficit of connective tissue. An age-related appearance of further risk factors, e.g. cardiovascular risk factors, low BP or vasospasm, may trigger reduced ONH circulation in these dangerous areas first as the final pathway in the multifactorial pathogenesis of the disease. Our long-term follow-up of 153 eyes/ patients with POAG and regulated IOP during the observation time showed that patients with high pre-existing VFD had a twofold probability of VF deterioration than patients with a beginning VFD (31 % vs 13 %). Patients with low systolic BP had a four times higher probability of VF deterioration than patients with normal or high systolic BP in spite of IOP regulation (34.9 % vs 9.2 %) [25]. Using regression analysis these risk factors were confirmed in a further study [34] showing that low systolic BP was the most important risk factor for VF deterioration in POAG with regulated IOP. This was followed by pre-existing VFD as the second most important risk factor in eyes with regulated IOP; maximum IOP before therapy was the third most important risk factor. These findings are also in accordance with the hypothesis of less connective tissue of the lamina cribosa. This additional risk factor does not change our therapeutic strategies, rather, a high level of pre-existing damage [25, 28, 31, 33, 49] needs a more aggressive IOP-lowering therapy and a subsequent therapy to treat systemic cardiovascular risk factors. There is a logical basis for the IOP-lowering therapy in the inverse relationship between IOP and perfusion pressure in the ONH [12, 49]. The higher the IOP the lower the perfusion pressure, the lower the perfusion pressure the lower blood flow if autoregulation is defective or if other local or systemic factors are involved. Other studies demonstrated that function of retinal nerve fibers depends on perfusion pressure [3, 54, 55]. Opinions differ about the benefit of IOP-lowering strategies. Eyes treated with laser trabeculoplasty had a decreased probability of successful filtration surgery but preoperative use of topical medication did not influence the outcome of surgery [61]. Therefore, IOP-lowering surgery should only by performed if medications fails, allergy exists or if, e.g., compliance for appropriate drug application is not sufficient. The development of combination preparations which leads to a more aggressive IOP-lowering therapy, a reduction of costs in the medical treatment of IOP, an improvement in compliance, and a decrease in the burden of preservatives is therefore an ethical and medical necessity [6, 7, 21, 51, 53].

Genetic Disposition of CDR

Studies of the prevalence and incidence of confirmed glaucoma in the relatives of glaucoma patients leave little room for doubt that genetic factors play a role. In patients with PG we found a family history of glaucoma (FHG) in 81 of 207 patients (39.1 %) [53]. Examining 443 patients with OH and POAG stage I we found a FHG in 17.1 % [38, 40]. For PG [53] and for OH [38, 40] we found that FHG does not influence the severity or the prognosis of the disease after regulation of IOP. FHG is a risk factor but not a prognostic indicator. In NTG we found a FHG in 40 % [25] but whether FHG in NTG is a prognostic indicator is not known so far and its evaluation is the aim of an ongoing study. For some of the different types of glaucoma differences in the gene locus of the disease have been mapped. In PG, the gene locus of the disease was localized to chromosome 7q35-36; and 1999 on 18q; in POAG to chromosome 3q21-24, in NTG to chromosome 2cen-q13, in juvenile glaucoma to chromosome 1q23-25, and in hydrophthalmia to chromosome 2p21, 1p36, 6p25. The gene locus on 18q is the first evidence we have for genetic heterogeneity of pigment dispersion syndrome and PG (Andersen et al. 1999, Invest Ophthalmol Vis Sci 40, No 4, Abstract 3128, p 596). Thus, new insights into the differences of the glaucomas described above can be expected (Table 4). However, we do not yet know what role these different gene loci of the disease play in the pathogenesis of the glaucomas. It may be possible that the gene defects mapped in NTG patients are responsible, e.g. for the connective tissue structure of the lamina cribosa and/or for the elasticity of the lamina cribosa, in juvenile glaucoma and POAG, e.g. for the outflow facility and in PG, e.g. for pigment liberation [26]. Genetic studies will hopefully find the protein defect which can target patients with a genetic disposition to less connective tissue of the lamina cribosa.

IOP is, in part, genetically determined. Graham [18] stated "if it be true that IOP is a cause of chronic glaucoma (surprisingly, although a widely accepted fact, this is actually still an unproven hypothesis), then this could well be one of the factors involved". There is a genetic disposition for anterior chamber depth, axial length of the eye, CDR and IOP, and possibly for the amount of connective tissue of the lamina cribosa. Armaly [4] showed that the CDR in normal persons is largely determined by genetic factors and, therefore, in some families, parents with large cups have off-

Table 4. Glaucoma-related loci and incidence of family history of glaucoma for the different types of glaucoma

Type of glaucoma	Family history of glaucoma	Gene locus	Gene symbol	Inheritance	Age of onset	IOP
Juvenile glaucoma		1q23-25	GLC 1A	Autosomal-dominant	5–45	High
NTG	40 %	2cen-q13	GLC 1B	Autosomal-dominant	> 40	Normal
POAG	17 %	3q21-24	GLC 1C	Autosomal-dominant	> 40	High
PG	39 %	7q35-36 18q	Not named	Autosomal-dominant	< 40	High
Hydrophthalmia	40 %	2p21 1p36 6p25	GLC 3A GLC 3B Not named	Autosomal-recessive	< 1	High

spring with large cups [4]. The exact pattern of inheritance has not yet been established. Our studies showed that unilateral NTG also has a large CDR in the fellow eye with normal VF. Further, there are studies showing that African-Americans, compared to Americans of European origin, have a larger CDR [11] and a thinner extracellular matrix of the lamina cribrosa, less collagen type I and less elastin [58]. These differences in the morphology of the optic disc could be an explanation for both why glaucoma is present at an earlier age in black persons that white persons, as well as why the disease has a much worse prognosis for black persons compared to white persons. Age-adjusted data show that the incidence of blindness from glaucoma is eight times greater for African-Americans. The confirmation of genetically determined differences in the extracellular matrix of the lamina cribosa might explain this difference in prognosis and may point the way to a more rational therapy in the different glaucomas. In contrast to Europe, NTG is the most common type of glaucoma in Japan, and CACG is the most common type of glaucoma found in Eskimos, suggesting again a genetically determined impact.

Conclusions

The differences in the morphology of the optic disc, the location of DHs in the inferior temporal quadrant in the initial stages of the disease and the occurrence of the first signs of glaucoma in the disc in the lower temporal disc quadrant (historically, the area with the weakest connective tissue structure of the lamina cribrosa) and the differences in the topography and progression of VFD lead us to the hypothesis that a genetic disposition to less connective tissue of the lamina cribrosa may be a further risk factor in glaucoma, and that this risk factor is more frequent in NTG than in other types of glaucomas. This may explain the biomorphometric difference found in eyes with NTG compared to different types of glaucomas with high IOP. Therefore, this hypothesis of primary less or changed connective tissue allows unification of the vascular and mechanical theories and conforms with the clinical features of the disease. Further investigations of the pathophysiological role played by the extracellular matrix of the lamina cribrosa, and the possible genetic disposition for less connective tissue of the lamina cribrosa, may contribute to the discovery of the origin and nature of glaucoma.

The relation of ONH appearance and stage of VFD in different types of glaucoma leads to the following conclusion regarding the diagnostic sensitivity of disc analysis: The difference in the mean CDR in relation to the stage of the VFL in the different types of glaucoma shows that it is not possible to conclude from the CDR alone about the onset or amount of VFL. Disc analysis is important for diagnosis to locate the damage, provide a differential diagnosis, detect prognostic disc parameters, e.g. DH, and detect other glaucomatous signs of the disc, e.g. pallor, rim notches, which are important predictors of the existence of a VFD [44]. Disc analysis and perimetry are, therefore, complimentary to each other, but disc analysis on its own will never replace perimetry for staging and follow-up of the glaucomas.

Acknowledgement. Dedicated to Professor Stephen Drance, Vancouver.

References

1. Airaksinen PJ, Mustonen E, Alanko HI (1981) Optic disc hemorrhages precede retinal nerve fiber layer defects in ocular hypertension. Acta Ophthalmol 59:627–641
2. Airaksinen PJ, Tuulonen A, Werner EB: Clinical evaluation of the optic disc and retinal nerve fiber layer. In: Ritch R, Shields MB, Krupin T (eds) The Glaucomas. C.V. Mosby, St Louis, pp 617–657
3. Andersson DR (1992) Autoregulation in glaucoma. In: Drance SM (ed) International Symposium on Glaucoma, Ocular Blood Flow, and Drug Treatment. Baltimore, Williams and Wilkins, pp 82–89
4. Armaly F (1967) Genetic Determination of Cup/Disc Ratio of the Optic Nerve. Arch Ophthalmol 78:35–43
5. Aulhorn E: Sensoric functional damage. In: Heilmann K, Richardson KT (eds) Glaucoma, Conception of a Disease. Georg Thieme Verlag, Stuttgart, p 158
6. Busche S, Gramer E (1995) Advantage of a new fixed combination preparation of carbachol and betablocker or carbachol and Dipivefrin: A pilot study. Invest Ophthalmol Vis Sci 36(4):736
7. Busche S, Gramer E (1997) Verbesserung der Augentropfenapplikation und Compliance bei Glaukompatienten. Eine klinische Studie. Klin Monatsbl Augenheilkd 1997, 211:257–262
8. Caprioli J (1992) Discrimination between normal and glaucomatous eyes. Invest Ophthalmol Vis Sci 33:153–159
9. Caprioli J, Spaeth GL (1985) Comparison of the optic nerve head in high- and low-tension glaucoma. Arch Ophthalmol 103:1145–1149
10. Caprioli J, Weinreb RN (1988) Measurements of the optic nerve head and retinal nerve fiber layer in glaucoma. In: Kaufmann PL, Mittag TW (eds) Glaucoma, Textbook of Ophthalmology. Mosby, St Louis 7:6.22–6.33
11. Chi T, Ritch R, Stickler D, Pitman B, Tsai C, Hsieh F (1989) Racial Differences in Optic Nerve Head Parameters. Arch Ophthalmol 107:836–839
12. Cunha L, Gramer E (1992) Intraocular pressure treatment in low tension glaucoma? Asymmetric visual field defects and its relation to unequal outflow facility in low tension glaucoma: A clinical study. In: Gramer E, Kampik A (eds) Pharmakotherapie am Auge. Springer Verlag, Heidelberg pp 19–28
13. Drance SM (1985) Low-tension glaucoma. Enigma and opportunity (editorial). Arch Ophthalmol 103:1131–1133
14. Drance SM (1993) Some risk factors in open-angle glaucoma. Aust N Z J Ophthalmol 21:67–69
15. Drance SM, Sweeney VP, Morgan RW, Feldman F (1973) Studies of factors involved in the production of low tension glaucoma. Arch Ophthalmol 89:457–465
16. Gasser P (1989) Ocular vasospasm. A risk factor in the pathogenesis of low-tension glaucoma. Int Ophthalmol 13:281–290
17. Goldberg T, Hollows FC, Kass MA, Becker B (1992) Systemic factors in patients with low tension glaucoma. Br J Ophthalmol 65:56
18. Graham PA (1986) Epidemiology of primary glaucoma. In: GLAUCOMA, Grune and Stratton, 5–16
19. Gramer E (1986) Quantitative Papillenanalyse mit dem Optic Nerve Head Analyzer. Z prakt Augenheilk 7:30–36
20. Gramer E (1990) Gesichtsfeldänderungen bei der Langzeittherapie des Glaukoms: Langzeitverlaufskontrolle glaukomatöser Gesichtsfeldausfälle bei Glaucoma simplex mit reguliertem intraokularem Druck und bei Glaukom ohne Hochdruck zur computerperimetrischen Quantifizierung des augeninnendruckunabhängigen Glaukomschadens. In: Metz H (Hrsg.) Neue Gesichtspunkte zur Entdeckung und Behandlung des Glaukoms. W. Zuckschwerd-Verlag, München, pp 19–41
21. Gramer E (1992) Neue Kombinationspräparate mit nur zwei Applikationen täglich als Bestandteil einer medikamentösen drei- oder vier-Komponententherapie des Glaukoms. In: Gramer E, Kampik A (eds) Pharmakotherapie am Auge. Springer-Verlag, Heidelberg, pp 134–157
22. Gramer E (1993) Automatische Perimetrie bei Glaukom ohne Hochdruck. In: B. Gloor (Hrsg.) Perimetrie mit besonderer Berücksichtigung der automatischen Perimetrie. Enke Verlag, Stuttgart, pp 325–343
23. Gramer E, Baßler M, Leydhecker W (1987) Cup/disc ratio, excavation volume, neuroretinal rim area of the optic disc in correlation to computer perimetric quantification of visual field defects in glaucoma with and without pressure: Clinical study with the Rodenstock Optic Nerve Head Analyzer and the program Delta of the Octopus Computer Perimetry 201. In: Greve EL, Heijl A (eds) Documenta Ophthalmologica Proceedings Series 49, Proceedings of the 7th International Visual Field Symposium, Amsterdam, 1986. Dr. W. Junk Publishers, Dordrecht, pp. 329–348

24. Gramer E (1995) General risk factors in glaucoma. Ger J Ophthalmol 4 (Suppl.1):37
25. Gramer E (1995) Risk factors in glaucoma. Clinical Studies. Glaucoma Update V, Proc Vol Closed Glaucoma Symp Glaucoma Soc Int Congr Ophthalmology, Quebec, June 22–24, 1994. Kaden Verlag, Heidelberg, pp 14–31
26. Gramer E (1997) Kriterien des operativen Erfolgs. In: Krieglstein GK (Hrsg.) Glaukom – eine Standortbestimmung. Kaden-Verlag, Heidelberg, pp 64–70
27. Gramer E (1997) Messung der Dicke der Nervenfaserschicht bei Glaukom. Klinische Studien. In: Prünte Ch, Flammer J (eds) Das Glaukom in der Praxis. Karger, Basel, pp. 86–102
28. Gramer E (1997) Calculation of a glaucoma progression risk index (GPI) In: M. Wall, A Heijl (eds) Proceedings of the XIIthe International Perimetric Society Meeting in Würzburg 1996. Kugler Publications, Amsterdam/New York, pp 321–327
29. Gramer E, Althaus G (1987) Quantifizierung und Progredienz des Gesichtsfeldschadens bei Glaukom ohne Hochdruck, Glaucoma simplex und Pigmentglaukom. Eine klinische Studie mit dem Programm Delta des Octopus-Perimeters 201. Klin Monatsbl Augenheilkd 191:184–198
30. Gramer E, Althaus G (1987) Risikofaktoren bei Niederdruckglaukom. Eine klinische Studie zur Progredienz des Gesichtsfeldausfalls bei Glaukom ohne Hochdruck. Z prakt Augenheilkd 8:388–399
31. Gramer E, Althaus G (1988) Zur Progredienz des glaukomatösen Gesichtsfeldschadens. Eine klinische Studie mit Programm Delta des Octopus-Perimeters 201 zum Einfluß des Vorschadens auf die Gesichtsfeldverschlechterung beim Glaucoma simplex. Fortschr Ophthalmol 85:620–625
32. Gramer E, Althaus G (1990) Bedeutung des erhöhten Augeninnendrucks für den Gesichtsfeldschaden. Eine klinische Studie. Klin Monatsbl Augenheilkd 197:218–224
33. Gramer E, Althaus G (1992) Risk factors for deterioration of visual field defects in primary open angle glaucoma. Invest Ophthalmol Vis Sci 33:1278
34. Gramer E, Althaus G (1993) Einfluß des systolischen Blutdrucks auf die Lage der Gesichtsfeldausfälle in oberer und unterer Gesichtsfeldhälfte bei Patienten mit Glaucoma chronicum simplex. Ophthalmologe 90:620–625
35. Gramer E, Althaus G (1994) Calculation of a glaucoma progression risk index (GPI) by an automated perimeter: A clinical study. Invest Ophthalmol Vis Sci 35:1283
36. Gramer E, Althaus G, Leydhecker W (1986) Lage und Tiefe glaukomatöser Gesichtsfeldausfälle in Abhängigkeit von der Fläche der neuroretinaler Randzone. Eine klinische Studie mit dem Octopus-Perimeter 201 und dem Optic Nerve Head Analyzer. Klin Monatsbl Augenheilkd 189:190–198
37. Gramer E, Althaus G, Leydhecker W (1987) Topography and progression of visual field damage in glaucoma simplex, low tension glaucoma and pigmentary glaucoma with program Delta of Octopus Perimeter 201. In: Greve EL, Heijl A (eds) Documenta Ophthalmological Proceeding Series 49, Proceedings of the 7th International Visual Field Symposium, Amsterdam, 1986. Dr. W. Junk Publishers, pp 349–363
38. Gramer E, Burkard G, Kimmich F (1998) Risikoprofil unbehandelter Patienten am Beginn der Glaukomerkrankung. Eine prospektive Studie. Ophthalmologe 95:61–62
39. Gramer E, Dirmeyer M (1998) Optical coherence tomography (OCT) to measure nerve fiber layer thickness in normal eyes. Invest Ophthalmol Vis Sci 39: Abstract No. 4296, p. 933
40. Gramer E, Gramer G, Kimmich F, Burkard G (1999) Visual field prognosis in patients with ocular hypertension and early glaucoma. A prospective study. Invest Ophthalmol Vis Sci: 40, No 4, Abstract No 367, p. 69
41. Gramer E, Lanzl M, Tausch M (1997) Optic disc hemorrhages in glaucoma. Invest Ophthalmol Vis Sci 38: No 4, Abstract No 1155, p. 249
42. Gramer E, Leydhecker W (1985) Glaukom ohne Hochdruck: Eine klinische Studie. Klin Monatsbl Augenheilkd 186:262–267
43. Gramer E, Leydhecker W (1984) Risikofaktoren glaukomatöser Gesichtsfeldschädigung bei Glaukom ohne Hochdruck, Glaucoma simplex mit niedrigem und hohem intraokularem Druck. [Abstract 25]. Tagung der Österreichischen Ophthalmologischen Gesellschaft Wien, Hofburg, 2. 6. 1984 (Österreich)
44. Gramer E, Leydhecker W (1985) Papillendiagnostik bei Glaukom. Z prakt Augenheilkd 6:294–302
45. Gramer E, Leydhecker W (1985) Zur Pathogenese des Glaukoms ohne Hochdruck. Z prakt Augenheilkd 6:329–333
46. Gramer E, Maier H., Messmer EM (1993) A measure for the thickness of the nerve fiber layer and the configuration of the optic disc excavation in glaucoma patients. A clinical study using the Laser Tomographic Scanner. Proceedings of the Xth International Perimetric Society Meeting in Kyoto. Kugler Publications, Amsterdam, 207–213
47. Gramer E, Mohamed J, Krieglstein GK (1982) Der Ort von Gesichtsfeldausfällen bei Glaucoma simplex, Glaukom ohne Hochdruck und ischämischer Neuropathie. Indikationen zur vasoaktiven Therapie. In: Krieglstein GK, Leydhecker W (Hrsg.) Medikamentöse Glaukomtherapie. J.F. Bergmann Verlag, München, pp 115–121

48. Gramer E, Siebert M (1989) Optic nerve head measurements: The Optic Nerve Head Analyzer – its advantages and its limitations. Int Ophthalmol 13: pp. 3–13 and 13: p. 235
49. Gramer E, Tausch M (1995) The risk profile of the glaucomatous patient. Curr Opin Ophthalmol 6:78–88
50. Gramer E, Tausch M (1998) Measurement of the retinal nerve fiber layer thickness in clinical routine. Curr Opin Ophthalmol 9:77–87
51. Gramer E, Tausch M, Kimmich F (1995) Efficacy of adding dipivefrin HCL 0.1 % to topical β1-β2 blocker therapy: A prospective clinical study. Invest Ophthalmol Vis Sci 36:736
52. Gramer E, Thiele H, Ritch R (1999) Risk factors for pigmentary glaucoma. In: Krieglstein GK (ed) Glaucoma Update VI, Proceeding Volume of the Closed Glaucoma Symposium of the Glaucoma Society of the International Congress of Ophthalmology, Edinburgh 16.–19-6-1998 Springer Verlag, Heidelberg Chapter 4, p. 27–33
53. Gramer E, Thiele H, Ritch R (1998) Familienanamnese Glaukom und Risikofaktoren bei Pigmentglaukom. Klin. Monatsbl. Augenheilkd 212:454–464
54. Grehn F (1990) Zur Pathogenese der glaukomatösen Opticusatrophie. Neurophysiologische und morphologische Untersuchungen von retinalen Ganglienzellen bei akuter Augeninnendruckerhöhung. In: Gramer E (ed) Glaukom – Diagnostik und Therapie. F. Enke-Verlag, Stuttgart, pp. 12–21
55. Grehn F, Prost M (1983) Function of retinal nerve fibers depends on perfusion pressure: Neurophysiologic investigations during acute intraocular pressure elevations. Invest Ophthalmol Vis Sci 24:347–353
56. Hamard P, Hamard H, Dufaux J, Quesnot S (1994) Optic nerve head blood flow using a laser Doppler velocimeter and haemorrheology in primary open glaucoma and normal pressure glaucoma. Br J Ophthalmol 78:449–453
57. Hayrey SS, Zimmermann MB, Podhajsky P, Alward WLM (1994) Nocturnal arterial hypotension and its role in optic nerve head and ocular ischemic disorders. Am J Ophthalmol 1994, 117:603–624
58. Hernandez MR, Andrzejewska WM, Neufeld AH (1990) Changes in the extracellular matrix of the human optic nerve head in primary open-angle glaucoma. Am J Ophthalmol 109:180–188
59. Hernandez MR, Pena J (1997) The Optic Nerve Head in Glaucomatous Optic Neuropathy. Arch Ophthalmol 1997, 115:389
60. Iwata K (1992) Is low tension glaucoma (LTG) a real glaucoma? Histopathological findings and their therapeutical suggestion. In: Gramer E, Kampik A (eds) Pharmakotherapie am Auge. Springer-Verlag, Heidelberg, pp 12–18
61. Johnson DH, Yoshikawa K, Brubaker PF, Hodge DO (1994) The effect of long-term medical therapy on the outcome of filtration surgery. Am J Ophthalmol 117:139–148
62. Katz J, Sommer A (1986) Asymmetry and variation in the normal hill of vision. Arch Ophthalmol 104:65–68
63. Kitazawa Y, Shirai H, Go FJ (1989) The effect of Ca^{2+}-antagonist on visual field in low tension glaucoma. Graefe's Arch Clin Exp Ophthalmol 227:408–412
64. Kraemer C, Gramer E, Maier H (1997) Comparison to disc size and disc diameter among healthy eyes and eyes with low-tension glaucoma, primary open-angle glaucoma and ocular hypertension. Proceedings of the XIIth International Perimetric Society Meeting in Würzburg 1996. Kugler Publications Amsterdam/New York, pp 355–362
65. Kraemer C, Gramer E (1998) Cup to dis ratio and stage of visual field loss in patients with Chronic Angle-Closure Glaucoma. Invest Ophthalmol Vis Sci 39:Abstract No. 119, p. 28
66. Krieglstein GK, Mittermaier E, Gramer E (1985) Zur Prognose der Filtrations-Chirurgie bei Glaukomspätstadien. Eine klinische Studie. Z prakt Augenheilkd 6:121–129
67. Leydhecker W, Gramer E (1989) Long-term studies of visual field changes by means of computerized perimetry (Octopus 201) in eyes with glaucomatous field defects after normalization of the intraocular pressure. Int. Ophthalmol 13:113–117
68. Lichter PR (1994) Genetic clues to glaucoma's secrets: The Edward Jackson Memorial Lecture. Am J Ophthalmol 117:706–727
69. Maier H, Serguhn S, Gramer E (1995) Sensitivität und Spezifität des Heidelberger Retina Tomographen für die Darstellung von Nervenfaserbündeldefekten bei Glaukompatienten mit lokalisierten Gesichtsfeldausfällen. Klinische Studie. Ophthalmologe 92:521–525
70. Maier H, Siebert M, Gramer E (1992) Unterschiede in der Form der Papillenexkavation bei Glaucoma chronicum simplex und Glaukom ohne Hochdruck. Eine klinische Studie mit dem Laser Tomographie Scanner. In: Gramer E, Kampik A (eds) Pharmakotherapie am Auge. Springer-Verlag, Heidelberg, pp 29–71
71. Maier H, Siebert M, Gramer E, Kampik A (1990) Eine Maßzahl für die Nervenfaserschichtdicke. Messungen mit dem Laser-Tomographie-Scanner (LTS). Eine klinische Studie. In: Gramer E (ed) GLAUKOM – Diagnostik und Therapie. F. Enke Verlag, Stuttgart, pp 120–145

72. Minckler DS (1993) Neuronal damage in glaucoma. In: Varma R, Spaeth GL (eds) The Optic Nerve in Glaucoma. J.B. Lippincott, Philadelphia, pp 51-59
73. Minckler DS (1980) The organization of nerve fiber bundles in the primate optic nerve head. Arch Ophthalmol 98:1630-1636
74. Minckler DS, Weinreb R (1990) Histology of optic nerve injury in experimental ocular hypertension and early glaucoma. In: Gramer E (ed) GLAUKOM - Diagnostik und Therapie. F. Enke Verlag, Stuttgart, pp 7-11
75. Minckler DS, Ogden TE (1987) Primate arcuate nerve fiber bundle anatomy. In: Greve EL, Heijl A (eds) Documenta Ophthalmologica Proceeding Series. Dr. W. Junk Publishers, Dordrecht, Nijhiff 49:605-612
76. Quigley H (1987) Are some retinal ganglion cells killed by glaucoma before others? In: Krieglstein GK (ed) Glaucoma Update III. Springer-Verlag, Berlin, pp 23-26
77. Quigley H, Pease ML, Thibault D (1994) Change in the appearance of elastin in the lamina cribosa of glaucomatous optic nerve heads. Graefe's Arch Clin Exp Ophthalmol 232:257-261
78. Quigley HA, Addicks AM (1981) Regional differences in the structure of the lamina cribosa and their relation to glaucomatous optic nerve damage. Arch Ophthalmol 99:137-143
79. Rojanapongpun P, Drance SM, Morrison BJ (1993) Ophthalmic artery flow velocity in normal subjects recorded by Doppler ultrasound. Am J Ophthalmol 77:25-29
80. Schwartz B (1990) Optic disc pallor: its measurement and clinical significance for open angle glaucoma. In: Gramer E (ed) GLAUKOM - Diagnostik und Therapie. F. Enke Verlag, Stuttgart, pp 66-72
81. Serguhn S, Gramer E (1996) Läßt sich mittels Laser-Polarimetrie durch in vivo Messung der retinalen Nervenfaser-Schichtdicke das Ausmaß des Glaukomschadens quantifizieren? Eine klinische Studie. Ophthalmologe 93:527-534
82. Serguhn S, Gramer E (1998) Läßt sich durch Messung der Asymmetrie des peripailliären Höhenprofils zwischen oberer und unterer Retinahälfte das Ausmaß des Glaukomschadens erfassen? Klin Monatsbl Augenheilkd 212:74-79 41
83. Shields B (1990) Disc topography: correlation of visual dysfunction and accuracy of measurements with the optic nerve head analyzer. In: Gramer E (ed) GLAUKOM - Diagnostik und Therapie. F. Enke Verlag, Stuttgart, pp 108-112
84. Shields MB, Krieglstein GK (1993) Glaukom. Springer-Verlag, Berlin/Heidelberg
85. Shiose Y (1992) Low tension glaucoma: Prevalence and background factors. In: Gramer E, Kampik A (eds) Pharmakotherapie am Auge. Springer-Verlag, Berlin/Heidelberg, pp 3-11
86. Shirato S, Adachi M, Koseki N, Yamagami J (1992) Optic disc findings and disc hemorrhages in low-tension glaucoma and their therapeutical suggestion. In: Gramer E, Kampik A (eds) Pharmakotherapie am Auge. Springer-Verlag, Heidelberg, pp 72-79
87. Siebert M, Gramer E (1990) Reproduzierbarkeit und klinische Anwendbarkeit der Meßergebnisse mit dem Optic Nerve Head Analyzer. In: Gramer E (ed) GLAUKOM - Diagnostik und Therapie. F. Enke Verlag, Stuttgart, pp 96-102
88. Siebert M, Gramer E, Leydhecker W (1989) Papillenabblassung - ein Frühzeichen des Glaukoms. Eine klinisch kontrollierte Untersuchung von Papillenblässe und Papillenexkavation bei Glaucoma simplex, okulärer Hypertension und gesunden Augen mit dem Optic Nerve Head Analyzer. Klin Monatsbl Augenheilkd 194:433-436
89. Sonnsjö B (1993) A study in scarlet. Disc haemorrhages and retinal vein occlusions in the natural history of glaucoma. Inaugaral dissertation. Malmö
90. Sugiyama K, Tomita G, Kitazawa Y, Onda E, Shinohara H, Park K (1997) The Associations of Optic Disc Hemorrhage with Retinal Nerve Fiber Layer Defect and Peripapillary Atrophy in Normal-Tension Glaucoma. Ophthalmology 104:1926-1933
91. Tausch M (1996) Den Glaukom-Genen auf der Spur. Internationaler Workshop "Genetics in Glaucoma" in Würzburg. Z Prakt Augenheilkd 17:448-452
92. Tjon-Fo-Sang MJ, de Vries J, Lemij HG (1996) Measurement by nerve fiber analysis of retinal nerve fiber layer thickness in normal subjects and patients with ocular hypertension. Am J Ophthalmol 122:220-227
93. Zulauf M (1994) Normal visual fields measured with Octopus Program G1. Graefe's Arch Clin Exp Ophthalmol 232:509-515

CHAPTER 21

The Intraocular Pressure as a Continuous Risk Factor for Glaucoma

C. E. Traverso

Introduction

Is the IOP the main problem in roughly 90 % of primary open-angle glaucomas? This is related to the following frequently asked question: Is IOP the cause, the effect or a sign of glaucoma? Unfortunately this is commonly incorrectly phrased, simply because we cannot talk about "glaucoma". One should define arbitrarily clinical types, including experimental models, and discuss each of them separately [1].

For the purpose of the present discussion I will restrict myself to POAG, and will base it on personal experience, literature, my own opinions and hopefully some common sense.

The Intraocular Pressure Is Useless

In the early 1980s, there was a substantial shift away from the concept of IOP as it was previously intended. On the one hand, clinical data demonstrated beyond doubt the existence of progressive POAG without a statistically abnormal IOP; this led to a variety of terms, like normal tension glaucoma or "glaucoma sine ipertensione". The belief that IOP might be irrelevant, at least for those eyes worsening at statistically normal IOP levels, cast doubt on the relevance of IOP for the whole spectrum of glaucoma. On the other hand, better, or perhaps just more standardized, perimetry methods and imaging techniques documented the absence of damage in many patients with prolonged, statistically elevated IOP. With fluorescein angiography, the role of perfusion problems in the optic nerve head (ONH) of POAG patients was confirmed. At the same time statistics to evaluate the success of medical, laser or surgical treatments became more sophisticated, and power sample calculations, Kaplan-Meyer survival curves and multiple stepwise regressions appeared more constantly in the literature. At that time we advocated "treat glaucoma, not just the IOP". However, over the years I changed my thought process. Up to the late 1980s I emphasized the concept of the multiplicity of etiologies for glaucomatous optic neuropathies (GON) and that we were unfortunate to have only the IOP to deal with therapeutically. In other words, many times, despite treatment, normalizing the IOP was of no use. In my teaching perimetry was suggested as a better method to assess what was happening, as it reflected ON status more appropriately and more directly than IOP.

The Intraocular Pressure Is Just One of the Risk Factors

In the 1990s I still found myself discussing the problem of not having other means for treatment other than to lower the IOP. Today, the focus has shifted from the IOP per se to the clinical course of the individual patient, considered as a person with a problem. What had occurred? Clinical data showed that, even for normal pressure glaucomas (NPG), there was an advantage in lowering the IOP well below statistically normal levels [2–3]; also, in many POAG patients with advanced disease, progression was less frequent if the IOP was likewise lowered drastically [4–7]. Many studies from different independent sources demonstrated the role of blood flow in ON health and disease. In the American Academy of Ophthalmology Preferred Practice Pattern for POAG the term "target IOP" was introduced by Paul Palmberg, setting a trend that continues. Last but not least, the ever more popular concept of apoptosis has entered the field of glaucomatology. According to the programmed cell death theory, as soon as any damage to the retinal ganglion cells (RGC) is triggered, it cannot be arrested no matter what is done; neurons might be spared from this external damage by neuroprotective molecules, some of which are also claimed to be of use for protecting neighboring healthy neurons from secondary, indirect, damage. This is now a driving force in glaucoma physiopathology. Apoptosis may be initiated by elevated IOP, ischemia/hypoxia, undersupply of growth factors or axonal transport block.

The Intraocular Pressure Is a Continuous Risk Factor the Individual

This wealth of new information has changed my approach of "treat glaucoma, not just the IOP". But treating glaucoma makes sense only if it preserves the well being, health and quality of life of the patient. We are now back to the question: is IOP the cause or the effect of glaucoma, or merely a risk factor? If apoptosis is indeed a major player, why does it occur only in the RGCs? Should this slow cell death also occur in TM cells; can it explain the progressive decrease in outflow facility seen in POAG? Nowadays, IOP is recognized as a major risk factor for the development of progressive glaucomatous damage. It is also the only risk factor directly affected by treatment. In most clinical studies on IOP-lowering methods, success is defined as reaching an IOP equal or below 21 mm Hg, or obtaining a percentage decrease from baseline, 20%–30% being the most popular range. A 30% decrease from 30 mm Hg as well as a 20% decrease from 26 mm Hg is still close to 21 mm Hg. One obvious problem is that no matter how success is defined now, historically the IOP criteria have been too high. Treatment is ineffective when it does not lower the IOP sufficiently; it is useless when there is no value in lowering the IOP. The confusion between those two terms contributed to the idea that glaucoma treatment was of no value; the wide-ranging implications of this thought process were dramatic in the USA, when ophthalmologists were challenged to produce better evidence for the efficacy of glaucoma management [8]. When the end point of a study on glaucoma treatment is an IOP level which is unlikely to prevent further damage, at least in eyes with evident GON, the results of such a study are going to be disappointing, confusing or both. Even today, surgical success is referred to as 21 mm Hg, sometimes with additional medication, in the latter case labeled as qualified success. If this figure is not at the statistical norm, why would anyone accept it for an eye where damage is already rampant, where apoptosis has already been triggered and where other risk factors might be present? There are now data showing a dose response curve for the effect of IOP on the course of POAG. Epidemiologists tell us that the higher the IOP, the more likely is GON [9]. Some of the relevant data taken from several clinical studies with medium to long term follow-up are summarized in Table 1 [4–5, 10–23]. We have observed, after filtration surgery, that lower IOPs were significantly associated with better preservation of visual function in patients with advanced damage [6]; our study, however, had a relatively short follow-up and a small sample size. What is striking is not the obvious positive relationship between IOP level and glaucoma damage, but rather what might be happening to those eyes still progressing at quite low IOP levels. There are possible explanations, as in patients in which the individualized target IOP was not met or was set too high, or when IOP peaks were not detected or not accounted for by the mean IOPs. These are the patients worth most of our attention as clinicians since they risk slipping towards visual handicap while under our care. Morton Grant wrote in an article 16 years ago "in most patients progression occurs because their IOP is not lowered sufficiently" [7]. This statement still holds true today. Also of great interest are the patients with POAG not getting worse despite their IOP remaining abnormally high. This group is a measurable percentage in all studies referred to in the table. Is this explainable by the unusually high resistance to IOP of some individuals? Should they be followed up long enough, would they invariably worsen? For patients in whom GON is already present, a continuous dose-response curve between IOP and progres-

Table 1. List of references on the clinical course of POAG as it relates to the IOP

Author	IOP mean or range	n	n, worse	Percent worse	Follow-up years
Lynn [4]	< 11	14	0	0	3.5
Lamping [10]	13.3	252	38	15	> 5
Roth [11]	14.4	33	2	6	> 5
Jay [12]	15	24	6	25	> 3
Odberg [5]	< 16	9	3	33	5–18
Kidd [13]	15.4	50	9	18	> 5
Chandler [14]	15.6	15	4	27	26
Watson [15]	16	62	4	7	3
Jerndal [16]	16	29	10	35	20
Werner [17]	16	24	10	42	3.5
Popovic [18]	16.9	54	15	28	5
Mao [19]	< 17	9	0	0	4–11
Burke [20]	17	48	24	50	5
Greve [21]	17.3	42	15	36	4
Kolker [22]	< 18	49	2	4	> 4
Jerndal [16]	18	102	17	18	5
Rollins [23]	18	31	9	29	5
Watson [15]	18.7	36	10	28	20
Roth [11]	19.1	19	11	58	> 5
Kolker [22]	> 22	35	11	29	> 4
Mao [19]	17–21	38	20	53	4–11
Odberg [5]	> 20	6	6	100	5–18
Mao [19]	> 21	8	8	100	4–11

sion of glaucoma damage has been established indirectly from the data of the clinical studies listed in the table mentioned. What is not known is the slope of the curve, nor where the curve starts in each individual. Data are difficult to interpret due to variable diagnostic definitions, follow-up criteria, sample composition and size, therapeutic modalities and study design. In the mid-section of the table, where IOPs are in the range between 16 and 19, the variability of reported worsening rates in very high. Even more complex is to try to correlate the onset of glaucoma damage in a normal individual as a consequence of elevated IOP.

Individualized Target Intraocular Pressure Makes Sense, But Needs To Be Proven Clinically

Target IOP is discussed by Zeyen, elsewhere in this volume. Target IOP, individualized to the stage of damage, rate of decay, life expectancy, baseline IOP and quality of life to be preserved, is the major advancement we can offer empirically to our patients. Time will tell if this approach will influence the clinical course and improve the quality of life. Thus the question remains: Is IOP the major risk factor, at least in caucasians with POAG is it relevant enough to be the sole risk factor responsible for GON in many individuals? The risk of a substantial decrease of quality of life is quantitatively related to the risk of persistently elevated IOP. Other risk factors cannot be ruled out and need to be weighted in each individual.

References

1. The European Glaucoma Society (1998) Terminology and Classification. In: Terminology and Guidelines for Glaucoma. Dogma srl, Savona, Italy, pp 62–80
2. Collaborative Normal-Tension Glaucoma Study Group (1998) Comparison of glaucoma progression between untreated patients with normal tension glaucoma and patients with therapeutically reduced intraocular pressures. Am J Ophthalmol 126:487–497
3. Collaborative Normal-Tension Glaucoma Study Group (1998) The effectiveness of intraocular pressure reduction in the treatment of normal-tension glaucoma. Am J Ophthalmol 126:498–505
4. Lynn JR, Swanson WH, Fellman RL, Starita RJ (1993) Does glaucomatous visual field loss continue despite surgically subnormal IOP? In: Mills RP (ed) Perimetry update 1992/1993. Kugler Publications, Amsterdam/New York, pp 129–135
5. Odberg T (1987) Visual field prognosis on advanced glaucoma. Acta Ophthalmol 65 (suppl) 182:27–29
6. Traverso CE, Semino E, Morescalchi S, Murialdo U, Zenzano D, Gandolfo E, Zingirian M (1995) Is the visual field of patients with advanced POAG protected by lowering the IOP? In: Mills RP, Wall M (eds) Perimetry update 1994/1995. Kugler, Amsterdam, pp 309–312
7. Grant WM, Burke JF (1982) Why do some people go blind for glaucoma? Ophthalmology 89:991–998
8. Eddy DM, Billings J (1988) The quality of medical evidence and medical evidence: Implications for quality of health care. Health Aff (Millwood) Spring: 19–32
9. Sommer AE (1991) Relationship between intraocular pressure and primary open – angle glaucoma among white and black americans. Arch Ophthalmol 109:1090–1095
10. Lamping KA, Belows AR, Hutchinson ST, Afran SI (1986) Long-term evaluation of initial filtration surgery. Ophthalmology 93:91–101
11. Roth SM, Spaeth GL, Starita RJ, Birbillis EM, Steinmann WC (1991) The effects of postoperative corticosteroids on trabeculectomy and the clinical course of glaucoma: five years follow up study. Ophthalmic Surgery 22:724–729
12. Jay JL, Murray SB (1989) Early trabeculectomy versus conventional management in primary open angle glaucoma. Br J Ophthalmol 72:881–889

13. Kidd MN, O'Connor M (1985) Progression of filed loss after trabeculectomy: a five year follow-up. Br J Ophthalmol 69:827–831
14. Chandler PA (1960) Long-term results in glaucoma therapy. Am J Ophthalmol 49:221–246
15. Watson PG, Jakeman C, Oztruk M, Barnett MF, Barnett F, Khaw KT (1990) The complications of trabeculectomy (a 20-years follow-up). Eye 4:425–438
16. Jerndal T, Lundström M (1980) 330 trabeculectomies: a long time study (3–5.5 years). Acta ophthalmol 58:947–956
17. Werner EB, Drance SM, Schultzer M (1977) Trabeculectomy and the progression of glaucomatous field loss. Arch Ophthalmol 95:1374–1377
18. Popovic V, Sjöstrand J (1991) Long-term outcome following trabeculectomy: II. Visual field survival. Acta ophthalmol 69:305–309
19. Mao LK, Steward LC, Shileds MD (1991) Correlation between intraocular pressure control and progressive glaucomatous damage in primary open-angle glaucoma. Am J Ophthalmol 111:51–55
20. Burke JW (1993) Field changes after satisfactory filtration operations for glaucoma. Trans Am Ophthalmol Soc 37:149–157
21. Greve EL, Dake CL (1979) Four year follow-up of a glaucoma operation. Prospective study of the double flap Scheie. Int Ophthalmol 1:139–145
22. Kolker AE (1977) Visual prognosis in advanced glaucoma: comparison of medical and surgical therapy for retention of vision in 101 eyes with advanced glaucoma. Trans Am Ophthalmol Soc 75:539–555
23. Rollins DF, Drance SM (1981) Five-year follow-up of trabeculectomy in the management of chronic open-angle glaucoma. In: Symposium on glaucoma. Transactions of New Orleans Academy of Ophthalmology. CV Mosby, St. Louis

CHAPTER 22

Target Pressures in Glaucoma

T. Zeyen

Background and Rationale

Despite exciting progress in the field of neuroprotection, lowering the intraocular pressure (IOP) is still the only available option to treat glaucoma patients. Several studies have shown that lowering the IOP is beneficial for glaucoma patients, even in normal tension glaucoma. It was even suggested that early surgery was more advantageous than medical treatment [1, 2]. Early surgery has the additional benefit of improving the lifestyle of the patient who does not have to adhere to a tight schedule of medication and is not exposed to the side-effects of the drugs. The American Ocular Hypertension Study and the European Glaucoma Prevention Study are currently testing the supposition that lowering the IOP is also beneficial for patients with ocular hypertension [3].

The rate of progression of glaucomatous damage is different fo each patient and is illustrated in Fig. 1. Mostly, progression is parabolic with a slow rate in the beginning and a much faster rate at the end of the disease [4]. Sometimes it is linear with a rate correlating with the level of IOP, but not necessarily leading to visual impairment. Sometimes the rate of progression can stop without noticeable change in the level of IOP. Conversely we also known that progression can continue, at least for a while, even after having drastically lowered the IOP, for example after filtering surgery. This is often the case in advanced glaucoma. It is therefore important to document progres-

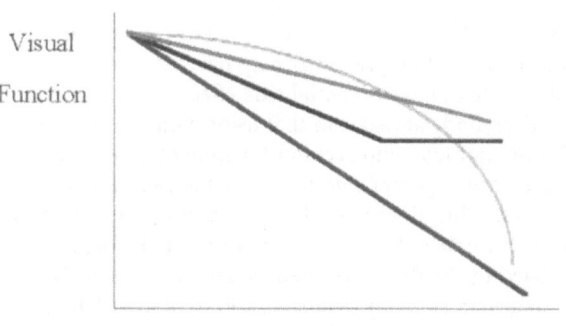

Fig. 1. Rates of progression of glaucomatous damage. Mostly, progression is parabolic with a slow rate in the beginning and a much faster rate at the end of the disease. Sometimes it is linear with a rate correlating with the level of IOP, but not necessarily leading to visual impairment. Sometimes the rate of progression can stop without noticeable change in the level of IOP

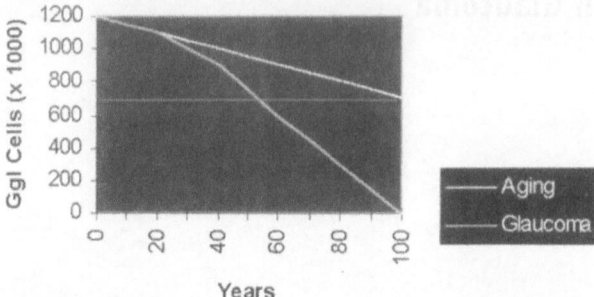

Years

Fig. 2. Rate of ganglion cell loss by aging compared to glaucoma. The natural loss of ganglion cells by aging is approximately 0.4 % loss per year. The rate of ganglion cell loss in glaucoma varies between 1 % and 4 % per year. Early visual field defects are usually detectable after a loss of 40 % of ganglion cells (horizontal line). This means that usually the visual field defects are detectable after 10 years of disease

sion as early as possible and to find out the rate of progression for every individual patient [5]. This information will allow the clinician to treat early and to know how aggressive one should be in lowering the IOP.

Figure 2 illustrates the rate of ganglion cell loss by aging compared to glaucoma. The natural loss of ganglion cells by aging is approximately 0.4 % loss per year. The rate of ganglion cell loss in glaucoma varies between 1 % and 4 % per year [4, 6]. Early visual field defects are usually detectable after a loss of 40 % of ganglion cells. This means that usually the visual field defects are detectable after 10 years of disease. This means also that every non-glaucomatous patient will ultimately develop glaucomatous visual field defects provided he or she will live at least for 100 years. By lowering the IOP one tries to bend the curve of glaucomatous loss towards the curve of loss by aging. The degree to which the IOP should be lowered to obtain this goal is unfortunately unknown. Until the day we can use optic disc or visual field improvement as endpoints we have no criterion for IOP reduction unless we set a target pressure [7].

How To Calculate a Target Pressure

Several methods have been used in practice and in clinical studies. Obviously the lowest possible pressure will be the safest for preventing further glaucomatous damage. But extreme low pressures may have drawbacks, and the medications necessary to obtain them have potential side effects.

Everybody agrees now that using a number (e.g. < 21 mm Hg) is obsolete, because is does not take into account the individual variability for each patient. Many studies have used a percentage (e.g. a reduction of at least 20 %) [8, 9]. This approach is attractive but does not take into account the risk of further damage. The greater the risk of further damage, the lower the IOP should be. The risk of further damage is related to the degree of damage already present and the IOP at which glaucomatous damage presumably occurred ("Presentation IOP").

A useful algorithm is a variation of the formula proposed by H. Jampel: "Target IOP = Presentation IOP – Presentation IOP % – Z", where Z is an optic nerve damage

Table 1. Grading scale to define the optic nerve damage severity factor Z

Z	Optic Nerve Damage
0	Normal disc and normal visual field
1	Abnormal disc and normal visual field
2	Visual field loss not threatening fixation
3	Visual field loss threatening or involving fixation

severity factor [10]. The grading scale used by H. Jampel to define the factor Z is shown in Table 1. For example an eye with a presentation IOP of 30 mm Hg, optic nerve damage and visual field loss not threatening fixation would have a target set at 19 mm Hg (30–30 %–2). The target pressure might be adjusted by including other risk factors such as age, race, burden of therapy, and IOP range.

How To Use a Target Pressure

It is recommended to record and highlight the target pressure in the chart of a patient. This is particularly useful when the care of the patient is shared by several ophthalmologists. If not written down there is a natural tendency to drift upward the target pressure. It is therefore very practical to draw an IOP curve for each glaucomatous patient and to highlight the target pressure on the curve.

The target pressure should be reevaluated periodically. It is clear that the target pressure needs to be lowered if glaucomatous damage is progressing despite IOPs below the initially set target. Conversely the target pressure may need to be adjusted upward, decreasing the side-effects of some medications, if the optic nerve and the visual field remain stable for a prolonged period.

It is probably wise to keep in mind a target range instead of a target pressure since it is unlikely that therapy will be modified on the basis of a 1 mm Hg change. For the same reasons it is judicious to use multiple IOP measurements before deciding that a modification of therapy is necessary. The IOP measurements should be taken at different hours of the day, especially when progression of damage is suspected. Let us also remember that IOP ranges of more than 5 mm Hg are considered as an additional risk factor. For those reasons home tonometry might be very useful [11].

We should also keep in mind that IOP readings can be over- or underestimated [12]. After refractive surgery for example the applanation tonometry is underestimated; because the cornea is thinner after excimer and lasik (laser in situ keratomileusis), and because the cornea is flatter after radial keratotomy. When the cornea is thicker the IOP may be overestimated. Hence pachymetry might be useful in patients with ocular hypertension [13].

Compliance is a limitation in using target pressures because the IOP measurements do not always reflect the real IOP fluctuations in a non-compliant patient. Fixed combinations of drugs are certainly beneficial for patients with poor compliance. Side-effects of the medication should always be taken into consideration, and if the target pressure cannot be reached with maximal tolerable medical therapy, surgery should be considered.

Conclusion

The concept of using a target pressure in glaucoma is based on the fact that no other treatment is available at this moment and that it is unknown to what extent the IOP should be lowered to stop progession for each individual patient. The target IOP is assessed by taking into account the risk of future damage and should be reevaluated periodically. If the pressure goal cannot be reached medically or if the drug or combination of drugs have side-effects, surgical treatment should be considered.

Above all it is important to estimate the slope of progression for each individual patient in order to minimize the risk of treatment being it medical or surgical. Hopefully, we shall have, in the near future, the means to treat the other risk factors resulting in optic nerve damage.

References

1. Migdal C, Gregory W, Hitchings R (1994) Long-term functional outcome after early surgery compared with laser and medecine in open-angle glaucoma. Ophthalmol 101:1651–1657
2. Jay J, Murray S (1988) Early trabeculectomy versus conventional management in primary open angle glaucoma. Br J Ophthalmol 72:881–889
3. Miglior S, Pfeiffer N, Cunha-Vaz J, Zeyen T, European Glaucoma Prevention Study Group (1999) The European Glaucoma Prevention Study. Objectives and Methods. Invest Ophthalmol Vis Sci Suppl 40 (4): S 566
4. Zeyen T, Caprioli J (1993) Progression of disc and field damage in early glaucoma. Arch Ophthalmol 111:62–65
5. Spaeth J (1997) Year book of ophthalmology 1997. R. Wilson, Mosby (ed) St. Louis, p 70
6. Airaksinen P, Tuulonen H, Alanko H (1992) Rate and pattern of neuroretinal rim area decrease in ocular hypertension and glaucoma. Arch Ophthalmol 110:206–210
7. Katz L, Spaeth G, Cantor L, Poryzees E, Steinmann W (1989) Reversible optic disc cupping and visual field improvement in adults with glaucoma. Am J Ophthalmol 107:485–492
8. The Fluorouracil Filtering Surgery Study Group (1989) Fluorouracil Filtering Surgery Study one year follow-up. Am J Ophthalmol 108:625–635
9. The Glaucoma Laser Trial Research Group. The Glaucoma Laser Trial (GLT) 2. Results of argon laser trabeculoplasty versus topical medicines. Ophthalmology 1990; 97:1403–1413
10. Jampel H (1997) Target pressure in glaucoma therapy. J Glaucoma 6:133–138
11. Zeimer R, Wilensky J, Gieser D, Viana M (1991) Association between intraocular pressure peaks and progression of visual field loss. Ophthalmology 98:64–69
12. Whitacre M, Stein R (1993) Sources of error with use of Goldmann-type tonometers. Surv Ophthalmol 8:1–30
13. Herndon L, Choudhri S, Cox T, Damji K, Shields M, Allingham R (1997) Central corneal thickness in normal, glaucomatous, and ocular hypertensive eyes. Arch Ophthalmol 115:1137–1141

CHAPTER 23

Relationship Between Transient or Permanent Low Blood Pressure and Glaucoma

A. Béchetoille and H. Bresson-Dumont

Introduction

Common sense tells us that a weakness of the pump which sends the blood to the peripheral circulation might be of importance, whatever the status of the vascular tree is, when assessing the causes leading to ischemia/reperfusion events at the optic disc microvasculature level.

Drance pointed out for the first time, in 1973, that a sudden and dramatic fall in blood pressure (BP) is able to produce the so-called shock-induced optic neuropathy, which resembles very much a glaucomatous optic neuropathy [1]. But, this is a caricature of glaucoma, and it is important to know if permanent low BP could be also harmful for the visual field, even when the intraocular pressure is low or controlled by adequate treatment. Permanent low BP can be primary, mainly in women, and is physiologically predominant at night, during sleep. Low BP can also be the consequence of some cardiac, low-noise pathological conditions, e.g. atrial fibrillation, other rhythm alterations, or silent myocardial ischemia. Variability of BP is also important to consider, as observed during the circadian cycle in overtreated arterial hypertension patients. Variability of BP can also be due to orthostatic hypotension, quite frequently observed in polymedicated elderly people.

Ambulantory Monitoring of Blood Pressure

Ambulatory monitoring of blood pressure (AMBP) is the method of choice to assess BP level during a 24-h period. A blood pressure cuff, applied to the patient's nondominant upper arm, just above the elbow, records automatically the humeral arterial tension at different intervals. The definitions of night time and day time, and of the intervals between measurements, are somewhat different among investigators, as is the choice whether to perform the measurement as an inpatient or outpatient procedure. However, in all cases, data are then processed by a computer program and reported as serial systolic, diastolic and mean BP values, which, in addition, allows the computer to calculate indices, such as pressure variability, and nocturnal dips (Table 1). The latter are defined as the percent decrease between mean BP at night time and mean BP during the day time. Nocturnal dips can be systolic and diastolic and are physiologic when they remain within certain limits, around 10 %.

"Dippers" are persons in whom dips are more than 10 %, a very frequent situation involving more than half of the population. Deep dips, i.e. deeper than 10 %, must be

Table 1. Parameters of ambulatory blood pressure monitoring

24 hour, nocturnal and diurnal, systolic diastolic and mean BP

BP variability
   Difference between the highest and the lowest blood pressure value
   Standard deviation of 24 hour, diurnal and nocturnal, systolic and diastolic, blood pressure values
   Systolic and diastolic dips (daytime mean BP – nighttime mean BP /nighttime mean BP) X 100

24 hour, nocturnal and diurnal, systolic and diastolic low readings (Percentage of low readings
when compared to the minimal normal readings indicated in the Staessen meta-analysis, i.e.,
inferior to 101/61 mm Hg at daytime and 86/48 mm Hg at nighttime

considered, as above 13 %, there is a decrease of perfusion pressure and consequently
a decrease in the posterior blood flow, of the eye.

Several quite recent surveys have shown a high association of glaucomatous optic
neuropathy with arterial hypotension [2–9]. Goldberg and Demailly found a lower
systolic BP in normal pressure glaucoma NPG than in high pressure glaucoma (HPG)
[2, 10]. Graham et al. found that all nocturnal blood pressure parameters were lowered in patients with progressive field defects compared to the patients whose visual
field parameters were stable, whereas the systolic, diastolic and mean arterial pressure dips were significantly larger [11]. Kaiser et al. and others showed that open
angle glaucoma patients with progression despite well controlled IOP, and patients
with normal pressure glaucoma had markedly and statistically significant lower systemic BP at night as well as during the day time [12].

Our group also performed 24-h blood pressure recording, using a Spacelab 90207
monitor, in more than 150 glaucoma patients. Subjects were hospitalized to get at the
same time an intraocular pressure (IOP) diurnal curve, but they were instructed to
take all their topical and systemic medications, given for any reason, on the same
schedule as prior to the observation period. The definition of day time was from
6 AM to 10 PM, during which period the brachial blood pressure level was monitored
every 20 min. At night time, from 10 PM to 6 AM, patients were allowed to go to bed
and to sleep at their convenience, with their BP monitored every 30 min. We compared AMBP parameters between a group of NPG and HPG patients (mean age:
54.1 years) in whom visual field losses were progessing despite good control of IOP
(progressors) ($n = 40$), and a similar group of patients (mean age: 67.4 years) whose
visual field remained stable (non-progressors) ($n = 43$). Progression, when identified
was confirmed by a second visual field test. IOP reduction in both groups was
obtained by maximum tolerated medical therapy and/or laser or surgical therapy.
Visual field performance was assessed over a minimum follow-up a 2 years using the
Humphrey field analyzer (HFA) or, occasionally (4.8 %), a Goldmann perimeter when
the visual field defects were too extreme. Progression was defined, when tested by
HFA, as a negative change of at least 15 % in the value of MD and/or CPSD. We found
that progressors were older women ($p = 0.017$) had deeper systolic ($p = 0.0375$) and
diastolic ($p = 0.0083$) dips, and had higher BP variability. No difference was found
between the two groups for diurnal and nocturnal, systolic and diastolic blood PP
(Fig. 1) [14].

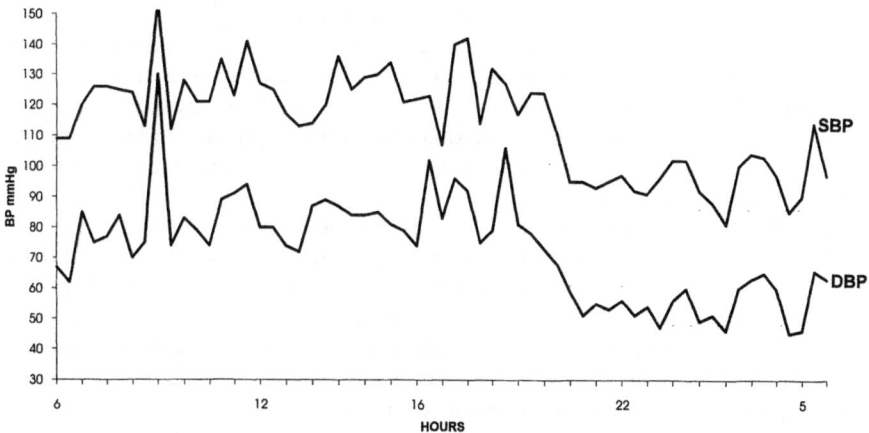

Fig. 1. Blood pressure ambulatory monitoring of a 79 year old woman with progressive focal ischemic glaucoma, characterized by an almost normal intra-ocular pressure and an arterial hypertension
treated by sotalol. She had also a Raynaud phenomena amplified by sotalol. She had aggravated left
eye optic disc cupping and visual field defect from –2.5 to 8.70 dB (MD) and 3 to 11.5 dB (CPSD) during a 4-year period where she was lost for follow-up. When she resumed follow-up, bilateral pressure
was still normal, around 16 mm Hg on systemic sotalol, and she had a bilateral optic disc rim hemorrhage along with the left cupping and the left visual field defect progression. Blood pressure monitoring showed at that time a mean systolic pressure at 136/77 mm Hg during daytime and 110/61 mm Hg
at nighttime; however the systolic dip was at 19.1 % and the diastolic dip at 33.8 %. The day time
blood pressure variability was underlined by the observation of a systolic blood pressure standard
deviation at 16 mm Hg and a diastolic blood pressure standard deviation at 14 mm Hg. This case
illustrates that the blood pressure variability, as seen in overtreated high blood pressure, can be a risk
factor for progression of glaucoma visual field defects

The Significance of Low Blood Pressure Findings in the Pathogenesis of Glaucomatous Optic Neuropathy

The fact that patients with Shy-Drager' syndrome, a disease of the autonomic system,
who have very low BP levels also have a normal incidence of glaucomatous lesions
prevalence raises the probability that something besides systemic hypotension must
be involved in causing such lesions through permanent or transient arterial hypotension. That the main difference in BP behavior between control and glaucomatous
patients is the presence of more and deeper nocturnal dips in the latter must be put
in perspective by another fact: IOP is increased at night, during sleep [15]. Factors
involved in BP autoregulation at the optic nerve head and pathological vasospasm
might also be of importance. Glaucoma patients, particularly older ones, may have
impaired BP autoregulation capabilities. Hayreh points out that autoregulation oper-
ates only over a critical range of perfusion pressure, so a fall perfusion pressure
beyond the critical range can make autoregulation ineffective [5]. The reason why a
fall in BP induces, in some individuals, a glaucomatous optic neuropathy instead of
AION is not fully known. Moreover, autoregulation functions when blood pressure
variations are relatively slow, but is less effective when variability is too high.

The treatment of arterial hypotension is somewhat disappointing. There are no
acceptable medications available to routinely increase BP, although Flammer recom-

mends, in the absence of contraindications, an oversalted regimen at the evening meal. However, some kind of therapy is possible in close coordination with the general practitioner, who can, in some cases, modify the treatment of arterial hypertension when it is overtreated. In an aging patient the approach may be to treat the varices or decrease then number of medications which might possibly to lead to orthostatic hypotension, and identify and treat some causes of permanent arterial hypotension, for instance atrial fibrillation.

AMBP studies should be an integral part of the workup of patients with normal, or moderately elevated, pressure glaucoma. Particular attention should be directed to BP variability and to the detection of nocturnal episodes of systemic arterial hypotension, including in those patients being treated for arterial hypotension. These investigations are particularly important in vascular forms of glaucoma. Further studies are needed to determine the prognostic value of the ambulatory brachial blood pressure profile in patients treated at an optimum IOP level.

References

1. Drance SM, Morgan SW, Sweeney VP (1973) Shock-induced optic neuropathy, a cause of non-progressive glaucoma. New England J Med 288:392
2. Goldberg I, Hollows FC, Kass MA, Becker B (1981) Systemic factors in patients with low-tension glaucoma. Br J Ophthalmol 65:56–62
3. Leighton D, Philips GI (1972) Systemic blood pressure in open angle glaucoma, low tension glaucoma, and the normal eye. Br J Ophthalmol 56:447–453
4. Hayreh SH, Zimmerman MB, Podhajsky P, Alward WL (1994) Nocturnal arterial hypotension and its role in optic nerve head and ocular ischemic disorders. Am J Ophthalmol 117:603–624
5. Hayreh SH (1997) Factors influencing blood flow in the optic nerve head. J Glaucoma 6:412–425
6. Peraesalo R, Raitta C (1990) Low blood pressure: a risk factor for nerve fiber loss in institutionalized geriatric glaucoma patients. Acta Ophthalmol 68 (suppl 195):65–67
7. Béchetoille A, Bresson-Dumont H (1994) Diurnal and nocturnal drops in patients with focal ischemic glaucoma. Graede Arch Clin Exp Ophthalmol 232:675–679
8. Staessen JA, Fagard RH, Lunen PJ (1991) Mean and range of the ambulatory pressure in normotensive subjects from a meta-analysis of 23 studies. Am J Cardiol 1:723–727
9. Bresson-Dumont H, Béchetoille A (1995) Hypotension artérielle dans le glaucoma à pression normale ou modérement élevée. J F Ophthalmol 18:128–134
10. Demailly Ph, Cambien F, Plouin PF, Baron P, Chevalier B (1984) Do patients with low tension glaucoma have particular cardiovascular characteristics? Ophthalmologica 188:65–75
11. Graham SL, Drance SM, Wijsman K, Douglas GR, Mikelberg FS (1995) Ambulatory blood pressure monitoring in glaucoma. Ophthalmology 102:61–69
12. Kaiser HJ, Flammer J (1991) Systemic hypotension: a risk factor for glaucomatous damage. Ophthalmologica 203:105–108
13. Kaiser HJ, Flammer J, Graft T, Stümpfig D (1993) Systemic blood pressure in glaucoma patients. Graefe's Arch Clin Exp Ophthalmol 231:677–680
14. Bresson-Dumont H, Béchetoille A (1996) Rôle de tension artérielle dans l'évolutivité des lésions glaucomateuses. J F Ophthalmol 19:435–442
15. Buguet A, Py P, Romanet JF (1994) 24-H (Nycthoemeral) and sleep related variations of intraocular pressure in healthy white individuals. Am J Ophthalmol 117:342–347

CHAPTER 24

Retinal Ischemia as a Risk Factor
for Secondary Glaucoma and Its Clinical Consequences

K. U. Bartz-Schmidt, A. Psichias, G. Thumann, K. Heimann, and G.K. Krieglstein

Introduction

Retinal ischemia represents the common property of all neovascular glaucoma. Retinal cells, especially the Müller cells [1, 2] and retinal pigment epithelial (RPE) cells [3, 4], are stimulated by hypoxia to produce growth factors such as vascular-endothelial growth factor (VEGF). The factors are then distributed by diffusion throughout the entire globe leading to neovascularisation.

The lens has a temporary limiting effect on this distribution but in the long-term neovascularisation is also formed on the iris. These neovascularisations are found from the pupillary rim to the chamber angle, transforming into fibrovascular tissue, which occludes the angle completely by contraction. The reduction of flow of aqueous humor leads to increases of the intraocular pressure. The increasing intraocular pressure worses the perfusion of the retina. The entire process leads to a self-enhancing circuit. Finally, after the ciliary body has been covered by fibrovascular membranes, the eye develops persisting hypotony and phthisis bulbi.

The only causative treatment consists in conversion of the relative hypoxia into total anoxia. Panretinal laser treatment destroys large areas of retinal tissue and RPE. These areas can no longer produce active growth factors and the remaining tissue disposes of more oxygen [5–7]. In advanced cases of neovascular glaucoma panretinal laser treatment is not possible because of opacification of the cornea and the lens or vitreous blood. To date, cryocoagulation of the ciliary body has been the method of choice to decrease the intraocular pressure in these eyes [8–10]. The decrease in intraocular pressure improves the retinal perfusion, but does not alter the pathomechanism. Therefore the therapeutic failure rate is quite high [9]. As long as the retinal ischemia persists new neovascularisations develop, leading to persisting hypotonia and phthisis bulbi by overgrowth of the ciliary body.

The therapeutic goal of our study was to employ panretinal laser treatment in eyes with neovascular glaucoma and opacification of the optic media (cornea, anterior chamber, lens, vitreous) by vitrectomy, if necessary with corneal abrasion and lensectomy. In the long run, this treatment inhibits the stimulus for neovascularisation. During surgery, we coagulate the ciliary processes to quickly decrease the pressure therefore improve the retinal perfusion. An intraocular tamponade with silicone oil is used in all eyes for the following reasons: (1) separation of the anterior from the posterior segment and therefore faster regression of the neovascularisation of the iris; (2) to prevent the occlusion of the chamber angle in some cases; (3) to achieve hemostasis, as silicone oil is not compressible and therefore stops postoperative bleedings; (4)

to get a clear view to the fundus, due to the hydrophobic characteristics of the tamponade so that postoperative complications can be detected sooner; (5) finally, the vitreous cavity is filled with an inert fluid, which prevents the accumulation of stimulating
factors, stabilizes the blood-retinal barrier, and decreases the risk of proliferative vitreoretinopathy (PVR), limiting the undesired event of a complicated retinal detachment.

Patients and Methods

We included patients with the following criteria into the study: (1) rubeosis iridis, (2)
neovascular glaucoma, (3) blood in the viterous cavity, (4) preceding central vein occlusion or, (5) advanced case of diabetic retinopathy, (6) follow-up 12 months and more.

We excluded patients with the following criteria: (1) all other glaucoma, (2) neovascular glaucoma not caused by central vein occlusion or diabetic retinopathy, (3)
follow-up less then 12 months. Patients with a history of chronic glaucoma were not
excluded from the study. Thirty-two eyes from 32 patients (17 female and 15 male)
were included in the study. These patients presented between January 1994 and
December 1996 in the department of Vitreoretinal Surgery for decompensated neovascular glaucoma. Eighteen eyes had a history of central vein occlusion and 14 eyes
had a history of advanced diabetic eye disease with proliferative diabetic retinopathy
(PDR). The mean age of the patients was 65.5 ± 14.5 years. Patients with diabetic retinopathy had a significantly lower mean age (53.9 ± 16.1 years) than patients with central vein occlusion (74.8 ± 9.8 years). The group of patients younger than 50 years was
exclusively represented by patients with diabetic retionpathy.

In all patients pars-plana vitrectomy with 3-port technique was performed. In phakic
eyes we also performed lensectomy by phakoemulsification. We also removed the lens
capsule completely. The artificial lens in pseudophacic eyes was left in place. During vitrectomy the posterior hyoloid separation was induced by suction with the outcome over
the optic nerve head. Fibrovascular tractive membranes at the posterior pole were dis-
sected and removed completely en bloc. After removal of the vitreous the cavity was filled
with perfluorodecaline. After this we performed panretinal laster treatment with at least
2000 laser spots and with indentation and precise coagulation of the ciliary processes.
Around 75 % of the ciliary processes were coagulated with a continuous green argon laser
beam (514 nm) at 100 MWatt until a solid white color and shrinkage of the processes was
achieved. After making an ando-iridectomy (in aphacic eyes) we exchanged the perfluorodecaline with silicone oil. All patients received 500 mg acetazolamide i.v. at the end of
surgery. The intraocular pressure was measured at 6 and 10 h in call cases, in some cases
in addition 14 h after surgery. At pressure levels over 40 mm Hg an additional 500 mg acetazolamide were given. At a pressure over 50 mm Hg or no light perception we also performed puncture of the anterior chamber to decrease the pressure instantly.

We planned the controls intervals at 1-3 days, 4-7 days, 3 months $\pm$ 14 days, 6
months $\pm$ 1 months, 12 months $\pm$ 2 months, 24 months $\pm$ 2 months, 36 months $\pm$ 2
months. Control parameters were visual acuity, intraocular pressure (applanatory),
ophthalmoscopy of anterior and posterior segment. We also monitored the systemic
and local medication for glaucoma and changed therapy depending on the therapeutic
results. The follow-up within the first 3 months was done by our department. Longer
follow-up results were obtained by ophthalmologists in private practice in some cases.

Table 1. Reasons for missing data in follow-up after antiproliferative surgery

	Day 3	Day 7	Month 3	Month 6	Year 1	Year 2	Year 3
Non-compliant	3	3	0	3	4	3	1
Follow-up too short	0	0	0	0	0	5	12 (17)
Died	0	0	0	2	0 (2)	2 (4)	0 (4)
Enucleation	0	0	0	0	1	0 (1)	0 (1)
Number of patients	29	29	32	27	25	19	9

Results

At the time of the antiproliferative surgery almost two thirds of the patients (63 % = 20/32) hade undergone one (n=15) or multiple (n=5) surgical interventions on that eye. In 12 patients cyclodestructive interventions had been performed. In two patients filtration surgery had been done for chronic glaucoma. The other interventions were cataract surgery or vitreoretinal surgery due to retinal detachment or vitreous hemorrhage in diabetes. Except 11 eyes, all patients received laser treatment of the retina for retinal ischemia prior to sugery.

All patients had a minimum follow-up of 1 year in December 1997. Due to several reasons we only obtained results of all study parameters in all patients for the 3-month interval. The reasons for drop-outs the follow-up (Table 1): In the period 3-6 months after surgery two patients died. These were two male patients with advanced diabetes, ages 62 and 69 years. The diabetes was known for 20 years in one case and for 28 years in the other. In addition the patients suffered from cardiovascular diseases at the time of surgery. One female patient, age 75 years, died 20 months after surgery. In these three patients the diagnosis of diabetic retinopathy was known for 2 years prior to surgery. One male patient, age 83 years, died 16 months after surgery. This patient had a 2 year history of central vein occlusion.

We enucleated one eye 6 months after surgery due to painful phthisi bulbi. This female patient was 81 years old and suffered from central vein occlusion. No more than four patients at each point of follow-up were non-compliant.

In five patients total follow-up was less than 2 years, in 12 patients less than 3 years.

Intraocular Pressure after Antiproliferative Surgery

The main criteria in follow-up was the intraocular pressure after 1 and to 3 years. In the box-plot diagram of Fig. 1) the reduction of the intraocular pressure becomes obvious as soon as 1 week after surgery (in the range of 50 % reduction).

After 1 week, 52 % (15/29 eyes); after 3 months, 50 % (16/32); after 6 months, 59 % (16/27); and after 1 year, 72 % (18/25 eyes) of the patients had normal intraocular pressure, between 8 and 21 mm Hg. After 2 years, 12 eyes and after 3 years, two eyes had normal intraocular pressure. In addition we performed Kaplan-Meier statistics to demonstrate the success in reduction of intraocular pressure (Statview version 4.55, Abacus, Berkely, USA). We calculated this for patients who did not achieve a reduction below 21 mm Hg. Figure 2 makes evident that about half of the patients

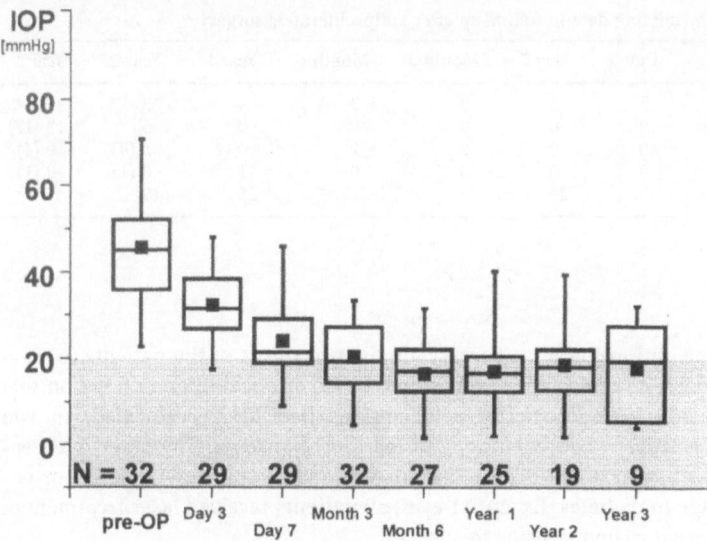

Fig. 1. Box-plot diagram of the intraocular pressure in flow-up

already achieved the reduction of pressure within the first few days after surgery. The other half achieved the aim within the following 6 months. The diagram does not show the incidence of patients with persisting hypotony and patients with recurrent intraocular pressure increases.

A hypotony was observed for the first time 3 months after surgery in 6% (2/32 eyes) of patients. After 6 months, 15% (4/27 eyes) and after 1 year, 12% (3/25 eyes) developed hypotony. After 2 years, one eye and after 3 years, three eyes had IOP lower than 8 mm Hg.

More information about the probability to develop a persisting hypotony after surgery is obtained by a Kaplan-Meier analysis. When the patients are split up after diag-

Fig. 2. Kaplan-Meier univariate estimates of the percent of patients without IOP ≤ 21 mm Hg statified by the diagnosis. Hash marks correspond to censored observations

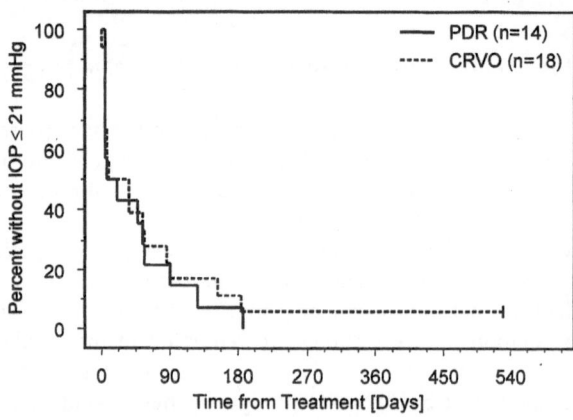

Fig. 3. Kaplan-Meier univariate estimates of the percent of patients without IOP ≤ 7 mm Hg statified by the diagnosis. Hash marks correspond to censored observations

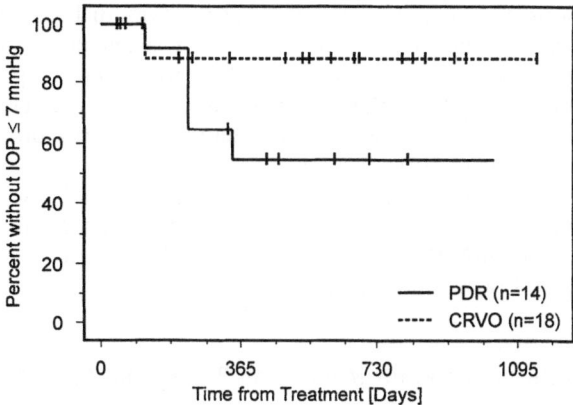

Table 2. Intraocular pressure (IOP) of all patients at the follow-up time points

Patient	Diagnosis	IOP pre-OP	IOP day 3	IOP day 7	IOP month 3	IOP month 6	IOP year 1	IOP year 2	IOP year 3	IOP final examination
1	CRVO	32	16	n.-c.	4	3	2	2	5	5
2	PDR	64	n.-c.	29	30	34	10	n.-c.	4	4
3	PDR	60	37	21	19	23	17	n.-c.	6	6
4	PDR	50	n.-c.	24	21	17	15	19	30	30
5	CRVO	55	31	23	17	13	20	22	17	17
6	CRVO	45	27	n.-c.	27	23	20	22	22	22
7	CRVO	64	48	18	29	20	22	15	32	32
8	CRVO	20	43	24	26	28	31	30	25	25
9	CRVO	31	35	21	14	9	13	13	19	19
10	CRVO	29	27	21	26	20	n.-c.	n.-c.	n.-c.	20
11	CRVO	50	39	20	15	19	20	22	--	22
12	PDR	45	28	50	26	8	11	8	--	8
13	CRVO	30	47	34	31	n.-c.	45	38	--	38
14	PDR	50	30	18	14	16	15	15	--	15
15	CRVO	45	31	30	13	20	21	19	--	19
16	PDR	52	34	30	25	25	22	17	--	17
17	PDR	42	42	27	36	14	6	8	--	8
18	PDR	64	24	8	15	17	16	18	--	18
19	CRVO	47	33	19	14	16	19	39	--	39
20	CRVO	35	33	20	14	16	13	12	--	12
21	CRVO	72	28	24	16	7	8	18	--	18
22	CRVO	39	n.-c.	n.-c.	28	n.-c.	n.-c.	16	--	16
23	PDR	24	23	21	5	13	15	--		15
24	CRVO	44	24	19	20	22	16	PD		16
25	CRVO	48	19	29	27	25	24	--		24
26	PDR	40	36	16	15	19	20	--		20
27	CRVO	50	41	36	24	17	19	--		19
28	CRVO	70	44	42	28	1	Enucleation			1
29	PDR	26	27	10	11	5	n.-c.	--		5
30	PDR	52	26	15	32	PD				32
31	PDR	38	27	21	16	n.-c.	n.-c.	PD		16
32	PDR	44	31	27	15	PD				15

(-- follow up too short, n.-c., non-compliant; PD, patient died)
CRVO, central retinal vein occlusion; PDR proliferative diabetic retinopathy.

nosis it becomes apparent that patients with diabetes carry a higher risk to develop persisting hypotony in the follow-up. This hypotony can become evident even after more than 6 months. Three out of the five hypotonic globes had undergone retinectomy after the antiproliferative surgery, due to initally high pressure levels. For patients with central vein occlusion the cumulative probability to develop persisting hypotony was 10 % (Fig. 3).

Elevated pressure (above 21 mm Hg) was found after 1 week, in 48 % (14/29 eyes); after 3 months, in 44 % (14/32 eyes); after 6 months, in 26 % (7/27 eyes); and after 1 year in 20 % (5/25 eyes). After 2 years the pressure was elevated in six patients and after 3 years in four patients (Table 2).

Antiglaucomatous Medication Before and After Antiproliferative Surgery

In order to control the IOP after surgery, patients were initially treated with local medication and only with IOP higher than 30 mm Hg systemically. In general we were able to abandon the systemic medication after antiproliferative surgery. In 17 out of 20 patients initially treated with systemic carbohydrase inhibitors (CA-I), this treatment was discontinued after surgery at the last control. At 3 months six patients; after 6 months two patients; and after 1 and 2 years, one patient still received systemic CA-I (Table 3).

Local medication was only discontinued in five out of 20 patients at the last control. The number of different drops was reduced from preoperative mean of 1.7 preparations (34/20) to 1.25 (25/20) after 3 months and 1.14 (16/14) after 6 months and 1.18 (13/11) after 1 year. After 2 years the ratio increased due to a therapeutic failure in a young patient with PDR and four local preparations to 1.63 (13/8) (Table 3).

Visual Acuity Before and After Antiproliferative Surgery

Ten eyes went blind after our antiproliferative intervention (Table 4). These included seven eyes with a history of central vein occlusion. One patient underwent surgery on a blind eye because of a painful neovascular glaucoma after central vein occlusion in order to relieve pain. This eye developed painful phthisis bulbi. Six months after surgery we had to enucleate the eye. Three patients went blind 3 months after surgery, an additional four patients went blind in the time between 3 and 6 months after surgery. In the following 6 months an additional two patients became blind and one last patient lost sight between 1 and 2 years after surgery. The cumulative survival statistic shows a probability to preserve vision for patients with diabetic retinopathy of 72 %, but for patients with central vein occlusion of 42 % (Fig. 4). After a follow-up of one year both groups are still similar (72 % for patients with PDR and 65 % for patients with CRVO) with the only difference that patients with CRVO go blind in closer association with the surgical intervention than patients with PDR. In addition patients with central vein occlusions lost light perception even after 1 year. This explains the difference in the final visual outcome of both groups. None of the patients with diabetic retinopathy went blind after more than 1 year after surgery (Fig. 4). In the direct comparison of initial vs final visual acuity (VA), 18 eyes shows

Table 3. Postoperative medication of all patients at the follow-up time points

ID	Diag-nosis	IOP pre-OP	pre-OP ED	pre-OP CA-I	Month 3 ED	Month 3 CA-I	Month 6 ED	Month 6 CA-I	Year 1 ED	Year 1 CA-I	Year 2 ED	Year 2 CA-I	Year 3 ED	Year 3 CA-I	Final exam. ED	Final exam. CA-I
1	CRVO	32	1	NM	0	NM	0	NM	0	NM	0	NM	0	NM	0	NM
2	PDR	64	1	M	1	M	1	M[a]	0	NM	0	NM	0	NM	0	NM
3	PDR	60	1	M	1	M	1	M[a]	0	NM	0	NM	0	NM	0	NM
4	PDR	50	1	M	1	NM	0	NM	0	NM	0	NM	2[b]	NM	2	NM
5	CRVO	55	1	M	0	NM	0	NM	0	NM	0	NM	0	NM	0	NM
6	CRVO	45	3	M	1	NM	1	NM	1	NM	1	NM	1	NM	1	NM
7	CRVO	64	1	NM	1	NM	1	NM	1	NM	1	NM	1	NM	1	NM
8	CRVO	20	0	NM	1	NM	2	NM[c]	1	NM	2	NM	2	NM	2	NM
9	CRVO	31	3	M	0	NM	0	NM	0	NM	0	NM	0	NM	0	NM
10	CRVO	29	1	NM	1	NM	1	NM	n.-c.		n.-c.		n.-c.		1	NM
11	CRVO	50	1	NM	1	NM	1	NM	1	NM	1	NM	--		1	NM
12	PDR	45	0	M	2	NM	0	NM[d]	0	NM	0	NM	--		0	NM
13	CRVO	30	3	NM	2	NM	n.-c.		2	NM	2	NM	--		2	NM
14	PDR	50	1	M	1	NM	1	NM	1	NM	1	NM	--		1	NM
15	CRVO	45	3	M	1	NM	1	NM[e]	0	NM	0	NM	--		0	NM
16	PDR	52	0	M	2	M[f]	1	NM	1	NM	1	NM	--		1	NM
17	PDR	42	0	M	2	M[g]	0	NM	0	NM	0	NM	--		0	NM
18	PDR	64	1	NM	0	NM	0	NM	0	NM	0	NM	--		0	NM
19	CRVO	47	3	NM	1	NM	1	NM	1	NM	4	M[h]	--		4	M
20	CRVO	35	0	NM	0	NM	0	NM	0	NM	0	NM	--		0	NM
21	CRVO	72	1	M	0	NM	0	NM	0	NM	0	NM	--		0	NM
22	CRVO	39	0	M	1	NM	n.-c.		n.-c-		1	NM	--		1	NM
23	PDR	24	0	NM					0	NM	--				0	NM
24	CRVO	44	3	M	0	NM	1	NM	1	NM	PD				1	NM
25	CRVO	48	0	M	2	NM	2	NM	2	M[i]	--				2	M
26	PDR	40	0	M	0	NM	0	NM	0	NM	--				0	NM
27	CRVO	50	2	M	1	NM	1	NM	1	NM	--				1	NM
28	CRVO	70	0	M	1	NM	0	NM[j]	Enucleation						0	NM
29	PDR	26	0	NM	0	NM	0	NM	n.-c.		--				0	NM
30	PDR	52	0	M	0	NM[k]	PD								0	NM
31	PDR	38	2	NM	0	NM[l]	n.-c.		n.-c.		PD				0	NM
32	PDR	44	1	M	1		PD								1	M
Σ	–	–	34 (20)	20	25 (20)	5	16 (14)	2	13 (11)	1	13 (8)	1	6 (4)	0	22 (15)	3

ED, number of glaucoma eye drops; CA-I, carboanhydrase-inhibitors; NM, no medication; M, medication; --, follow up too short; n.-c., non-compliant; PD, patient died.
CRVO, central retinal vein occlusion, PDR, proliferative diabetic retinopathy.
[a] Revision-vitrectomy with retinectomy and gas tamponade 6 months after antiproliferative surgery.
[b] Relapse of rubeosis iridis with recurrent pressure increase despite permanent silicone oil tamponade.
[c] Transscleral cyclophotocoagulation 10 months after antiprofilerative surgery.
[d] Phthisis bulbi due to violent disturbance of the blood-ocular barrier after surgery with development of cyclitic membranes.
[e] Removal of silicone oil 6 months after surgery.
[f] Revision vitrectomy for silicone oil removal, complementary panretinal laser treatment, complementary external cyclocryotherapy 4 months after surgery, 1 month later recurrent vitreous hemorrhage, again revision vitrectomy with silicone oil tamponade, 7 months later revision vitrectomy and silicone oil removal, since then stable situation.
[g] Revision vitrectomy with retinectomy and gas tamponade 3 months after antiproliferative surgery, 6 weeks later revision vitrectomy with silicone oil filling because of vitreous hemorrhage final situation: no light perception.
[h] Decompensated intraocular pressure 13 months after surgery, patient refused further interventions.
[i] Central vein occlusion with history of PEX glaucoma, during follow-up IOP increases caused by the PEX glaucoma, no signs of reactivation of the proliferative disease, patient refused further surgical treatments
[j] Enucleation 6 months after surgery because of painful phthisis bulbi due to violent disturbance of the blood-ocular barrier, with development of cyclitis membranes and anterior PVR.
[k] Transscleral cyclophotocoagulation 2 months after antiproliferative surgery, until then therapy with CA-I.
[l] Revision vitrectomy for silicone oil removal combined with phacoemulsification of the lens and posterior chamber lens implantation 3 months after surgery, patient then non-compliant (no ophthalmic controls at all), patient died 20 months after surgery.

Fig. 4. Kaplan-Meier univariate estimates of the percent
of patients without loss of
light perception statified by
the diagnosis. Hash marks
correspond to censored
observations

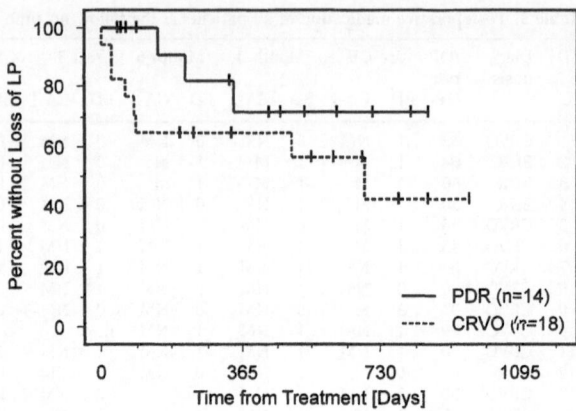

Table 4. Visual acuity before and after antiproliferative surgery

	pre-OP	Month 3	Month 6	Year 1	Year 2	Year 3	final examination
NL	1	+3 (4)	+4 (8)	+2 (10)	+1 (11)	+0 (11)	11
LP	9	12	6	7	4	3	7
HM	15	6	6	3	1	1	6
CF	1	6	3	4	3	0	3
≥ 20/400	6	4	5	4	3	1	5
No data	0	0	4	4	10	16	0

Table 5. Number of changes in Visual acuity, values prior to surgery compared with last follow-up

Δ VA	ADED (PDR)	CRVO	All
Better	3	2	5
Same	5	4	9
Worse	6	12	18
Σ	14	18	32

VA, visual acuity; ADED, advanced diabetic eye disease; PDR, proliferative diabetic retinoparthy;
CRVO, central retinal vein occlusion.

a worsening compared to initial vision. Twelve of these 18 eyes had a history of central vein occlusion. Nine eyes showed stable vision, and five patients (three of these with PDR) improved their VA (Table 5).

Revision Procedures Following Antiproliferative Surgery: Latest Findings and Subjective Complaints

Because of persisting high intraocular pressure despite systemic treatment with CA-I we performed silicone oil removal and retinectomy with temporary gas tamponade in three patients [11]. This intervention became necessary in one patient after 2 months and in the other two patients after 6 months. The early intervention was complicated by the development of a macular pucker, which made an additional revision surgery necessary. Intraocular pressure in these three patients at their last follow-up was between 4 and 8 mm Hg, without any local or systemic antiglaucomatous treatment.

In one patient with IOP over 30 mm Hg and local medication we performed external cyclophotocoagulation. With local medication the IOP was then kept below 30 mm Hg. In two patients with good VA results (better than counting fingers) we removed silicone oil 2 and 6 months after surgery. The aim was to relieve discomfort due to anisometropia caused by the silicone oil.

In one patient with persistent active diabetic retiopathy we performed revision surgery with complimentary laser treatment but without silicone oil tamponade. One month later, this patient developed a recurrent vitreous hemorrhage indicating the necessity of silicone oil tamponade. One year after the initial procedure we removed the silicone oil and the eye has remained without any complications since then.

Due to intense fibrinous exudations we injected recombinant tissue plasminogen activator (rTPA) into the anterior chamber in the early postoperative course (day 4–7) in three patients. With this treatment fibrinous membranes dissolved quickly. One of these patients developed epiretinal membranes at the posterior pole later on.

One patient had an occlusion of the ando-iridectomy due to fibrinous membrane formation indicating revision surgery of the anterior segment. The silicone oil had contact to the corneal endothelium, but intraocular pressure was normal. After the reopening of the ando-iridectomy, the eye developed hypotonia.

Phthisis bulbi occurred in two eyes. One eye became enucleated due to persistent pain 6 months after the initial surgery.

Other abnormal findings at the last control of each patient were: recurrent neovascularisation of the papilla in two diabetic patients, persisting macular edema, persisting intraretinal bleedings, anterior proliferations with tractional retinal detachment, reactivated iris neovascularisation, intraocular lens (IOL) dislocation and subepithelial corneal stroma opacification after epithelial abrasion (Table 6). A total of three patients complained about pain in the eye at their last control.

Discussion

Neovascular glaucoma most likely develops following central retinal vein occlusion (CRVO) or in patients with advanced diabetic retinopathy. Numerous other rare pathologies may lead primarily or secondarily to this disease. In order to increase the significance of this study, we limited the possible different pathomechanisms to patients with history of CRVO and advanced diabetic eye disease.

In the early 1980s Magaral showed areas of retinal ischemia of ten disc areas by fluorescence angiography in 90 % of eyes with neovascular glaucoma after CRVO. In addition he was able to demonstrate in 100 consecutive patients with acute ischemic central vein occlusion, that prophylactic laser treatment could almost eliminate the risk of development of neovascular glaucoma [12]. Another study showed that visual acuity is not reduced by panretinal laser treatment [13]. Jacobson and coworkers showed the regression of iris neovascularisation with the help of laser treatment in eyes with central vein occlusion [14]. The same finding was described for patients

Table 6. Revision surgery after antiproliferative procedure and final control

ID	Revision procedure	Time interval (Days)	Reason	Anterior segment final clinical finding	Posterior segment final clinical finding
2	Retinectomy	181	IOP 34 with CA-I	OK	OK
3	Retinectomy	187	IOP 23 with CA-I	OK	OK
4	--	--		Iris neovascularisation, Silicone oil emulsification	NVD with silicone oil
8	CPC external	309	IOP between month 6 and year 1 >30	OK	OK
12	rTPA injection	7	Fibrin formation	Corneal decompensation	Phthisis bulbi
13	rTPA injection	4	Fibrin formation	IOP >30, corneal edema	OK
15	Silicone oil removal	183	Anisometropia	OK	OK
16	Revision vitrectomy + silicone oil removal	118	Persistent active retinopathy		
	Revision vitrectomy + silicone oil injection	149	Vitreous hemorrhage		
	Silicone oil removal	368	Functional improvement	OK	OK
17	Retinectomy	70	IOP >30 under CA-I	OK	OK
	Revision vitrectomy + gas	147	Macular pucker		
21	--	--		OK	anterior PVR
22	--	--		Corneal decompensation	Persistent entmacular edema
23	--	--		IOL subluxation	OK
28	rTPA injection	4	Fibrin formation	Corneal decompensation	Phthisis bulbi
	Enucleation	185	Painful phthisis bulbi		
	Sec. Gutthoff-implant	211	Cosmetic improvement		
29	Ando revision	72	Silicone oil endothelial contact due to closed ando-iridectomy	OK	Pre-retinal fibrin membrane

CA-I, carbonic anhydrase inhibitor; CPC, cyclophotocoagulation; rTPA, recombinant tissue plasminogen activator; NVD, neovascularisation of the optic disc

with PDR by Wand [15]. In his study 93 PDR patients were treated with panretinal laser coagulation on one eye, the fellow eye served as control. The mean follow-up was 7.1 years (range 5–9 years). Fourteen patients developed rubeosis iridis at the non-treated eye with additional neovascularisation in the chamber angle in seven patients, but none of the laser treated eyes developed any neovascularisation of the anterior segment. In a recent paper Ohnishi shows the regression of neovascularisation of the chamber angle in 68 % of his patients after panretinal laser treatment [16]. In addition the laser treatment was followed by normalization of the intraocular pressure in 41 % of those patients with initially elevated IOP without any specific antiglaucomatous treatment. The benefit of the laser treatment can be explained by numerous experimental studies. Stefansson and Machemer [5] examined the oxygen concentration in the preretinal vitreous in patients who underwent vitrectomy due to proliferative vitreoretinopathy. They have found significantly higher oxygen concentrations over areas with panretinal laser treatment than non-treated areas in the same eye. Panretinal laser treatment therefore most likely has a beneficial effect on the oxygenation of the inner retina. On the other hand this also means that in not-treated eyes the retinal ischemia supports the cellular hypoxia. The influence of cellular hypoxia has been studied in animal models and cell culture experiments [2, 3, 17–19]. In 1995 Stone and coworkers were able to show the suppression of formation of VEGF and angiogenesis in an oxygen enriched environment in neonatal rats and cats [2]. Pierce [17] localized the site of VEGF synthesis by in situ hybridization in the inner nuclear layer of the mice retina. He also demonstrated increasing VEGF levels depending on increasing mRNA expression in northern blots. These results were confirmed in albino rats by Robbins in 1997 [18]. In cell cultures of retinal glia cells Sueishi [19] showed an increase in VEGF protein level under hypoxia and constant basic fibroblast growth factor levels (bFGF). The conditioned media induced higher thymidine incorporation rates in cultures of retinal endothelial cells and increased in vitro angiogenesis with formation of capillary tubuli. In addition he showed in rats 6 months after streptomycin induced diabetes, increased expression of VEGF mRNA and protein in retinal glia cells by in situ hybridization and immunohistochemistry. He also demonstrated increased permeability for albumin without formation of proliferative (angiogenic) retinopathy. Following application of toxic oxygen concentrations in neonatal rats, Dorey and coworkers [3] showed a quantitative and localized relation between VEGF mRNA expression and neovascularization. This was limited to areas with avascular retina and stopped at the border of the vascularized retina. Amin [20] showed in histologic sections of human eyes that increased VEGF expression in retina and optic nerve precedes neovascularization. He interpreted these results carefully, saying that ischemia induced increased expression of VEGF may not represent the only stimulus for retinal neovascularization. In the same year Hirata and coworkers [1] demonstrated in cell culture experiments with Müller cells the angiogenic influence of advanced glycation products (AGEs) extracted from the vitreous of patients with proliferative diabetic vitreoretinopathy.

Aiello [21] was able to show in an experiment the intracellular effect of elevated levels of VEGF. He showed fast activation of protein kinase C in the retina following intravitreal injection of VEGF due to induction of membrane translocation of the protein kinase isoform α, β and δ. The highest effect was seen after selective inhibition of the β-isoform. The detection of this interrelation led to speculation about the possibility of medicamentous treatment by protein kinase C β-isoform-specific antibodies [22].

Nevertheless, neither a medicamentous inhibition of the mediator nor blockage of the VEGF receptor or VEGF neutralizing antibodies change the underlying pathomechanisms [21–24]. Even an ideal euglycemia in an experimentally induced diabetes cannot induce complete recovery of the pathologic changes due to hyperglycemia with loss of pericytes in the retinal capillaries [25]. For this reason discontinuation of the medication would result in the reactivation of the neovascularisation due to the subsisting retinal hypoxia. Therefore, destructive therapy (panretinal photocoagulation) will continue to represent an important part in the therapy of neovascular glaucoma. The use of new antiproliferative drugs may possibly improve the therapy by inhibiting activity until the coagulation is completed. The aim of the therapy in neovascular glaucoma nowadays is to combine maximum comfort (no pain) with good cosmetic aspect and best functional results in the long run.

The quantification of treatment results in neovascular glaucoma is very difficulty [26]. In contrast to patients with chronic glaucoma, the eyes of these patients provide initially a very limited or absent view to the fundus. Therefore, visual field analysis or topography of the optic nerve head is impossible. The remaining criteria for therapeutic success are IOP, avoidance of blindness and the rate of phthisis bulbi or severe hypotonia. The comparison with the results of other treatment concepts (cyclodestructive therapy, shunt implantation, filtrating surgery with antimetabolites or combined procedures) is often complicated. In many reports patient groups are too small [27–29] or to heterogenous [30, 31] or follow-up is too short or not synchronized [32].

Cyclocryotherapy for the Treatment of Neovascular Glaucoma

There are contradictory reports concerning treatment of neovascular glaucoma. The aim of the treatment is the destruction of the nonpigmented ciliary body epithelium, which is responsible for the production of the aqueous humor. This most internal structure is reached last by an external treatment. Therefore, also the ciliary body muscle is coagulated. This might be a reason for the high rate of phthisis in this treatment method [8]. Cyclocryotherapy results in an at least temporary decrease of IOP by functional destruction of the inner ciliary body epthelium but does not change the underlying pathology. The decrease of the IOP improves temporarily the retinal perfusion; however, the underlying pathology persists and permeability factors are released again, and the neovascularisation is reactivated. Possibly, ethnic differences exist in the response to cryotherapy in neovascular glaucoma. In a retrospective Indian study [33] a regression of neovascularization in over 90 % and normalization of IOP in over 80 % is reported following anterior retinal cryocoagulation only.

Tube Shunt Implantation for the Treatment of Neovascular Glaucoma

Besides the neovascular glaucoma, there are a number of other glaucoma types which are not treatable by conventional methods, in the 1970s [26] drainage implants first were applied. Mermoud published in 1993 [34] his long term results following implantation of such a tube shunt in a prospective consecutive study including 60 eyes with neovascular glaucoma. Success was defined as IOP equal or less than 21 mm Hg and sustained light perception. After 1 year, his success rate was 62.1 %, after 2 years, 52 %, after 3 years, 43.1 %, after 4 years, 30.8 %; and after 5 years 10.3 %. Using the same criteria the success rate of our antiproliferative approach is, with 56 %, in the same range after 1 year. The long term results of our patient group are still open. The main reason for therapy failure in the study of Mermoud was loss of light perception in 48 % (compared to 31 % in our study, six out of these ten patients had normalized IOP), progression of the disease to phthisis in 18 % (6 % in our study) and scarification of the filtering bleb in 10 %. Mermoud also found a significantly better prognosis for eyes with diabetic disease compared to eyes after CRVO. This is accordance with our findings (out of the 10 eyes which lost light perception during the follow-up, seven eyes had a history of CRVO).

In another study Lloyd and coworkers [34] reported their results of combined Molteno implantation and pars-plana vitrectomy for neovascular glaucoma of different ethiology. Only four out of ten eyes were treated successfully. The remaining six eyes suffered from postoperative complications such as recurrent bleeding into the vitreous cavity and retinal detachment three eyes each), hyphema (two eyes), tube shunt blockage, severe fibrin formation, epiretinal membrane formation and total retina necrosis (one eye each). These complications can be expected due to the severely altered blood-retina barrier prior to surgery. For this reason we performed primarily a silicone oil endotamponade in our extensive surgical procedure. The positive effects of the silicone oil tamponade consist in the inhibition or limitation of postoperative bleedings, the avoidance of accumulation of active factors in the vitreous cavity and the limitation of a possible retinal detachment. In addition the silicone oil tamponade allows the patient fast visual rehabilitation. Certainly silicone oil tamponade and implantation of a drainage shunt cannot be combined. Due to the free flow of aqueous humor through the tube shunt, the silicone oil would prolapse into the anterior chamber and result in permanent silicone oil endothelial contact. Furthermore, silicone oil could enter the tube and drainage system and therefore completely block the outflow of aqueous humor. Comparable problems would occur after filtrating surgery. In our model there were only two possibilities remaining for reduction of the intraocular pressure: cyclodestruction with decreased production of aqueous humor or improvement of the outflow by creation of an internal fistula by a retinectomy procedure [11]. Based on our experience with retinectomy in eyes with active neovascular glaucoma, we decided on a two step procedure. In the primary surgery we performed vitrectomy, panretinal laser treatment, coagulation of the ciliary body processes over 180°-270° and silicone oil tamponade. If the intraocular pressure remained elevated, we performed retinectomy in combination with silicone oil removal after regression of the active neovascular compenent [35] with a gas tamponade in two patients. After this second surgical step in two patients the intraocular pressure was in the low normal level, without the development of phthisis of the globe. One patient underwent revision vitrectomy because of the development of recurrent bleeding into the vitreous cavity. At the last control the intraocular pressure of this patient was still elevated. One of the eyes went blind after retinectomy.

Filtrating Surgery in the Treatment of Neovascular Glaucoma

Conventional filtrating surgery for neovascular glaucoma without restoring the retinal pathology always results in failure. Active factors which reach the filtrating area and the surrounding conjunctiva by the aqueous humor induce proliferation and finally occlusion of the artificial outflow channel. Attempts were made to inhibit this mechanism with the use of antimetabolites (5-fluouracil). In a prospective study of Tsai and coworkers [35] the Kaplan-Meyer survival statistics of 34 patients over a follow-up of 5 years showed a success rate of 71 % after 1 year, 67 % after 2 years, 61 %

after 3 years, 41 % after 4 years and 28 % after 5 years. Twelve eyes went blind (35 %) and eight eyes (24 %) developed phthisis bulbi. Over the long-term, antimetabolites were not able to provide a sufficient solution.

Endophotocoagulation of the Ciliary Processes in the Treatment of Neovascular Glaucoma

The chamber angle in advanced neovascular glaucoma is completely occluded in most cases; therefore the panretinal photocoagulation itself cannot induce sufficient IOP regulation, even if good regression of the rubeosis iridis is achieved. Direct precise coagulation of the ciliary processes was developed because external cyclodestruction carries a high risk of phthisis, and fistulating surgery in the long run showed disappointing results. The advantage of this method is the aimed and controlled character of the procedure. With the aid of an endoscope ciliary processes can be coagulated directly over the pars plana under visual guidance. Uram and coworkers [36] were able to achieve a mean IOP reduction of 65 % in ten patients. In our patients the mean IOP before treatment was 45.5 ± 13.2 mm Hg and after 1 year 17 ± 18.7 mm Hg, corresponding to an absolute reduction by 28.5 mm Hg or 63 %, therefore confirming the results of Tsai also in a larger group of patients.

In summary we performed with the panretinal laser treatment in combination with vitrectomy a cauative treatment of the underlying pathology in neovascular glaucoma. During surgery it is possible to perform aimed cyclodestruction for fast IOP reduction by direct coagulation of the ciliary processes with the help of scleral indentation. In order to avoid postoperative vitreoretinal complications and to achieve a fast regression of active rubeosis we used, for the first time, silicone oil as a vitreous substitute in the entity. In case of insufficient IOP regulation the silicone oil removal can be combined with retinectomy. With this procedure we were able to not only save IOP reduction but also to preserve the globe with a certain remaining function and a significant reduction in systemic medication.

References

1. Hirata C, Nakano K, Nakamura N, Kitagawa Y, Shigeta H, Hasegawa G, Ogata M, Ikeda T, Sawa H, Nakamura K, Ineaga K, Obayashi H, Kondo M (1997) Advanced glycation end products induce expression of vascular endothelial growth factor by retinal Muller cells. Biochem Biophys Res Commun 236:712–715
2. Stone J, Itin A, Alon T, Pe, Gnessin H, Chan-Ling T, Keshet E (1995) Development of retinal vasculature is mediated by hypoxia-induces vascular endothelial growth factor (VEGF) expression by neuroglia. J Neurosci 15:4738–4747
3. Dorey CK, Aouididi S, Reynaud X, Dvorak HF, Brown LF (1996) Correlation of vascular permeability factor/vascular endothelial growth factor with extraretinal neovascularization in the rat [see comments] [published erratum appears in Arch Ophthalmol 1997 Feb; 115(2):192]. Arch Ophthalmol 114:1210–1217
4. Ishibashi T, Hata Y, Yoshikawa H, Nakagawa K, Sueishi K, Inomata H (1997) Expression of vascular endothelial growth factor in experimental choroidal neovascularization. Graefes. Arch Clin Exp Ophthalmol 235:159–167
5. Stefansson E, Machemer R, de JEJ, McCuen BW II, Peterson J (1992) Retinal oxygenation and laser treatment in patients with diabetic retinopathy. Am J Ophthalmol 113:36–38

6. Pournaras CJ, Ilic J, Gilodi N, Tsacopoulos M, Leuenberger MP (1985) [Experimental venous thrombosis: prrential PO2 before and after photocoagulation]. Klin Monatsbl Augenheilkd 186(6):500–501

7. Ernest JZ, Archer DB (1979) Vitreous body oxygen tension following experimental branch retinal vein obstruction. Invest Ophthalmol Vis Sci 18:1025–1029

8. Benson MT, Nelson ME (1990) Cyclocryotherapy: a review of cases over a 10-year period. Br J Ophthalmol 74:103–105

9. Rehak J, Vymazal M (1994) Cryotherapy in treatment of neovascular glaucoma with closed chamber angle. Klin Monatsbl Augenheilkd 204:20–23

10. Vest E, Rong-Guang W, Raitta C (1992) Transillumination guided cyclocryotherapy in the treatment of secondary glaucoma. Eur J Ophthalmol 2:190–195

11. Kirchhof B (1994) Retinectomy lowers intraocular pressure in otherwise intractable glaucoma: preliminary results [see comments]. Ophthalmic Surg 25:262–267

12. Magargal LE, Brown GC, Augsburg JJ, Donoso LA (1982) Effiancy of panretinal photocoagulation in preventing neovascular glaucoma following ischemic central retinal vein obstruction. Ophthalmology. 89:780–784

13. Laatikainen, L, Kohner EM, Khoury D, Black RK (1977) Panretinal photocoagulation in central retinal vein occlusion: A randomised controlled clinical study. Br J Ophthalmol 61:741–753

14. Jacobson DR, Murphy RP, Rosenthal AR (1979) The treatment of angle neovascularization with panretinal photocoagulation. Ophthalmology 86:1270–1277

15. Wand M, Dueker DK, Aiello LM, Grant WM (1978) Effects of panretinal photocoagulation on rubeosis iridis, angle neovascularization, and neovascular glaucoma. Am J Ophthalmol 86:332–339

16. Ohnishi Y, Ishibashi T, Sagawa T (1994) Fluorescein gonioangiography in diabetic neovascularisation. Graefes Arch Clin Exp Ophthalmol 232:199–204

17. Pierce EA, Avery RL, Foley ED, Aiello LP, Smith LE (1995) Vascular endothelial growth factor/vascular permeability factor expression in a mouse model of retinal neovascularization. Proc Natl Acad Sci USA 92:905–909

18. Robbins SG, Conaway JR, Ford BL, Roberto KA, Penn JS (1997) Detection of vascular endothelial growth factor (VEGF) protein in vascular and non-vascular cells of the normal and oxygen-injured rat retina. Growth Factors 14:229–24

19. Sueishi K, Hata Y, Murata T, Nakagawa K, Ishibashi T, Inomata H (1996) Endothelial and glial cell interaction in diabetic retinopathy via the function of vascular endothelial growth factor (VEGF). Pol J Pharmacol 48:307–316

20. Amin RH, Frank RN, Kennedy A, Eliott D, Puklin JE, Abrams GW (1997) Vascular endothelial growth factor is present in glial cells of the retina and optic nerve of human subjects with nonproliferative diabetic retinopathy. Invest Ophthalmol Vis Sci 38:36–47

21. Aiello LP, Brusell SE, Clermont A, Duh E, Ishii H, Takagi C, Mori F, Ciulla TA, Ways K, Jirousek M, Smith LE, King GL (1997) Vascular endothelial growth factor-induced retinal permeability is mediated by protein kinase C in vivo and suppressed by an orally effective beta-isoform-selective inhibitor. Diabetes 46:1473–1480

22. Aiello LP (1997) Vascular endothelial growth factor and the eye: biochemical mechanisms of action and implications for novel therapies. Ophthalmic Res 29:354–362

23. Aiello LP, Avery RL, Arrigg PG, Keyt BA, Jampel HD, Shah ST, Pasquale LR, Thieme H, Iwamoto MA, Park JE (1994) Vascular endothelial growth factor in ocular fluid of patients with diabetic retinopathy and other retinal disorders [see comments]. N Engl J Med 331:1480–1487

24. Aiello LP, Pierce EA, Foley ED, Takagi H, Chen H, Riddle L, Ferrara N, King GL, Smith LE (1995) Suppression of retinal neovascularization in vivo by inhibition of vascular endothelial growth factor (VEGF) using soluble VEGF-receptor chimeric proteins. Proc Natl Acad Sci USA 92:10457–10461

25. Aiello LP, Robinson GS, Lin YW, Nishio Y, King GL (1994) Identification of multiple genes in bovine retinal pericytes altered by exposure to elevated levels of glucose by using mRNA differential display. Proc Natl Acad Sci USA 91:6231–6235

26. Molteno AC, Van RM, Bartholomew RS (1977) Implants for draining neovascular glaucoma. Br J Ophthalmol 61:120–125

27. Haicl P, Boguszakova J (1991) Cryotherapy of neovascular glaucoma in diabetics. Cesk Oftalmol 47:241–245

28. Bohnke M, Sayar RB (1990) Clinical results following cyclo-cryocoagulation with a nitrogen cooled probe. Fortschr Ophthalmol 87:134–137

29. Lloyd MA, Heuer DK, Baerveldt G, Minckler DS, Martone JF, Lean JS, Liggett PE (1991) Combined Molteno implantation and pars plana vitrectomy for neovascular glaucomas. Ophthalmology 98:1401–1405

232   K. U. Bartz-Schmidt et al.: **Retinal Ischemia as a Risk Factor for Secondary Glaucoma**

30. Airaksinen PJ, Aisala P, Tuulonen A (1990) Molteno implant surgery in uncontrolled glaucoma. Acta Ophthalmol (Copenh) 68:690–694
31. Uva MG, Gagliano C, Ott JP, Ferrigno G, Sciacca S, Reibaldi A (1994) Experiences with sclerostomy with the Holmium laser. Ophthalmologe 91:592–594
32. Eid TE, Katz LJ, Spaeth GL, Augsburger JJ (1997) Tube-shunt surgery versus neodymium: YAG cyclophotocoagulation in the management of neovascular glaucoma. Ophthalmology 104:1692–1700
33. Sihota R, Sandramouli S, Sood NN (1991) A prospective evaluation of anterior retinal cryoablation in neovascular glaucoma. Ophthalmic Surg 22:256–259
34. Mermoud A, Salmon JF, Alexander P, Straker C, Murray AD (1993) Molteno tube implanation for neovascular glaucoma. Long-term results and factors influencing the outcome. Ophthalmology 100:897–902
35. Tsai JC, Feuer WJ, Parrish RK2, Grajewski AL (1995) 5-Fluorouracil filtering surgery and neovascular glaucoma. Long-term follow-up of the original pilot study. Ophthalmology 102:887–892; discussion 892-3
36. Uram M (1992) Ophthalmic laser microendoscope ciliary process ablation in the management of neovascular glaucoma. Ophthalmology 99:1823–1828

CHAPTER 25

Specific Treatment of Causal Factors in Glaucoma

J. Thygesen

Introduction

In order to achieve the most effective approach to glaucoma, a better definition of the disease in mandatory. Glaucoma is not a single condition caused by an elevation of the intraocular pressure (IOP) but a progressive bilateral optic neuropathy, often asymmetric, with a particular pattern of optic and visual field damage that results from different diseases affecting the eye, often but not always associated with the main causal factor, elevated IOP.

Each of these conditions has a specific aetiology, pathophysiology and natural course. Understanding them as specific entities allows us to use specific treatments, not only aimed at lowering the IOP, but also focused at treatment of the causal factor in the development of the disease. A precise evaluation of all the risk factors is therefore mandatory.

In many cases the IOP is certainly the main risk factor, but not the only one. Main risk factors are age, race and family history. Other factors, besides myopia, that have

Table 1. Risk factors in glaucoma

Ocular
IOP
Disk hemorrhage
Myopia
Pseudoexfoliation
Pigmentary dispersion
Sytemic
Age
Race
Positive family history
Arterial hypertension
Arterial hypotension (particularly at night)
Migraine headaches
Vasospasm (associated with cold extremities)
Raynaud's phenomenon
Abnormalities of bloodflow to the optic nerve and posterior segment
Haematological abnormalities
Defects in autoregulation
Abnormality of extracellular matrix
Diabetes mellitus (?)
Obesity?
Smoking?

been currently identified, include abnormalities of blood flow to the optic nerve and posterior segment, haematological abnormalities, defects in the autoregulation, low intracranial pressure, low blood pressure, autonomic insufficiency, abnormalities of the extracellular matric and autoimmune phenomena. The rate of progression of the disease may also be influenced by external factors such as obesity, smoking and exercise (Table 1). Our increasing knowledge on glaucoma risk factors has oriented research towards new treatments of glaucoma.

Treatment of Risk Factors

Glaucoma is a diabling disease not only from a functional point of view, but also because it may cause a general decrease in the quality of life, often also related to the treatment. Current therapy does not yet treat the cause of the disease but is mainly directed toward the reduction of the introacular pressure. Much research is now directed towards improving optic nerve head blood flow, neuroprotection, neuroregeneration and gene therapy.

IOP Lowering Treatment

Elevated IOP is generally accepted as one of the most important risk factors for chronic primary open-angle glaucoma (POAG) (Table 2).

The current treatment for glaucoma is directed toward the regulation of aqueous humor formation by the ciliary body, and increased outflow of aqueous humor through the trabecular meshwork, uveoscleral passage (Table 3) or alternative pathways created by laser or surgical procedures. The patient must be followed long term with routine IOP, optic disc, and visual field examinations to rule out progressive glaucomatous damage.

As it is crusial to know whether the therapeutic intervention alters the natural course of the disease in the typical glaucoma patient The National Eye Institute currently supports the Early Manifest Glaucoma Trial (EMGT), a prospective clinical trial

Table 2. Relative risk of developing glaucoma

IOP (mm Hg)	Relative risk (%)
< 16	0.8
16–19	1.7
20–23	4.0
> 23	10.5

(Armaly)

Table 3. Aqueous humor dynamics and control of IOP

May be influenced by:
- Aqueous secretion: β-blockers, CAI, α-2-agonists
- Trabecular outflow: miotics, epinephrine
- Uveoscleral outflow: prostaglandins
- Episcleral venous pressure: α-2-agonists with α-1-agonist properties

Table 4. Agents to be avoided in these conditions

β-blocker: asthma, brady arrythmia, low blood pressure
Epinephrine: chronic conjunctivitis, tachyarrythmia, high blood pressure
Pilocarpine: age below 40 years
α-2-agonists: severe hypotony, ortostatic dysregulation
Carbonic anhydrase inhibitors: allergy to sulfonamide, nephrolithiasis

Table 5. Medical therapy

What relative IOP reduction can approx imately be expected?	
Monotherapy:	25 %
Combination therapy:	35 %
Maximum/Multipharmacy:	40 %

in Sweden, in which patients who have definite early-to-moderate glaucomatous damage are randomized to treatment (medicine or laser) or observation. It is hoped that the result from the study will determine whether currently available glaucoma treatments are efficacious in POAG.

Based on current practice, the β-blockers remain the most common first-line medical agent in the treatment of glaucoma. However it is evident that many patients should not receive these drugs because of the potential for pulmonary, vascular or central nervous system side effects. For such patients some of the medications introduced more recently, such as the topical carbonic anhydrase inhibitors like dorzolamide and brinzolamide, the α-2-agonist brimonidine, or the prostaglandin latanoprost, may be excellent as alternative that have good efficacy as initial therapy and potentially enhanced safety profiles compared to β-blocker (Table 4).

Since up to 50 % of glaucoma patients take more than one class of agents, these recently developed agents are often preferred in the additive regimen as second-line agents. Having six different classes of glaucoma medications it is now mandatory to include the patient in the decision-making process in choosing the optimal therapy and in discussing the safety and tolerability of the treatment options. Considerations on switching medical therapy in stead of add-on therapy should be made. Polypharmacy should be avoided by switching to other pressure lowering methods like laser trabeculoplasty or filtering surgery as further pressure reduction should no be expected by polypharmacy (Table 5). Early laser trabeculoplasty may be considered in the elderly who cannot tolerate medical therapy or in patients who are controlled inadequately on medication or who will not undergo surgery. Patients with pseudoexfoliation glaucoma may also benefit from early or primary laser trabeculoplasty. Early surgery may be considered if the IOP is not controlled by two to three drugs, if a low target pressure is required or if compliance is a problem.

Improving Optic Nerve Head Blood Flow

Current studies indicate that mean blood flow velocity in patients who have chronic open angle and normal pressure glaucoma is impaired. Blood flow modifications and disturbances of the optic nerve head (ONH) autoregulatory mechanisms have been incriminated. Also vasospasm may occur in some patients with normal pressure glaucoma. Additionally, evidence exists that ocular hypertensive patients who progress to glaucoma are more likely to have reduced blood flow velocity and increased vascular resistance [1]. Consequently, an increase in blood flow in these patients may help to stabilize glaucomatous progression through a reversal of any optic nerve ischemia induced by elevated IOP or specific vascular factors. The questions remain, however, what is the exact role of blood flow in glaucomatous ONH cupping and does the improvement in ONH blood flow preserve the nerve from further glaucomatous damage? But still, increase of blood supply to the optic nerve to reduce the effect of ischemia (axonal rescue) is one of the main goals in future glaucoma treatment in patients with disk hemorrhage, arterial hypertension, arterial hypotension (particularly at night), migraine headache, vasospasm with cold extremities. Raynaud's phenomenon, abnormalities of bloodflow to the optic nerve and posterior segment, haematological abnormalities and defects in autoregulation. In patients with diabetes mellitus, obesity and smoking no clear association has been found with glaucoma.

The optic nerve, as a part of the nervous system has a high oxygen consumption and metabolic activity, both of which are required for the neuronal transport process. Nutrition and oxygenation of the ONH depend on blood flow. Blood flow can be calculated by the equation: blood flow = perfusion pressure/resistance to flow. The value of the perfusion pressure equals the difference between the mean blood pressure and the intraocular pressure. The resistance to flow depends on the contractile state of the smooth muscle of the arterioles irrigating the ONH and potentially the pericytes of the ONH capillary network. It is probably regulated by the interaction of multiple factors such as neurotransmittors, circulating vasoactive substances, local metabolic factors (partial pressure of oxygen and carbon dioxide, pH, metabolic products) and endothelium derived substances like endothelin, prostaglandins (PGs) or nitric oxide (NO).

Autoregulatory mechanisms insure the constant supply of oxygen and nutritional elements of the ONH, despite variations in the parameters that influence ONH blood supply. Variations in the perfusion pressure at the ONH are implicated in the pathogenesis of glaucomatous optic neuropathy. In the normal human eye, the ONH blood flow usually shows autoregulation, within a range of IOP, but there is a decline in blood flow when the IOP reaches 45-55 mm Hg. However some glaucoma individuals do not show this autoregulation, but exhibit a decline in blood flow linearly related to IOP, even at moderate increases in IOP to, for example, 25 mm Hg [2]. Local transient tissue hypoxia affecting ONH neuronal function may occur during systemic hypotensive or hypertensive episodes, overloading the ONH autoregulatory mechanisms.

The vasoactive substances may interfere with nerve head autoregulation in response to elevated IOP, and this may result in reduced blood flow. The potential then exists for vasodilating substances, such as calcium channel blocking agents, selective for the central nervous system, to reduce susceptibility of the optic nerve to pressure [3]. Further work is needed to define the risk-benefit ratio of such treatment in long-term clinical trials.

Current evidence indicates that NO and endothelin are involved in maintaining basal vascular tone in uveal, retinal and choroidal circulations [4,5]. In this context NO donors could potentially have positive actions in pathologies, such as glaucomatous optic neuropathy. A better understanding of NO transduction pathway may lead to more efficient nitrovasodilators or agents which mimic or modulate the role of NO in vasodilation. Other experiments have reported that NO was able to decrease IOP in normal eyes [6]. During glaucoma, the application of non-toxic oxide-generating compounds could restore a normal IOP, and then present a new class of antiglaucomatous treatment. However many experiments must be conducted to demonstrate the lack of toxicity of such NO generating compounds in the anterior segment of the eye.

Neuroprotection

Among various research projects, the most fascinating are undoubtedly those examining therapies affecting the site of glaucomatous damage (the optic nerve) using neuroprotective and neuroregenerative agents. Recent neurobiological research has given us better understanding of neural cell death. Unlike necrosis, this can be a "programmed cell death", called apoptosis, which is genetically determined. It may occur spontaneously or secondary to an injury. It can follow increased concentrations for excitatory amino acids, free radicals, NO, potassium or calcium. It has been shown that, after an acute injury, the exent of damage exceeds that expected for the initial insult. It appears that neuronal damage in the central nervous system progresses even when the primary cause is alleviated. In fact, injured cells release various components, e.g. glutamate, inducing a secondary degeneration in the surrounding neurons. The level of glutamate may be elevated in the vitreous in glaucoma patients as compared to cataract patients [7]. Besides increasing the blood supply to the optic nerve, a number of different compounds that reduce the effect of ischemia on the optic nerve (axonal rescue) have been evaluated, which include those that limit the effect of excitotoxins, free radicals and abnormal calcium fluxes. Thus glutamate blockers may help limit penumbral nerve damage in an animal model of stroke. Another approach would be using medications that act directly on the optic nerve by using trophic factors, like growth factors, that would improve the metabolism of the optic nerve and help it better withstand the insults from chronic open angle glaucoma.

The development of specific nerve protection may be difficult because the events that initiate the cell death (apoptosis) still remain unknown. How to deliver drug to the optic nerve in such a way as to assure clinical efficacy without clinical side effects? How to measure physiologic improvement in vision and in ocular blood flow?

Gene Therapy

Gene therapy in glaucoma may be available in the early next millenium in the treatment of risk factors like age, race, positive family history, myopia, pseudoexfoliation, pigmentary dispersion and abnormality of the extracellular matrix.

To clone the genes responsible for glaucoma development and determine the functions of the normal and abnormal protein products of these genes will identify the processes that can results in glaucoma. This information will lead to the development of novel treatments designed to eradicate the abnormal molecular and cellular processes that may cause the disease. In addition to the development of new medical treatments for glaucoma, isolation of genes responsible for the disease also may result in the development of gene therapy, in which damaged genes are replaced and the underlying defects are corrected.

Isolation of genes responsible for glaucoma will also lead to new methods for diagnosis of the conditions, based on the DNA sequence changes the result in defective gene protein products. Such DNA-based diagnostic tests can identify individuals at risk for the disease before any visual deterioration has occurred.

The map of genes responsible for certain glaucoma subtypes, such as congenital glaucoma, Rieger's syndrome, juvenile and adult-onset POAG, pigmentary glaucoma and pseudoexfoliation syndrome, has influenced the widespread acceptance of glaucoma as a genetic or partly genetic disorder. Juvenile glaucomas, Rieger's syndrome, and pigment dispersion syndrome can be inherited as an autosomal dominant trait. Large pedigrees have been identified and used for genetic linkage analysis. One gene responsible for juvenile-onset glaucoma was located initially on chromosome 1q23 (GLCIA) and this gene has been identified recently. The gene codes for a protein referred to as TIGR (trabecular meshwork glucocorticoid response protein) [8]. Mutations in this gene have been associated with juvenile-onset POAG, and with some cases of adult-onset POAG. Patients affected POAG are more likely to develop an increase in IOP in response to dexamethasone eye drops, a trait shown to be inherited [9].

The origins of the genetic complexity of POAG are likely to stem from the diversity of ocular tissue and cell types potentially involved in the disease process. Many studies suggest that defects in the trabecular outflow pathways are responsible for the elevation of the IOP associated with the majority of cases of POAG. However, the cell types and biochemical processes that are altered in the disease have not yet been identified. It is possible that mutations in a number of genes that encode for different proteins may alter the normal function of the ocular outflow pathway.

The identification of genes and loci involved in disease enables Studies to evaluate the clinical features of the disorder with respect to molecular information. It will be possible to determine if cases of glaucoma caused by a specific gene share common features that can be recognized clinically. Similarly it will be possible to determine if molecular subclasses of the disease respond similarly to specific treatment modalities. A potential use for gene therapy is a drug delivery system to help minimize the influence of axonal injury at the ONH and to change the effect of the glaucoma gene on the trabecular meshwork. This could be performed by encoding external genes to the patient's own genome, which would produce protective trophic factors intracellularly.

Problems with genetic therapy in the eye include drug delivery and the potential carcinogenic effects of the implantation of new genomes inside the cell.

References

1. Hamzavi S, Stewart WC, Hamzavi SL, Stroman GL (1996) Transcranial Doppler in progressed and stable ocular hypertensive patients. Invest Ophthalmol Vis Sci (Suppl.):31
2. Pillunat LE, Anderson DR, Knighton RW, Joos KM, Feuer WJ (1997) Autoregulation of human optic nerve head circulation in response to intraocular pressure. Exp Eye Res 64:737–744
3. Netland PA, Erickson KA (1995) Calcium channel blockers in glaucoma management. Ophthalmol Clin North Am 8:327–334

4. Becquet F, Courtois Y, Gourneau O (1997) Nitric oxide in the eye: Multifaceted roles and diverse outcomes. Surv Ophthalmol 42:71–82
5. Haefliger IO, Flammer J (1998) Nitric oxide and endothelin in the pathogenesis of glaucoma. Lippincott-Raven, Philadelphia. New York
6. Nathanson JA (1992) Nitrovasodilators as a new class of ocular hypotensive agents. J Pharmacol Exp Ter 260:956–965
7. Dryer EB, Zurakowski D, Schumer RA, Podos SM, Lipton SA (1996) Elevated glutamate levels in the vitreous body of humans and monkeys with glaucoma. Arch Ophthalmol 114:299–305
8. Stone EM; Fingert JH, Wallace LM et al. (1997) Identification of a gene that causes primary open angle glaucoma. Science 275:668–670
9. Schwarz JR, Reuling FH, Feinleib M, Garrison RJ, Collie DJ (1972) Twin herability study of the effect of corticosteroids on intraocular pressure. J Med Genet 9:137–143

Subject Index